Deaf Culture

Exploring Deaf Communities
in the United States

Second Edition

Deaf Culture

Exploring Deaf Communities in the United States

Second Edition

Irene W. Leigh, PhD
Jean F. Andrews, PhD
Raychelle L. Harris, PhD
Topher González Ávila, MA

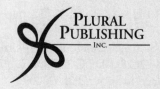

PLURAL
PUBLISHING
INC.

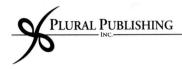

5521 Ruffin Road
San Diego, CA 92123

e-mail: information@pluralpublishing.com
Website: https://www.pluralpublishing.com

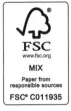

Copyright © 2022 by Plural Publishing, Inc.

Typeset in 10.5/13 Palatino by Flanagan's Publishing Services, Inc.
Printed in the United States of America by McNaughton & Gunn, Inc.
25 24 23 22   2 3 4 5

Library of Congress Cataloging-in-Publication Data

Names: Leigh, Irene, author. | Andrews, Jean F., author. | Harris,
  Raychelle L., author. | González Ávila, Topher, author.
Title: Deaf culture: exploring deaf communities in the United States /
  Irene W. Leigh, PhD, Jean F. Andrews, PhD, Raychelle Harris, PhD, Topher
  González Ávila.
Description: Second edition. | San Diego, CA : Plural Publishing, [2022] |
  Includes bibliographical references and index.
Identifiers: LCCN 2020027009 | ISBN 9781635501735 (paperback) | ISBN
  9781635501803 (ebook)
Subjects: LCSH: Deaf—United States. | Deaf culture—United States.
Classification: LCC HV2545 .L45 2022 | DDC 305.9/0820973—dc23
LC record available at https://lccn.loc.gov/2020027009

Contents

Preface

Deaf culture has been around for centuries, definitely since the 1700s and perhaps even earlier. Deaf people have always been on this earth. When schools for the deaf were started, deaf people began coming together. The ways they communicated and interacted with each other planted the seeds of Deaf culture that have grown to what it is today: a vibrant culture with a diverse membership.

Many books have been written about Deaf culture. Our book takes a different approach. Yes, we explain what Deaf culture is all about. We describe the Deaf community, its history and contemporary perspectives, and what Deaf culture has to offer. Looking at the Table of Contents, you may wonder: What are some of those chapters doing in a book on Deaf culture? Auditory Innovations? Deaf Education? How Deaf Children Think, Learn, and Read? Technology and Accessibility? Careers? As you continue to read this Preface, you will see why we address these issues.

These chapters are a testimony to how Deaf culture has been influenced by experiences related to each area and how culturally Deaf individuals have influenced new approaches in each area that have taken Deaf people's perspectives into account. We four authors, three Deaf and one hearing, teamed up to work on revisions for this second edition and agreed that we needed to present the Deaf experience in areas that have profoundly influenced the lives of Deaf people. We have had close connections with each of these areas and want to share what we have learned with you, the reader. As three white cisgender, abled women, two

Deaf and one hearing, working with a Latino Queer Deaf man, we have collaborated to give you a perspective of how complex the Deaf experience is and how it is transitioning from the framework of a purely white straight Deaf experience to one that reflects the reality of diversity with the multiple communities within the greater Deaf community, including DeafDisabled individuals. Following, we describe our backgrounds.

Irene W. Leigh's parents, stateless refugees who ended up in Great Britain during World War II and survived the bombing, found out their daughter was deaf on her second birthday. Her hearing mother repeatedly told her how she responded to the news, grieved, and then after one week pulled herself together and started to get information on how to give her daughter access to language. After the family emigrated from Great Britain to the United States, they were detained at Ellis Island for questioning because it was thought Irene as a 4-year-old deaf person would be a burden to the government of the United States. Her parents were able to demonstrate her mastery of language, which exceeded that of the immigration officer's 4-year-old grandson. Upon release, they moved to Chicago, Illinois, where she eventually attended the Bell School, a Chicago public school that had a day school for the deaf as part of an elementary school with hearing pupils. She was able to play with and learn with both Deaf and hearing peers. Nonetheless, she was consistently aware of her immigrant status and her subtle sense of difference compared to her American peers. She witnessed firsthand how Deaf students struggled to master the educational curriculum without teachers who could use American Sign Language (ASL) and without ASL interpreters in the classroom. She herself had to prove to educators in high school and college and supervisors at work that as a Deaf person, she was able to keep up with hearing peers and surpass them or perform jobs at work as well as hearing peers. She saw Deaf people going to Deaf friends' houses, hoping they were at home because there was no way they could have phoned ahead of time. From talking to parents and from her own parents' experiences, she understood what hearing parents go through with their Deaf children. She herself has gone through the parenting experience, having raised two children, one hearing and one Deaf, possibly due to a recessive gene. She saw Deaf people explaining how they became deaf. She saw how difficult it was for Deaf people with mental health issues to get help from signing mental health clinicians who could provide culturally affirmative services. These formative experiences led her to become a teacher of the deaf and a counselor before entering the clinical psychology doctoral program at New York University to become a psychologist. Again and again, both socially and at work, she encountered Deaf people who told of how they had to work extra hard to overcome the disbelief of well-intentioned, unenlightened hearing people that they could be competent workers. And she saw how Deaf people went about solving life problems and living productive and happy lives. All of these experiences reinforced her desire to explain to you, the reader, Deaf lives and how Deaf people navigate the early years, the educational system, and the world of home and work. At Gallaudet University, the world's only liberal arts university for

Deaf and hard-of-hearing people, she has trained or supervised numerous doctoral-level psychologists to work with Deaf people in culturally affirmative ways. She has also written extensively on the subject of Deaf people, with particular focus on deaf identities and multiculturalism, and has produced research in the areas of depression, attachment, mental health, cochlear implants, and deaf identities. She has also presented at numerous national and international conferences on these topics. She sees herself as a bicultural individual, comfortable in the Deaf community and comfortable with hearing individuals, thanks to the positive upbringing she received from her hearing parents who supported her as a Deaf person.

Jean F. Andrews is a hearing educator who early on immersed herself in the Deaf community as a young adult. During her graduate studies, she learned about Deaf culture and ASL by socializing with Deaf classmates and working on class projects with Deaf/hearing collaborative teams. She continued her learning of ASL with Deaf faculty at the Maryland School for the Deaf in the teachers' workroom and during after school social activities. While in the classroom, she explored the best ways to teach her Deaf students English reading skills by observing how they used ASL and English to understand print. Throughout her professional life, she continually connected with the Deaf community. She has spent extensive time in more than 20 Deaf schools and mainstreamed schools, researching how to best teach Deaf children using ASL/English bilingual methodology and developing alternative frameworks to teach reading using ASL English, and fingerspelling. Throughout her 45-year career, she has prepared teachers, administrators, and doctoral-level educators to understand

Deaf culture; welcomed Deaf teachers, administrators, and graduate students; and worked to give Deaf students the best academic experience possible in culturally Deaf ways. Along the way, she attended educational conferences and saw how hearing researchers dominated the podium, lecturing about how they think Deaf people should be taught to read, write, and be educated. She often wondered why more culturally Deaf professionals, with their culturally affirming insights, were not invited to participate in federally funded research teams on language, literacy, and educationally related issues. She also has experienced firsthand many Deaf people who have had significant difficulty learning in school due to language deprivation, but they somehow made it through graduate school and got into professions when accommodations were provided. But she has also seen many other Deaf adults at the lower end of the achievement spectrum who have ended up in jails and prisons without being able to communicate with their attorneys or signing interpreters. Her philosophy has been to make sure that the education and forensic fields are culturally affirmative for Deaf people. On the international front, she has collaborated on teaching classes in the Gaza Strip, Jordan, Mexico, Brazil, Morocco, and Taiwan. With international colleagues, she has published research to develop language and reading strategies for Deaf children learning alphabetic and nonalphabetic scripts.

Raychelle Harris grew up with Deaf parents and one Deaf and one hearing sister. Her parents, her mother's parents and aunt, and some relatives are Deaf, making her third-generation Deaf. The sisters learned ASL as their first language from their Deaf father, who graduated from the Florida School for the Deaf and Blind (FSDB), and their Deaf mother, who graduated from North Carolina School for the Deaf (NCSD). They met at Gallaudet College (before Gallaudet became a university in 1986) and married in 1972. Her Deaf sister met her Deaf husband at a Deaf Awareness Day event at Six Flags in New Jersey. Her husband comes from a Deaf Lithuanian family that immigrated to the United States in adulthood, and all of them learned ASL and English as their third and fourth languages in addition to Lithuanian Sign Language and both written and spoken Lithuanian. All of them are connexin 26 recipients (see Chapter 2) and/or carriers. A geneticist at Gallaudet informed her sister and her husband, both carriers of the connexin 26 mutation, that all of the children they have would be Deaf. They now have two beautiful Deaf children, who are fourth-generation Deaf. Raychelle's hearing sister, an OHCODA (only-hearing Child of Deaf Adults), fluent in ASL, married a hearing man who learned to sign. They have a beautiful hearing and signing daughter.

Growing up, Raychelle never had an opportunity to study her language or culture until a historic Deaf Studies course was offered at her Deaf high school, taught by two Deaf teachers in 1989. The experience was mind-blowing for Raychelle. When she enrolled at Gallaudet University, she met many Deaf people who did not think ASL was a language. They did not think there was a Deaf culture either. This bothered Raychelle. Her mother was the principal of a Deaf school that was the first public Deaf school to adopt the bilingual-bicultural philosophy, teaching using ASL and written English from kindergarten through high school. This inspired Raychelle to establish the first bilingual-bicultural week with all Deaf presenters explaining about ASL and

Deaf culture at Gallaudet in 1992, which then led to the establishment of a Student Body Government position focused on ASL and Deaf culture.

For a long time, Raychelle has been passionately involved in teaching ASL as well as Deaf culture to her students both at the precollege and college levels. She has researched how ASL is used in the classroom in different school settings. She has worked to include ASL and Deaf Studies in school systems. Her research found that kindergarteners who arrive at school already fluent in ASL are better able to participate in academic discussions. She has found that teachers can promote higher-order thinking skills to very young preschool children through the use of complex Academic ASL techniques and principles. Her research provides innovative approaches for ASL/English bilingual preschools and kindergartens to lay the foundation for lifelong literacy in ASL and English.

In 2011, Raychelle established the Masters in Sign Language Education (MASLED) program for teachers of signed languages and cultures. Notable alumni include numerous graduates who teach their own native sign languages such as Saudi Sign Language (SSL), Hong Kong Sign Language (HKSL), and Lengua de Señas Mexicana (LSM). Over hundreds of alumni are now teaching at the University of California, Los Angeles; Harvard University; Gallaudet University; Cornell University; Boston University; Austin Community College; Georgia State University, and many more, transforming their students' perceptions of Deaf people, Deaf cultures and Deaf communities, and hopefully yours, as you read this book.

Topher González Ávila was born in Mexico City, Mexico, to Patty Avila, a Deaf Latina woman. Patty and her eight siblings grew up in poverty in Mexico. Patty's dad worked as a taxi driver. Patty's mom stayed at home and took care of everyone. Patty wasn't able to attend what is the equivalent of high school in the United States because at the time, schools in Mexico were not required to provide access to communication. This means schools in Mexico were not obligated to provide interpreters and accommodations for Deaf and Disabled students to have equal access as other students. Instead, Patty went to trade school and completed a certification program in sewing.

Patty experienced language deprivation and severe economic hardships as a Deaf Latina woman and did not want the same for Topher, so Patty and some of her siblings moved to the United States. Most moved to Texas, California, New York, and even Canada. Patty stayed in Dallas, Texas, and had two more children, who both are Deaf. Patty learned two languages: American Sign Language (ASL) and English while navigating through a new country. Thanks to her dedication to her children, Topher and his siblings all were able to have education. They all graduated from high school and went to college. Thanks to Patty, Topher became the first one in his family to get a bachelor's degree as well as a master's degree.

Topher grew up in public schools in Dallas while his siblings attended Texas School for the Deaf (TSD). They all had choices when it came to the school they attended. Topher was new to the United States and stayed with his mom. Topher graduated and went to the University of North Texas (UNT). He completed his dual degrees in Radio, Television, and Film (RTVF) and Criminal Justice in 2015. Following graduation, Topher joined Deaf Action Center (DAC), a local Deaf-run nonprofit with services and programs available to support the Deaf communities in Dallas–Fort Worth (DFW).

DAC has been instrumental in Patty and her family's transition to the United States, and this was Topher's way of giving back to the Deaf communities. For 2 years, Topher worked in the interpreting department as their Scheduling Coordinator Assistant and then as their Training & Outreach Liaison. Topher became familiar with the interpreting field. He took the BEI exams and became one of the first known Latinx Deaf interpreters in Texas. The more Topher worked for the Deaf communities, the more Topher realized that it starts with schools. Changes need to start in school. So he went to Gallaudet University for their Masters in Sign Language Education (MASLED) program and graduated in 2018.

In the program, Topher studied teaching methods and approaches, assessment tools and strategies, and curriculum development and implementation. Topher completed his MASLED internship with Nozomi Tomita, a Japanese Deaf woman who taught Japanese Sign Language. Through her skills and expertise, Topher was able to co-develop and co-teach Gallaudet University's first hybrid Lengua de Señas Mexicana (LSM) course with Armando Castro-Osnaya. During his studies at Gallaudet, he also did two other internships.

He did an Accelator internship with Mitú in Los Angeles, California. Mitú is an online entertainment channel by Latinx people and for Latinx people. There, he worked with some of the industry's writers, filmmakers, and editors. He completed his internship with a short film, *Connected Manos* (2018), on his mom. Lastly but certainly not least, he worked with HEARD (Helping Educate to Advance the Rights of Deaf Communities),

an all-volunteer nonprofit organization that works for Deaf and Disabled people who are impacted by mass incarceration. Topher believes that one can never stop learning, and he hopes to continue working with and for our Deaf communities to bring long-term positive changes.

For Ayisha Knight-Shaw, being asked to create the cover art for this book has truly been an honor. The beautiful collaboration between Ayisha Knight-Shaw, Topher González Ávila, and fellow Deaf artist Jessica Arevalo has made this a reality. Ayisha is a Deaf California-based multimedia artist, poet, educator, and Reiki Master Teacher. The daughter of a white Jewish mother and Black Cherokee father, she was raised by her mother in an ethnically diverse community of poets, painters, sculptors, photographers, and storytellers who taught her that creating and sharing art is as much a political act as a thing of beauty. These intersectional identities have been at the forefront of her art since she began exploring photography at age 13 and have evolved over the years. Her life as a Deaf woman in California, Washington, DC, and Massachusetts, as well as visits to Cuba, Mexico City, and Oaxaca have given Ayisha the opportunity to create a tapestry of many cultures in her work. Her solo and shared photo exhibits have been showcased at Very Special Arts Boston, the Boston Public Library, the Cambridge Center for Adult Education, Salem Access TV, Espresso Royale Café, Two Dogs Working, Galant Gallery, North Shore Career Center, Deaf Expo, Disability Expo, Maine Deaf Expo, and Dorian's in Provincetown, Massachusetts.

As a poet, Ayisha has been seen at the Lincoln Center for the Performing Arts, Teatro Pregones, La Mama theater in New York City, Rhode Island School of Design, Amherst 20th Anniversary of the ADA, Northampton Pride, and Wake Up The Earth. Television and other video appearances include HBO Def Poetry Jam Season 4 as the first Deaf poet, Basic Black, and Urban Update, The Museum of Fine Arts Boston, Gore House Museum, and Culture Coach International. Her 2004 show at Wheelock Family Theater, "Hey Sistah, Welcome Home," led to a grant by the Cambridge Arts Council. She holds a BA degree in Theater Arts from UC Santa Cruz, and a master's degree in Sign Language Education from Gallaudet University. Over the years, her passion for art, storytelling, theater, Reiki, and education has been forming a tapestry that continues today. If you would like to see more of her work, you can visit her website (http://www.deafayisha.com).

While we focus strongly on Deaf culture in this book, we also write about persons who do not identify with Deaf culture. Why do we write about these individuals? We contrast their experiences with the experiences of people who grow up either exposed to Deaf culture or who become part of the culturally Deaf community after their school years. We feel this will help you understand more fully how persons who are deaf experience their lives, whether culturally Deaf or not.

Exactly what have we done for this second edition? Each chapter has been significantly updated. In Part I, "Deaf Culture: Yesterday and Today," we have two chapters. Chapter 1 covers the past and present of the Deaf community. It consists of an introduction that reports on the Deaf community, who its members are, how large the community is, its history, and the different ways to explain the Deaf experience.

What is a chapter on "Causes of Being Deaf and the Auditory Field" doing in Part I? Deaf people themselves *are* interested in genetics. And, contrary to popular belief, many do not necessarily want to become hearing. They are proud of themselves as Deaf people. But they are interested in how genes that cause differences in hearing are transmitted from generation to generation. We assume you readers will be interested, too. Deaf people also talk about how they became deaf from nongenetic causes such as diseases, and we explain this. Everyone with hearing differences has been through hearing testing and different ways to get access to hearing through auditory aids. They all have experiences with audiologists. Culturally Deaf people, including those who want to use hearing aids and cochlear implants (devices to help people hear), have their own perspective on experiences in hearing and speech centers. It is part of their lives, and they have been working to make such experiences more culturally sensitive.

Moving on to Part II, we learn about "Signed Languages and Learning." This gets to the heart of Deaf culture. In this section, we include information that shows how signed languages and learning continue to evolve. In Chapter 3, "American Sign Language," you will learn that despite centuries of linguistic imperialism oppression, ASL and other signed languages remain a vibrant marker of Deaf communities worldwide who cherish and celebrate its use. Here we explore the following: What is a signed language? How do culturally Deaf people, for whom ASL is their unique language and bond, use ASL to communicate? What is the difference between sign language and sign communication? Yes, there is a difference! Do Deaf people all over the world use the same sign language? Read this chapter to find out.

In Chapter 4, "How Deaf Children Think, Learn, and Read," we explore how Deaf and DeafDisabled students develop their cognitive abilities, world knowledge, and literacy through their different life experiences at home and school with the resources of a sign language, Deaf culture, multiculturalism, and auditory, tactile, and visual technologies.

And in Chapter 5, "Deaf Education, Deaf Culture, and Multiculturalism," we learn how Deaf, DeafBlind, and Deaf-Disabled people from different cultural backgrounds have been educated and what they have learned. There are laws about educating children with disabilities, including deaf children. Do you know how much input culturally Deaf people had into their own education? What was the education system like for them? We also examine learner factors in Deaf education related to Deaf culture and multiculturalism and note disruptive dynamics such as institutional and individual racism, linguicism, and audism. What do we know from research about what works and does not work? Get the answers in this chapter!

Moving on to Part III, "Deaf Lives, Technology, Arts, and Career Opportunities," we get more into how Deaf people live their lives. Chapter 6, "Deaf Identities," covers different theories and ways that identity develops in Deaf people and how culturally Deaf people may see themselves. When scholars began to explore Deaf culture, they based their conclusions on white Deaf people. What about Deaf people of color? What about Lesbians, Gays, Bisexual, Transgender, and Queer culturally Deaf people? What about Deaf-Disabled people? The field of intersectionality, or how different identities interact with each other and how these interactions are compounded by oppression, is

growing fast. Scholars are finally paying attention to these different Deaf groups and how their identities intersect. In this edition, we pay more attention to issues of intersectionality.

The Deaf community is not just one big white Deaf community, just as hearing society is not one huge hearing community. Both consist of multiple communities. In Chapter 7, written for this edition, we take an in-depth look at exactly what these communities are as represented by various Deaf individuals and what they have done in view of their unique identities. We also present how the disenfranchised communities experience discrimination and oppression.

What life issues do culturally Deaf people confront? How do they deal with these life issues? Do they feel equal to hearing people? When they face discrimination by hearing people, whether in school, on the playground, at work, or in the community, how do they stand up for themselves? That is the focus of Chapter 8, "Navigating Lives ." Many Deaf people do just fine. But others struggle in the world of work. They may also face health and mental health issues and can get caught in the criminal justice system. When they search for help, are the available services Deaf culturally affirmative?

Deaf people have made their mark in technology and access. In Chapter 9, "Technology and Accessibility," we provide a historical background to explain the access issues Deaf people had to struggle with. When technology finally caught up enough to enable Deaf people to have functional equivalence (this means they can access technical devices just like hearing people can), their lives were transformed in positive ways. In this chapter, new information has been added so that you can learn how Deaf people currently use and benefit from captions, telephones, alarm systems, and other types of innovative technology. Deaf people have worked to invent much of the technology that they now benefit from.

Laws, legislation, and Deaf communities are the focus of Chapter 10, a new addition to this edition. You may ask what it is about laws and legislation that is so important for the Deaf community. This chapter explains the significant and protective impact these laws have had on the lives of Deaf people. They have used the legal powers of these laws to counteract discrimination and achieve functional equivalence with their hearing counterparts in areas such as education, health care, employment, and the criminal justice system that includes both victims of crime and offenders.

Chapter 11, "Arts, Literature, and Media," provides a window to the arts and literature that is a vital part of Deaf culture. This chapter reflects new work that has emerged since the first edition. We show you how Deaf culture has contributed to the arts through visual means. There are plays, sculptures, paintings, and literary renderings, among others, that have been produced by culturally Deaf people. You will get a taste of sign language literature and written literature that shows how Deaf people express themselves. We also provide information on how Deaf people have been and are being portrayed in the arts, literature, and media. There are Deaf people in Hollywood, on Broadway, and in multiple television shows, including reality shows.

Chapter 12, "Advocating and Career Opportunities," was written with you, the reader, in mind. We present ways in which

hearing people can work together with Deaf people as advocates and allies while minimizing potential pitfalls in working together. There is new emphasis on the importance of mutual respect and awareness of hearing privilege. We also provide information on different career opportunities that allow you to be involved with Deaf people. Hopefully, it will help you decide where you want to go with what you have learned from this book. There are many other possibilities beyond the careers we write about where you can be involved in working with and for Deaf people, if that interests you.

And finally, in Chapter 13, we present "Final Thoughts on Deaf Culture and Its Future." What impact will all the technology and genetic advances have on Deaf culture and ASL? Does the Deaf community have a future? What is the legacy of the Deaf community and Deaf culture? Has sufficient attention been paid to the diversity of the Deaf community considering that earlier Deaf culture scholarship has been described through a white lens? How can hearing parents benefit from knowledge about Deaf culture? Having a deaf child does not have to be anxiety ridden and problem filled; it can be a joyful experience to support a Deaf child, understand the world of this child, and provide ways to be bicultural as this child connects with both hearing and Deaf societies.

We hope you, the reader, enjoy the book as much as we have enjoyed writing it for you. We hope you will get a sense of Deaf culture and the different ways Deaf people have worked to improve their quality of life and to show they are an important part of the diversity of the human race.

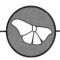

Acknowledgments

We acknowledge the assistance of those individuals who eased the process of our work, starting with Gallaudet University graduate research assistants Alexander Wilkins, Amanda Strasser, and, particularly for this second edition, Erin Timberlake. They ably contributed reference sources that ensured we had updated information. Alexander Wilkins went beyond the call of duty in creating images and ensuring that photographs selected for this book were prepared for publication. We also gratefully acknowledge Ayisha Knight-Shaw's new design work for the book cover. To them we express appreciation.

Ashley L. Dockens, AuD, PhD, and James G. Phelan, AuD, made sure that the information on audiology was accurately and impeccably presented. From Lamar University, we thank Brian Sattler for his photographs and Chatman Sieben for his editorial support. Diane Clark, PhD., chairperson of the Department of Deaf Studies and Deaf Education at Lamar provided resources via access to doctoral research in her Cognition in Context (C'nC) Research Laboratory. Brian Greenwald, PhD, of Gallaudet University provided valuable information regarding the eugenics controversy we cover in Chapter 9. We could not have obtained some of our photographs and permissions to use these without the assistance of Susan Flanigan, Coordinator of Public Relations and Communications in the Laurent Clerc National Deaf Education Center at Gallaudet University, and Michael Olson, former Interim Director, Gallaudet University Archives. And we thank the anonymous reviewers for their comments, which enabled us to polish this second edition. Also, we give profound thanks to Kalie Koscielak, our first editor, and to Christina Gunning, who replaced her, for responding promptly to our requests for information and providing encouragement as we worked to bring this book to fruition. As our copyeditor, Gillian Dickens cast a sharp eye on the manuscript. And finally, researching sources went that much faster thanks to the Internet, which in fact was created by a deaf man!

We cannot leave the Acknowledgment section without thanking our families, who patiently endured our long hours on the computer as we worked to meet deadlines. They understood the importance of getting this book out to you, the readers, so that you can learn what Deaf culture is all about. And finally, we express our appreciation to everyone who has shared or written about perspectives on Deaf culture, without which we could never have written this book.

Irene W. Leigh
Jean F. Andrews
Raychelle L. Harris
Topher González Ávila

About the Authors

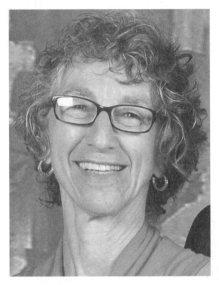

Irene W. Leigh, PhD, is a Deaf psychologist with an undergraduate degree in Deaf Education from Northwestern University, a master's degree in Rehabilitation Counseling, and a doctorate in Clinical Psychology, both from New York University. Her experience includes high school teaching at a school for the deaf, psychological assessment, psychotherapy, and private practice. From 1985 to 1991, she was a psychologist and assistant director at the Lexington Center for Mental Health Services in Queens, New York. She taught in the Gallaudet University Clinical Psychology Doctoral Program from 1992 to 2012, was Psychology Department Chair from 2008 to 2012, and attained professor emerita status in 2012. Dr. Leigh serves on review boards of professional journals and was associate editor of the *Journal of Deaf Studies and Deaf Education* from 2005 to 2011. She has presented nationally and internationally on identity, multiculturalism, depression, mental health, parenting, attachment, cochlear implants, and psychosocial adjustment and has published more than 50 articles and book chapters in addition to authoring, coauthoring, and editing or coediting several books. As a Fellow of the American Psychological Association, she served on two task forces, chaired the Committee on Disability Issues in Psychology, and was on the Board for the Advancement of Psychology in the Public Interest. She also maintains a private practice and has received multiple awards for her work.

Jean F. Andrews, PhD, received a bachelor's degree in English language and literature from Catholic University, in Washington, DC; a master's in education in Deaf Education from McDaniel College (formerly Western Maryland College) in Westminster, Maryland; and a doctorate in Speech and Hearing Sciences from the University of Illinois, Champaign-Urbana, Illinois. Dr. Andrews was a classroom teacher of reading at the Maryland School for the Deaf in Frederick, Maryland. From 1983 to 1988, she prepared educational interpreters and teachers of Deaf students at Eastern Kentucky University, Richmond, Kentucky. From 1988 to 2015 at Lamar University in Beaumont, Texas, she taught classes, prepared

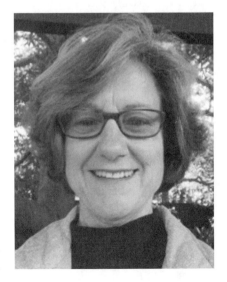

teachers and doctoral-level leaders, and conducted applied research. Dr. Andrews has been recognized by the Kentucky Association for the Deaf and the Texas Association for the Deaf for her contributions to deaf education. She has also served on the governing board of the Texas School for the Deaf. Her research interests include language and literacy, Deaf Studies, ASL/English bilingualism, and forensic issues with Deaf individuals. For 20 years, she has been involved as an expert witness and has educated judges, lawyers, and criminal justice officials about Deaf culture and the language and communication needs of Deaf, DeafDisabled, and DeafBlind individuals caught up in the criminal justice system. Dr. Andrews has coauthored several academic texts related to psychology, education, and Deaf people. She has also written fiction and nonfiction for young Deaf readers.

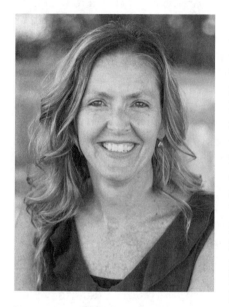

Raychelle L. Harris, PhD, a third-generation Deaf and a native ASL signer, received her bachelor's degree in American Sign Language (ASL) from Gallaudet University in 1995 and master's degree in Deaf Education from Western Maryland College in 2000. Dr. Harris has been teaching ASL as a first and second language since 1993. She returned to Gallaudet University for her doctoral studies in the areas of education and linguistics, with her dissertation topic focused on ASL discourse in academic settings. In 2008, she joined Gallaudet University's Department of Interpretation as a faculty member. Since 2009, she has been teaching in the Department of ASL. Dr. Harris holds professional certification with the American Sign Language Teachers Association and is a Certified Deaf Interpreter with the Board for Evaluation of Interpreters (BEI) and is court certified in the state of Texas. She is also one of five coauthors of TRUE+WAY ASL, an innovative and digitally based ASL curriculum, along with Dr. Nathie L. Marbury, Lisa Gelineau, Ritchie Bryant, and Tracy Shannon.

Topher González Ávila, MA, was born in Mexico City, Mexico. He moved to Dallas, Texas, when he was a baby. His Deaf mom raised Topher and his two Deaf siblings in a multilingual family of Lengua de Señas Mexicana (LSM), American Sign Language (ASL), English, and Spanish. Topher graduated from University of North Texas with bachelor's degrees in Criminal Justice and Radio, Television, and Film (RTVF) in 2015. He continued his education at Gallaudet University and graduated in 2018 with a master's in Sign Language Education. Topher has been a Certified Deaf Interpreter with the Board for Evaluation of Interpreters (BEI) since 2016. He is the first Deaf Latinx interpreter in the state of Texas to hold a BEI Court Interpretation certification. Topher teaches for Gallaudet University's Masters in Sign

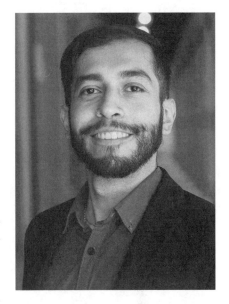

Language Education program. Topher works as a community interpreter and a freelance video editor. Topher is proud to be Brown, Queer, and Deaf. It was and still is a journey for him to finally embrace the person he is. He works with and for his communities especially, BIPOC Deaf youth and Queer Deaf youth, through local, state, and national organizational advocacy efforts.

PART I

Deaf Culture:
Yesterday and Today

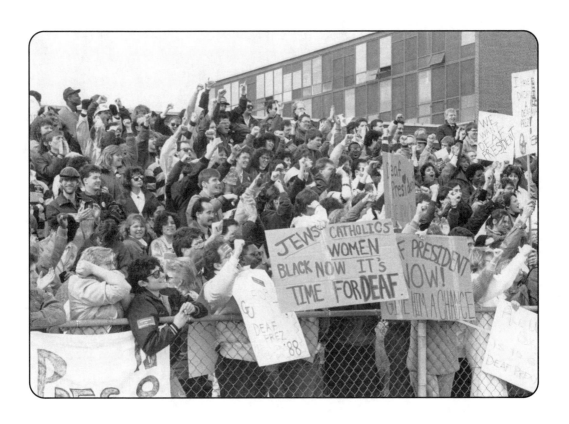

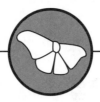

CHAPTER 1

Deaf Community:
Past and Present

INTRODUCTION

If you are a hearing person or, in other words, a person who is not deaf and who just happens to bump into a stranger and start talking, how do you react when that person says, "I am deaf" and points to his or her ears while shaking his or her head? Many of you likely will blurt out loud, "Oh, I'm so sorry." This has happened time and time again.

What does this mean? Were you sorry because you were not aware and are apologizing for your mistake? Or were you sorry because that person cannot hear, cannot easily understand spoken language, and has to struggle to communicate?

Many people have created a vision of "deaf" as meaning limited and unable to communicate with hearing people around them. They think deaf people are limited in what they can learn in school and in the kind of jobs they can do. They see deaf people as isolated and unable to connect with the world. This may be why many people look to medicine to "cure" hearing loss. They believe that surgery to insert a cochlear implant as a means for deaf people to gain access to the sensations of sound (see Chapter 2 for details), or the use of hearing aids to amplify sounds, will "help" deaf people "hear" and understand people who speak. People in general often want deaf people to learn how to speak and hear so that they are a part of their hearing families and their environment.

We've also seen people using sign language on the street or in a restaurant. All over the United States, American Sign Language (ASL) courses are very popular. On TV and in the movies, there are deaf actors and actresses using sign language. One example is that of Shoshannah Stern, pictured in Figure 1–1, who is well known especially for TV roles in programs such as *Threat Matrix*, *Providence*, *ER*, and *This Close*. Her colleague, Josh Feldman (Figure 1–2), who cowrote the script for *This Close* and acted with her in this series, is yet another example. Their parents and siblings are Deaf. They attended schools for the deaf and grew up always connected to culturally Deaf people. Read on, and in a few paragraphs, you will see

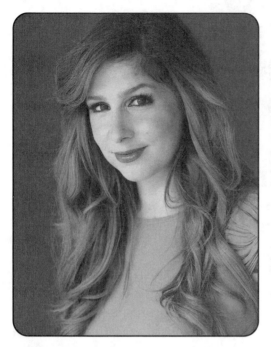

Figure 1–1. Shoshannah Stern, Deaf actress. Photo credit: Tate Tullier. Used with permission of Shoshannah Stern.

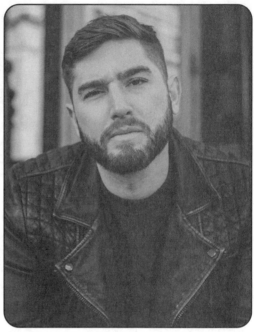

Figure 1–2. Josh Feldman, Deaf actor. Photo credit: Tiffany Saccente. Used with permission of Josh Feldman.

an explanation of the difference between deaf and Deaf.

In the music field, we have Sean Forbes, a popular deaf rapper who was selected as outstanding hip-hop artist of the year at the Detroit Music Awards (Stone, 2015). And there is Aarron Loggins, who signed the National Anthem with singer Gladys Knight, while sisters Chloe and Halle Bailey signed "America the Beautiful" along with her at the LIII Super Bowl (Slane, 2019). There are talented Deaf artists working in every possible media, as noted in Chapter 11. Every now and then, newspapers will include information about Gallaudet University, the world's only liberal arts university for deaf and hard-of-hearing students. Deaf people's opinions are often included in media articles about the cochlear implant. Their opinions cover two contrasting

perspectives. One perspective is that cochlear implants support access to the hearing world and help with hearing and speaking. The other perspective is that cochlear implants hurt the Deaf community because the focus is on hearing and speaking and not on sign language, which is visual and accessible. These perspectives are elaborated further in Chapter 2.

You may even have a deaf medical doctor or a deaf lawyer! Deaf people have made inroads in many careers and organizations. For example, we have Suzy Rosen Singleton, pictured in Figure 1–3. She is a Deaf lawyer who serves as Chief of the Disability Rights Office of the Consumer and Governmental Affairs of the Federal Communications Commission. Her parents are Deaf, as are her two siblings, one of whom is also a lawyer while the other is a mechanical engineer. She uses sign

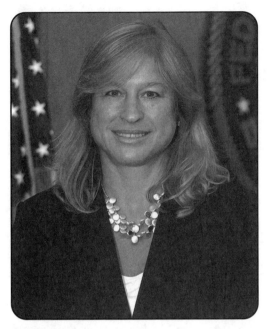

Figure 1–3. Suzy Rosen Singleton, Chief, Disability Rights Office. Photo credit: Steven Balderson. Used with permission of Suzy Rosen Singleton.

NEGATIVE LABELS

Auditory Handicap

Hearing Impaired

Hearing Handicapped

Deaf Mute

Prelingually Deaf

Deaf and Dumb

language interpreters during scheduled meetings. Among her responsibilities is that of helping to implement the Commission's goal of ensuring accessibility of modern communications services and technologies for persons with disabilities.

Google "Deaf" and you will find hundreds, even thousands, of references. Because of this explosion of information, many more people than ever before are aware of deaf people, deaf communities, and Deaf culture. But often the lay public is not aware of the many nuances or details of this unique population. They may not know that being deaf may have more meanings than just "cannot hear." They may use different phrases to describe deaf people, such as auditory handicap, hearing impaired, hearing handicapped, deaf mute, prelingually deaf, or deaf and dumb.

Deaf people will often interpret these terms as negative because they focus on the disability and what the deaf person cannot do. *Deaf* and *hard of hearing* tend to be the preferred terms, although *hearing impaired* is also frequently used throughout the United States but not by culturally Deaf people themselves (Holcomb, 2013). Commonly and culturally, Deaf people feel that *hearing impaired* means that something is wrong, broken, impaired, or not working, and they don't see themselves as wrong, broken, impaired, or not working.

It helps to understand that being deaf can reflect a meaningful and productive way of life. Deaf people who identify with Deaf culture want to be labeled as people who are normal in their own way, primarily use vision, sometimes supported by audition (through hearing aids or cochlear implants), to communicate and interact with others. They describe Deaf as a positive way of life, not as something "impaired." Interestingly and in contrast, the term *deaf impaired* is sometimes used to denote hearing people who do not understand Deaf culture or ASL. You can decide whether the use of the word *impaired*, whether deaf or hearing, makes sense after looking at this list of possible types of impairments and considering how subjectively negative these are.

Thin impaired

Tall impaired

Hair impaired

So our purpose in this book is to provide information to help you understand deaf people and their vibrant deaf community. You may have noticed that we use the terms *deaf* and *Deaf*. What is this all about? The term *deaf* refers to individuals whose hearing loss makes it very hard or impossible to understand spoken language through hearing alone, with or without the use of auditory devices (hearing aids, cochlear implants, FM systems, etc.). Many of those individuals who call themselves "deaf" tend to rely on auditory assistance devices, prefer to use spoken language, and tend to socialize more often with hearing people than with deaf people.

"Deaf" represents what we see as the culture of Deaf people. These people use sign language and share beliefs, values, customs, and experiences that create a very strong bond and group identity (Holcomb, 2013). They often prefer to socialize with other culturally Deaf people and do not see themselves as tragically isolated from society, contrary to what many hearing people think. They see benefits to being deaf that many are unaware of.

Here you see the term *culture* used.

What is your definition of culture?

Culture is a term that has been debated for a long time and has multiple definitions (Eagleton, 2013). One way to define culture is that it includes the values, beliefs, social forms, and traits of a group of people. These values represent specific meanings, beliefs, and practices that guide the group in individual and social development. It is common to think of culture as representing the many observable characteristics of a group that can be seen, most obviously their behavior. We need to understand the reality that cultural behavior is only an external representation of the deeper and broader concepts of culture, specifically the complex ideas, attitudes, and values (Languageandculture.com, 2015). As seen in Figure 1–4, the image of a cultural iceberg helps us to understand what aspects reflect cultures. The observable part of the iceberg includes behaviors and practices that can be seen or observed, while the buried or hidden part of the iceberg incorporates how the core values (learned ideas of what is acceptable or desirable, including religion, family practices, and so on) are shown in specific situations such as working or socializing. Although different cultural groups may share similar core values, such as respect, such values may be interpreted differently in different situations and incorporated differently into specific attitudes for daily situations. These internal core values may become visible to the casual observer who sees the observable behaviors such as the words that are used, the ways people in the culture act, and so on.

Can you think of examples that show how respect is demonstrated in different cultures?

Now consider this: What is your definition of Deaf culture?

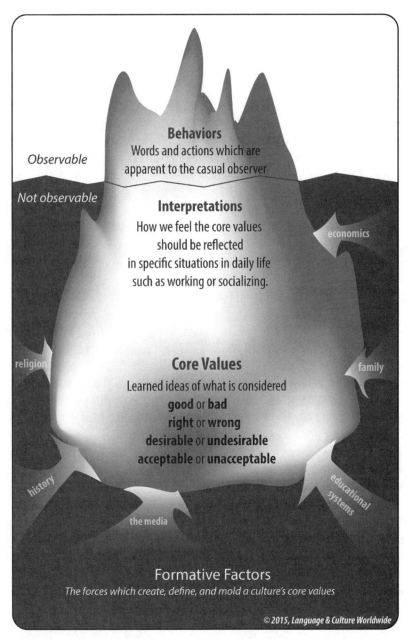

Figure 1–4. The Cultural Iceberg. Used with permission of Language & Culture Worldwide, LLC. http://www.languageandculture.com

A lot of people have no idea that there is such a thing as Deaf culture (see, for example, Jassal, 2017; Solomon, 2014). When we write about Deaf culture, we are writing about the beliefs, mores, artistic expressions, behaviors, understanding, and sign language expressions that Deaf people use (e.g., Holcomb, 2013; Padden & Humphries, 1988). Atherton (2016) states that Deaf culture reflects "those activities and behaviours deaf people share when they gather together" (p. 14). It is a culture that people are either born into or join later after meeting culturally Deaf people. It can mean participating in events that include Deaf people. Culturally Deaf people tend to view being Deaf as a positive attribute or as a gain, not as something negative or pathological that needs to be fixed (Bauman & Murray, 2014). This gain reflects the attributes of enhanced and prolonged eye contact, ways of engaging with others, collectivist ways of socializing, ability to engage with Deaf individuals from other countries, less auditory distraction, and ability to maximize the use of vision to understand space (visuospatial aptitudes), among others. Deaf gain is a perspective that promotes resiliency in the face of difficult experiences, using cultural capital (Yosso, 2005). Cultural capital involves the use of cultural knowledge and cultural competencies, including skills and abilities. In turn, social capital reflects socialization, networking, reciprocity, trust, and shared norms and values (M. Kusters, 2017). As M. Kusters explains, Deaf community cultural and social capital wealth includes the use of visual language, visual learning, navigating and negotiating society as a deaf person, being Deaf as a way of life, having access to information about deaf events and networks, and the connections with Deaf people who are leading full lives. Such capital lends support to a protective factor when Deaf people work to maximize their opportunities even while experiencing lower expectations on the part of hearing people. The development of cultural and social capital is facilitated when Deaf role models are available to help young people navigate developmental processes, life challenges, and ways of communicating both information

and emotional expressions (Cawthon, Johnson, Garberoglio, & Schoffstall, 2016; Gala, 2017).

Instead of the medical model that frames deaf people as having a medically based issue that is viewed as pathological and thereby needing to be fixed, specifically ears that are ineffective or nonfunctional in processing sound stimuli, we can place the Deaf culture paradigm within the social-minority or sociocultural model. This theoretical model posits that life with a "difference" reflects a different way of being, not a deficit, that grants Deaf people minority group status (Leigh, 2009).

When did deaf communities begin to exist? Many people do not realize that deaf communities in different countries have existed for centuries (e.g., Bauman, 2008; Branson & Miller, 2002; Eriksson, 1993; Van Cleve & Crouch, 1989). An examination of biblical lore has encouraged Gulliver and Lyons (2018) to believe that there likely were signing deaf communities in ancient Israel. However, the term *Deaf culture* became popular only in the 1980s, after the book *Deaf in America: Voices From a Culture* (Padden & Humphries, 1988) was published. Why talk about Deaf culture when Deaf people often use the very popular term *deaf community*?

Although the deaf community brings up a picture of how people interact within this community, Deaf culture is a different and unique way of looking at deaf people (Holcomb, 2013; A. Kusters, De Meulder, & O'Brien, 2017a; Padden & Humphries, 1988). This focus on Deaf culture instead of "deaf community" legitimizes how Deaf people look at life, how they function, and how they define themselves, not by how hearing people define them. This is a different "center" from how hearing people define being deaf. Culturally Deaf people often have little interest in knowing how well one can hear or speak or how one became deaf. This is similarly true for culturally DeafBlind individuals who have little interest in knowing how much one can see or how one became DeafBlind. They see themselves as individuals who develop as others develop, who naturally learn their signed language and culture in a normal way that is different from the typical hearing way, or easily learn both as they transition to their local Deaf or DeafBlind community. They use their signed or tactile languages to pass on social norms, values, language, and technology to new entrees and to the next generation. Simply put, using the term *Deaf culture* is a search for the Deaf self, the ways of being Deaf, through analyzing what it means to be a complete Deaf person, not a person who is incomplete because of the lack of hearing. This represents the value of living full, rewarding Deaf lives instead of struggling to compensate for being "incomplete." Most deaf people are not born into Deaf culture because they have hearing parents, but rather enter the culture later. This is analogous to individuals who affirm a Lesbian or Gay identity while growing up and then connect with Queer communities.

The field of Deaf Studies has encouraged deeper study of cultural ways of being Deaf, with more research into what Deaf culture is all about and an increasing research base created by Deaf scholars themselves (A. Kusters, De Meulder, & O'Brien, 2017a, 2017b). Deaf culture was formerly viewed as a culture with specific rules regarding language and behavior that contrasts with the "hearing world"

culture. Now that scholars are increasingly aware of and have studied the multiple cultures within the "hearing world" of the United States and abroad, Deaf Studies scholars are examining how truly diverse Deaf culture is when looking at the Black, Native American or Indigenous, Latinx,[1] and Asian groups within the Deaf culture in the United States as well as the different cultural groups in other parts of the international Deaf community. Below and throughout this book, readers will begin to understand the truly diverse and evolving nature of Deaf culture.

THE DEAF COMMUNITY AND ITS MEMBERS

Who are the members of the deaf community? Atherton (2016) defines the deaf community as consisting of members "whose deafness gives rise to interests and experiences that they actively share and participate in with other deaf people" (p. 27). He asserts that audiological status is not a necessary criterion. Hearing people have often participated in deaf community events, as have deaf individuals who vary in their use of sign language, those who become deaf later in childhood or adulthood, and, of course, members of Deaf culture.

The deaf community is not just one community. Again, just look at the Latinx, Native American or Indigenous, Asian, or Black communities. Each has its own diverse groups and cultures. For instance, Indigenous communities have multiple tribes. Similarly, Deaf communities not only have diverse deaf members; they also

---

[1]"Latinx" is a term that is neutral in terms of gender (Reichard, 2015). It includes both Latina and Latino terms, thereby being more inclusive without having to specify whether female, male, or nonbinary.

have diverse groups of members within the culture (Padden & Humphries, 1988). There is much ethnic and racial diversity both within groups and across groups. This diversity includes both those born in the United States and those born in other countries and who have immigrated at different periods of their lives ranging from childhood to adulthood.

These diverse groups also show differences in their use of language, either spoken or signed. Furthermore, there are differences in hearing levels that range from those individuals with minor hearing losses to individuals who hear absolutely nothing. There are also differences across religions, in political opinions, in socioeconomic status, and in sexual orientation, among others. Deaf people attain different levels of education, ranging from elementary through secondary, post-secondary, and higher education. Deaf people may or may not have additional disabilities, including sensory, physical, cognitive, learning, reading, or psychosocial disabilities.

However, even within this diversity of characteristics, there are fundamental similarities. For example, becoming culturally Deaf means using signed languages, being upfront as a Deaf person, being comfortable with other Deaf people, and wanting to interact with them. We provide descriptive characteristics of groups that are typically viewed as part of the deaf community below. Please keep in mind that all these individuals are part of the racial and/or ethnic diversity spectrum as well, as is emphasized throughout this book.

Deaf Children of Culturally Deaf Parents

These individuals tend to be seen as those who pass on Deaf culture from genera-

tion to generation (Padden & Humphries, 1988). They often grow up immersed in the Deaf cultural community and using sign language. Culturally Deaf children often attend schools where sign language is used. They may attend camps with other Deaf children. They also go to Deaf social events such as Deaf festivals, conventions, religious services, or sporting events. Here they learn the values of Deaf culture through everyday experiences interacting with other culturally Deaf people. Shoshannah Stern, Josh Feldman, and Suzy Rosen Singleton, each of whom was mentioned earlier, are prime examples who have achieved well in life. Some culturally Deaf parents do see spoken languages as important so that their children can be both bilingual, bimodal, and bicultural (Mitchiner, 2014). This makes it easier for them to interact with both hearing and Deaf cultural groups. It is helpful to keep in mind that, in addition, there are deaf parents who prefer to use only spoken language and communicate in this way with their deaf children.

Deaf Children of Hearing Parents

Approximately 96% of deaf children are born to hearing parents (Mitchell & Karchmer, 2004). These parents are often shocked when they find out that their new baby has not passed the hearing screening test done at the hospital. After going through stages such as shock, anger, grief, denial, and possibly doctor shopping, they finally accept the reality of the permanence of their child's deafness (Leigh & Andrews, 2017; Sass-Lehrer, 2016). In contrast, Deaf parents tend to focus on wanting a healthy child. If they find out their new baby has passed what they call the Deaf test rather than "failed the hearing test," they tend to be comfortable with this finding.

These hearing parents have to start learning about how to communicate with their babies and what it means to have a deaf child (Leigh & Andrews, 2017; Sass-Lehrer, 2016). Most do not know sign language. Some will learn, but many do not master the language. Their children will often learn about Deaf culture later, perhaps from their teacher or other Deaf adults in school, go to summer camps where there are Deaf children who use sign language, when attending Deaf cultural festivals or conferences, or even when working with sign language users. If they attend Gallaudet University; the National Technical Institute for the Deaf at the Rochester Institute of Technology; California State University, Northridge; or other colleges/universities where there is a large population of deaf college students, they are going to be exposed to peers with information about Deaf culture. If they are at mainstream community colleges or universities where there are sign language interpreters, they may learn about Deaf culture from the sign language interpret-ers. Many will connect with the deaf community, while others will remain comfortably within their hearing communities.

Darby's mother mourned the loss of her "hearing daughter" after she stopped denying that her child was deaf. After intensive research and speaking with people about what to do, she decided to start communicating with Darby using ASL. She felt that she was able to learn ASL and felt comfortable about creating a bilingual (ASL and English) family because she and her husband came from bilingual homes. She took ASL classes and a parent/infant teacher came weekly to help with ASL learning. She also went to Darby's school for the deaf daily to maintain exposure to ASL. When Darby was in fifth grade, the mother proudly reported that Darby was at or above grade level for reading (Layton, 2007).

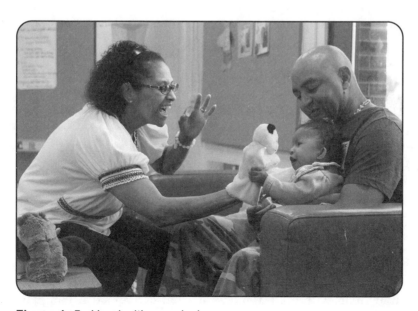

Figure 1–5. Used with permission.

Hearing Members in Deaf Families

Hearing siblings of deaf children, hearing children of deaf adults (CODAs), and hearing people who marry or partner with deaf persons may connect with the Deaf community and/or identify with Deaf culture, especially if they are very comfortable using sign language (e.g., Berkowitz & Jonas, 2014; Hoffmeister, 2008; Torres, 2009). These hearing members often are bilingual, knowing both a spoken and a signed language. For example, the Deaf parents may voice in English, or bring in hearing family members to expose the hearing child to spoken English, while using ASL at other times. If they use only spoken English with their hearing child, that language will be the child's primary language. If you are interested in how deaf and hearing siblings relate to each other, the book, *Deaf and Hearing Siblings in Conversation* (Berkowitz & Jonas, 2014), illustrates the perspectives hearing and deaf siblings have for each other, especially in how they communicate and how their families interact with each other. For example, some hearing siblings learn ASL and develop close bonds with their deaf siblings while others do not. How close they are depends on their level of comfort with each other's language and communication needs as well as individual characteristics. As one sibling commented on her perspective of an exemplary relationship: "Your brothers and your sisters—they're all no different than you are. We all have our own needs. You know, we all want to be included. We all want to be accepted." (Berkowitz & Jonas, 2014, pp. 167–168)

Hard-of-Hearing Individuals

These are individuals with mild or moderate hearing levels who will rely more on what they can hear with hearing aids (Leigh, 2009). Speechreading or lipreading the spoken language is less important for them. If they have deaf parents who use ASL, they will naturally be acculturated to Deaf culture. If they have hearing parents, they will likely follow the hearing culture of their families. They often will want to just "be hearing" and not differ from their families or friends. Because of this, they sometimes will avoid meeting other deaf people. They may struggle in communicating with others due to their difficulties in hearing. Some may learn ASL in high school or college and start to get involved in Deaf sports or groups if they are welcomed and show eagerness to sign. Some become part of the Deaf community.

> Kathy Vesey and Beth Wilson (2003), pictured in Figures 1–6 and 1–7, both grew up hard of hearing in the mainstream. They felt something was missing. As adults, they learned sign language. They write about feeling fortunate to be part of the richness of Deaf culture while still being accepted in hearing society. They also note that it is sad to see hard-of-hearing adults trying to be "hearing" or to "pass as hearing." They know what a struggle that is.

Late-Deafened Individuals

These are individuals who became deaf after the age of 18 due to illness, sustained or acute exposure to workplace noise, accident, genetic predisposition, medication allergy, or other unknown cause (American Speech-Language-Hearing Association, 2019). The hearing loss may

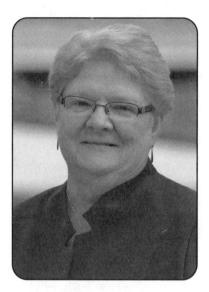

Figure 1–6. Kathy Vesey. Used with permission of Kathy Vesey.

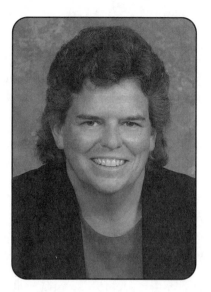

Figure 1–7. Beth Wilson. Used with permission of Beth Wilson.

be gradual or sudden. It affects communication, making it hard for these individuals to communicate with their families, coworkers, or friends. They may grieve for their lost hearing and often will try hearing aids or cochlear implants in order to be able to hear again, but that technology still is not the same as typical hearing. Some may try to learn ASL and interact with the Deaf community if they feel comfortable doing so.

DeafBlind Individuals

Some of you may know of Helen Keller and how she became both deaf and blind at the age of 2 due to illness. How she learned to communicate using finger-spelling is shown in *The Miracle Worker*, a film released in 1962. Other DeafBlind persons are born with these dual-sensory disabilities. Alternatively, some deaf people gradually lose some of their sight in childhood or adolescence, due to a genetic condition called Usher syndrome (Bailey

& Miner, 2010). Others are born blind and become deaf later in life. Or they may lose their sight and hearing in early childhood or adulthood due to illness. Within these groups of individuals who are DeafBlind, there are many who can be successful in school and in the workforce with accommodations. There are also DeafBlind persons who have cognitive or learning disabilities. Some DeafBlind individuals will learn tactile ASL and become part of a vibrant DeafBlind community with its own unique social networks and support systems. They find a home in this community compared with the possibility that they may not be as welcomed in the larger Deaf community. Hearing and Deaf people may feel uncomfortable with DeafBlind individuals because of the need to touch them for communication, which can create feelings of awkwardness (Bailey & Miner, 2010). Individuals who gradually lose their sight and hearing due to aging typically do not join the Deaf community and remain in their hearing communities.

Multiple Communities

Although we may often talk or write about "the Deaf community," it is important to keep in mind that the groups described above are not all inclusive of the Deaf community. The deaf community is not just one huge international or national community. There are many communities within these communities that make up the larger Deaf community (Van Cleve & Crouch, 1989) that we are interested in learning about. There are international organizations such as the World Federation of the Deaf, an organization in Great Britain called deafPlus, and national organizations in the United States such as the National Association of the Deaf and the National Black Deaf Advocates. Also, there are state associations, many church groups, sports organizations, theater groups, groups of individuals who are Deaf and may have additional specific conditions, and so on. Many of these groups have common goals, including improving the quality of life and creating communication access in schools, the workplace, the theater and arts, and other places that hearing people have easy access to. On the Internet, you will find websites full of information about all the diverse groups in the deaf community.

DEMOGRAPHICS

How many deaf people are there?

The World Health Organization (2019) reports that approximately 466 million people worldwide have "disabling" hearing loss (meaning they are hard of hearing or deaf). Of this group, 34 million are children. Roughly 2 to 3 of every 1,000 children in the United States are born deaf or hard of hearing. About 96% of deaf children are born to hearing parents (Mitchell & Karchmer, 2004). The National Institute on Deafness and Other Communication Disorders (NIDCD, 2016) reports that approximately 15% of the U.S. popula-

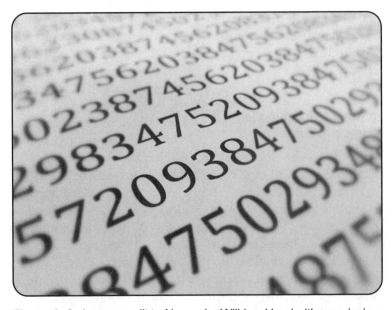

Figure 1–8. Image credit to Alexander Wilkins. Used with permission.

tion, or 37.5 million adults, report some degree of hearing loss. There is a strong relationship between age and hearing loss. As people age, more and more of them will experience hearing loss.

What about deaf people who use ASL? There have been no actual data collected on deaf users of ASL since 1974, when a study of the deaf population of the United States was conducted (Schein & Delk, 1974). These numbers are clearly out of date but still are useful for estimated purposes. Here we explain. Based on the 1974 data, Schein (1989) estimates that there are over 400,000 individuals who became deaf before age 19. Mitchell, Young, Bachleda, and Karchmer (2006) explored that 1974 study of the deaf population of the United States as well as other data. They used that information to roughly estimate that there are approximately 360,000 to 517,000 deaf ASL users (Mitchell, 2005). However, if you include individuals such as sign language interpreters, hearing children in families with deaf members (parents, grandparents, or siblings) who use ASL, hearing parents who have learned ASL to communicate with their deaf children, hearing spouses and partners who use ASL with their deaf spouses/partners, and those who have studied ASL in school and are fluent in ASL, the statistics on ASL users would be far greater. We can see that the deaf children born to Deaf parents (approximately 4% of deaf children; Mitchell & Karchmer, 2004) are likely to learn ASL from them.

We need to know more about the number of deaf people of color or in ethnic minority groups. Our best data came from annual surveys of deaf children in schools and programs for the deaf in the United States (Gallaudet Research Institute, 2011). Unfortunately, that data include only approximately 60% of the deaf student population. That is because not all schools replied to the survey to report their numbers. As the annual surveys were not being conducted at the time of this writing, we need to rely on the 2011 survey results. What we know from schools that reported to that survey is that there are increasing numbers of deaf Latinx and Asian students, while the numbers of African American and Native American deaf students are stable. Overall, it is expected that all these minority groups will constitute the majority of deaf persons within the next few decades, similar to U.S. demographics on the major ethnic groups that show significant increases in Latinx and Asian populations with comparatively more modest growth for African American and other ethnic groups (Frey, 2018). Statistically, the white population is on the way to becoming the minority group in comparison to the larger group of people of color or ethnic minority groups.

HISTORICAL HIGHLIGHTS

How did the deaf community start? As previously mentioned, there have been deaf people going as far back as the start of historical records. First of all, the physical fact of not hearing is the first way we can identify these deaf people. There are a few records of deaf people in the times of ancient Egypt, Greece, and Rome and in the geographical areas where the Old and New Testaments were created (e.g., Abrams, 1998; Bauman, 2008; Buchholtz & Leigh, 2020; Eriksson, 1993; Gulliver & Lyons, 2018; Rée, 1999).

The writings we have today show that sometimes these deaf people were accepted in their society and sometimes they were rejected. For example, Aristotle, the Greek philosopher, thought that deaf people lacked reason and therefore could not learn. During the early Roman times, deaf people could not own property. This was true during the Middle Ages when deaf people were also not permitted to marry or do legal transactions. However, there are records from that time that describe signing deaf people working as farmers, painters, and craftspeople. And in Turkey, the Ottoman Court used "mutes" to provide services because they could get instructions through the use of signs and keep secrets (Miles, 2000). In addition to the sources cited in this paragraph, there are books on deaf history if you want to learn more. Examples of deaf history books are shown in Figure 1–9.

Change started to come in the 1500s. In Spain, and later in France, Great Britain, Germany, and other European countries, people began to realize that deaf persons could be educated (e.g., Branson & Miller, 2002; Rée, 1999; Van Cleve & Crouch, 1989). This possibility started with individual tutoring and then expanded to

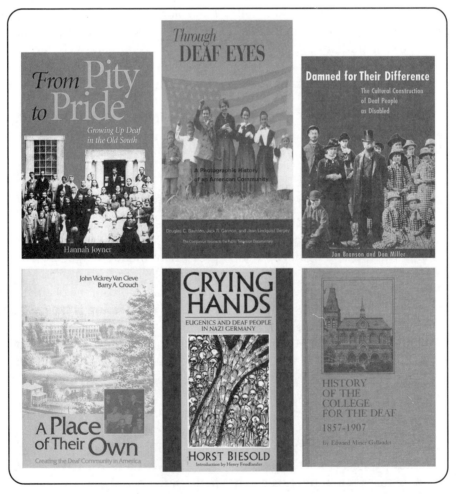

Figure 1–9. Covers of Gallaudet University Press books reprinted by permission of the publisher.

include small groups, which then led to the establishment of schools for deaf students. Since technology that enabled deaf people to hear sound did not exist, language was usually taught using manual alphabets or signs, often with efforts to teach speech through visual means, using speechreading, gestures, pictures, and objects. In Chapter 3, you will find information on leaders in deaf education who used fingerspelling and signs to teach deaf students.

In the 1700s, families in the United States who could afford it sent their deaf children to schools in Europe. Finally, in 1817, the first formal school for the deaf was established in Connecticut. It was called the American Asylum for the Education and Instruction of Deaf and Dumb Persons. This school still exists as the American School for the Deaf, pictured in Figure 1–10.

As time went on, more schools for the deaf were founded to teach both basic academic subjects and vocational training. Often, deaf teachers in the schools provided vocational training in the areas of farming, tailoring, shoemaking, and printing. Figure 1–11 shows a typical print shop where training was provided.

These training experiences encouraged the development of occupations that provided employment opportunities for deaf people. These experiences also encouraged togetherness since Deaf people working in the same fields had a lot in common and could share knowledge and job strategies through ASL, especially with employers who were not sure Deaf people could do the work. Deaf people often had to prove themselves against discrimination by employers who thought Deaf people were deficient in their ability to work.

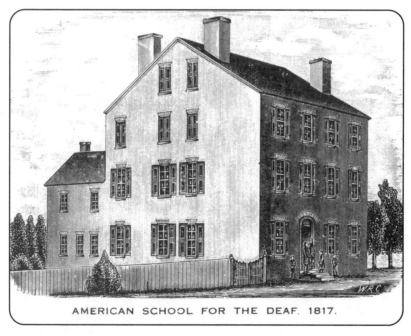

AMERICAN SCHOOL FOR THE DEAF. 1817.

Figure 1–10. American School for the Deaf, circa 1800s. Courtesy of Gallaudet University Archives.

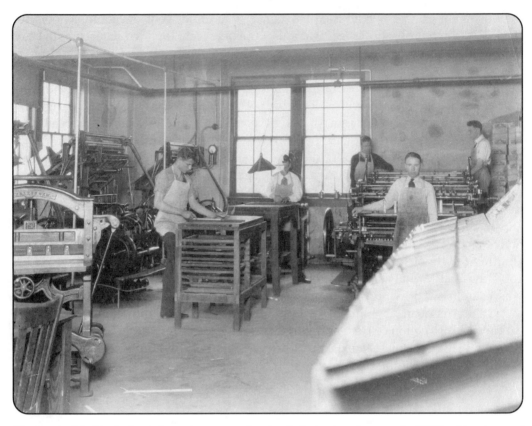

Figure 1–11. Typical printing classroom for deaf students, circa early 1900s. Courtesy of Gallaudet University Archives.

At first, most of the schools for the deaf used sign language, but as time went on, there were arguments about whether to use signed or spoken languages, as well as which signed approach to take (either as a language, following spoken word order, or using fingerspelling alone; Burch, 2002). Toward the end of the 1800s, the supporters of spoken language promoted the philosophy that sign language was a primitive language and spoken language was far superior to sign language, being viewed as a higher level linguistically. Mabel Hubbard Bell, pictured with her family in Figure 1–12, became deaf at age 5. She was the wife of Alexander Graham Bell, who patented the invention of the telephone. She has been described as having strong speaking and speechreading capabilities and frequently associating with hearing individuals (Winefield, 1987). Very little is mentioned regarding how much she associated with signing deaf people. This is an example of those deaf individuals who wanted to fit in with hearing society and be "as normal as possible." There were other deaf people like her who openly objected to sign language and avoided being part of deaf communities. In contrast, Deaf communities with a strong sense of their identity and signed language at that time strongly advocated for their sign language to be used as a teaching tool (Burch, 2002).

At the 1880 International Congress on the Education of the Deaf in Milan, Italy,

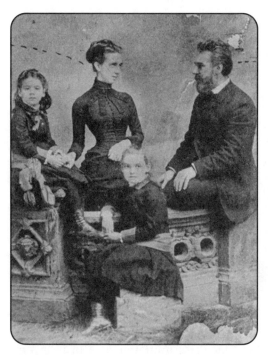

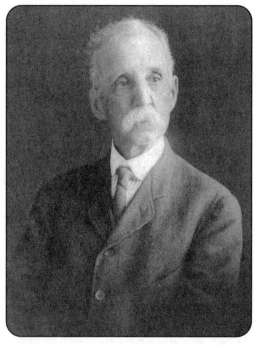

Figure 1–12. Mabel Hubbard Bell with her husband, Alexander Graham Bell, and her two daughters. Courtesy of Gallaudet University Archives.

Figure 1–13. James Denison. Courtesy of Gallaudet University Archives.

where only one of the 164 participants was Deaf (Figure 1–13), the decision was to confirm the spread of spoken language education in schools for the deaf (Van Cleve & Crouch, 1989). This decision reflected a blatant disregard for users of sign language who believed that focus on speech would take time away from learning academic subjects and that too many deaf children would have difficulty learning to speak.

James Denison was the principal of the Kendall School in Washington, DC. He was the only Deaf delegate to the 1880 International Congress on Education of the Deaf and voted against the motion to support only spoken language for deaf students.

This is an example of how hearing educators decided what was best for deaf people (Burch, 2002). They tended not to involve and/or listen to deaf people who themselves had experiences with which communication or language worked best and in which settings.

In the United States at that time, most of the schools were residential since travel took a long time. Because of this, deaf students lived together in dormitories at the schools and came home only for winter and summer breaks. This meant that they felt most comfortable with their deaf friends. When they completed their education and migrated into outside communities, they often made sure they lived in areas where there were deaf people so that they could keep their social connections, often with old school friends. This trend continued even as schools confirmed their mission to integrate their deaf students into mainstream society (Van Cleve & Crouch, 1989).

That is how Deaf communities spread throughout the United States. Deaf people connected with these communities through friendship, the use of a common visual language (sign language), and social gatherings sponsored by religious institutions, sports areas, and Deaf clubs, for example. However, keep in mind that schools for the deaf were segregated until after the U.S. Supreme Court's 1954 *Brown v. Board of Education* decision that separate educational institutions are basically unequal. As a result, the Black American Deaf community rarely mingled with the white American Deaf community until the schools were desegregated (Padden & Humphries, 2005). Only recently has it been acknowledged that Black Deaf people have been neglected in Deaf history, and scholars are beginning to address this neglect (Dunn & Anderson, 2020).

In religious settings, services were often led by Deaf ministers and conducted in sign language. An important belief was that God had created deaf people and sign language was a way to direct access to religious doctrines. Because Deaf people tended to congregate in religious settings, this reinforced a strong sense of community. For example, the Chicago Mission for the Deaf was a Christian religious setting that was managed by Deaf members (Olney, 2007). Founded in the late 1800s, it was very popular for more than 50 years. In these settings, Deaf people felt they were really part of the services and not marginalized as they might have been in hearing congregations (Buchholtz & Leigh, 2020). This was a critical part of the foundation for Deaf cultural ways of socializing and connecting.

Deaf people also socialized in many other places of their own, at banquets, Deaf clubs, Deaf associations, conventions for Deaf people, sports events, and deaf schools in areas with large Deaf communities. They had their unique ways of communicating and interacting with each other, ways that we now describe as Deaf culture. Hearing participants were often not welcomed at these sites so that Deaf people could feel they had control, and it was safe to share common experiences and concerns about hearing society (Burch, 2002; Rée, 1999; Van Cleve & Crouch, 1989).

In the United States, the National Association of the Deaf was founded in 1880. This is a national organization that has worked to advocate for deaf people who face discrimination in education, employment, politics, and language choices. This organization and many others at the national, state, and local levels, as well as similar organizations all over the world, demonstrated that deaf people could advocate for common interests in their lives. These organizations tend to have Deaf leaders and members who use sign language (ASL) as central to their identity, and this has become a significant part of Deaf culture. Members feel that belonging to these organizations not only has expanded their connection with others but also has enhanced their ability to communicate, participate, and contribute to society in meaningful ways. Indeed, Deaf people show that in this way, they are not isolated and limited. This is in contrast to what many hearing people thought—that deaf people were alone, isolated, and separated from mainstream society.

Sports organizations and events offer wonderful opportunities for deaf people to get together, compete, and socialize (Stewart, 1991/1993). There are Deaf people who love sports, just as hearing people do, and join sports organizations for that reason. Not only that, many of them want to show that they are as athletic as their hearing peers and that they can be competitive. It can be difficult for them to join hearing athletic groups because of the difficulty in communicating and socializing. Also, hearing members may not always feel comfortable with deaf people for the same reason.

David Stewart (1991/1993) views deaf sports as a portrait of the Deaf community. In his writing, he stated that "Essentially, Deaf sport emphasizes the honor of being Deaf, whereas hearing society tends to focus on the adversity of deafness" (p. 1). There have been Deaf sports teams since the 1800s. Figure 1–14 shows a deaf baseball team from the year 1898.

In 1924, the French Deaf Sports Federation held the first International Silent Games in Paris, France. Since then, every few years there have been Deaflympic games (International Committee of Sports for the Deaf, 2019). Currently, there are 108 national sports federation members, representing different countries all over the world.

We cannot leave the history section without mentioning the Deaf President Now (DPN) movement (Christiansen & Barnartt, 1995). During the 1988 search for a new president at Gallaudet University, the world's only liberal arts university for deaf students, the Board of Trustees selected a hearing person even though qualified deaf applicants were also finalists for the position. Gallaudet University had never had a deaf president. The message was that deaf people could not lead their own university. Considering that Howard University, a predominantly Black university, has had a Black president

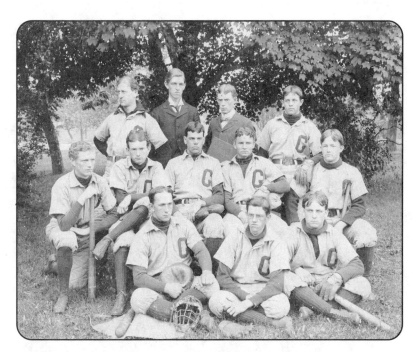

Figure 1–14. Deaf baseball team, circa 1898. Courtesy of Gallaudet University Archives.

since 1926, deaf people felt this to be a great injustice. There was an uprising to protest this selection of a hearing person. Figure 1–15 depicts a rally that was part of this uprising.

This uprising was publicized all over the world through television and newspapers (the Internet was not in existence at that time). After the hearing candidate resigned and I. King Jordan, a late-deafened professor and dean, became the first deaf president of Gallaudet University, the uprising ended. This was a very important historical event that showed the power of the Deaf community to get together and advocate for significant change, including putting Deaf people in charge of not only Gallaudet University but also other major institutions. This event also created strong symbolic visibility for the Deaf community. The Deaf community showed that

"Deaf" could mean empowerment, solidarity, pride in the use of ASL, and ability to work within the political process.

In conclusion, the history of deaf people and the DPN protest showed that Deaf people could face up to and contradict hearing society attitudes that Deaf people were deficient because they could not hear. The repercussions resulting from the DPN protest were felt not only nationally but also internationally. For example, in South Africa, Deaf people mobilized to start advocating for policy decisions that affirmed their civil rights (Druchen, 2014).

CONTEMPORARY DESCRIPTIONS

Just like any other culture, Deaf culture is constantly evolving in how it is represented. One term that has been frequently

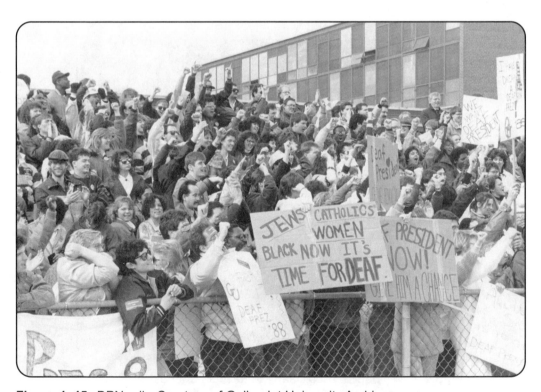

Figure 1–15. DPN rally. Courtesy of Gallaudet University Archives.

used is that of *Deaf-World* (Lane, Hoff-meister, & Bahan, 1996). This term does not refer to a geographical location but rather encompasses Deaf people who share common characteristics or pursuits as part of a particular way of life that involves social networks. Members of the Deaf-World communicate using the sign language of their country as part of their culture.

Scholars have recently developed new terms to illustrate different aspects of Deaf culture. We now explore some of those terms and how they represent culturally Deaf people.

Deafhood

Google Deafhood and you will find a long list of explanations. That is because this term has become very popular ever since Paddy Ladd (2003) first wrote about it in his book, *Understanding Deaf Culture*. He defines Deafhood as a Deaf consciousness concept that involves the processing and reconstructing of Deaf traditions related to becoming and staying "Deaf." It is a way of actualizing oneself as a Deaf person. Because Deafhood is always changing, Ladd sees it as preventing Deaf culture from having a strict list of criteria for membership.

Deafhood is a concept that Deaf people have embraced as a way of defining themselves in a positive sense. Some people have broadened this concept to include all the diverse ways of being deaf, not just in the cultural Deaf sense. The key issue is however one experiences being deaf, which is ever-changing depending on if one is in a hearing or Deaf situation, the person is aware of it in a positive sense. There are different ways to describe Deafhood, as noted in the list provided

here. A. Kusters and DeMeulder (2013) write that even though the Deafhood concept is very wide and vague, that is a strength. They make the point that Deafhood focuses on the self-exploration of deaf individuals and how they explore themselves and their groups. Deafhood lends itself to exploration by a wide variety of deaf people.

Descriptions of Deafhood

The process individuals undergo to accept themselves as being Deaf

Has to do with the positive of being Deaf

Personal journey to understand themselves as Deaf persons

To evaluate themselves and liberate themselves from oppression by hearing people

Deepens understanding of the Deaf self

Feeling at home as a Deaf person

Note. Paraphrased from various blogs and vlogs (video blogs).

Deaf Gain

Deaf gain is a more recent concept than Deafhood. It has received attention within Deaf Studies. The term *Deaf gain* makes the point that there IS a gain to being deaf. Being deaf is not all about hearing loss or being isolated in society. Deaf gain is the opposite of hearing loss (Bauman & Murray, 2014). It is about the benefits of being deaf. You may think: What benefits are there?

Highly visual and spatial ways of thinking can contribute to the richness of life. The sense of hearing is not the only way of knowing and understanding the world. Deaf people have been able to adapt to the world around them in positive ways, largely through visual processing of information and language. They wonder why seeing the world is perceived as not good enough compared to hearing the world. Deaf people feel that seeing the world works for them. Seeing the world adds a different dimension to human experience. The gain is in how nuances of communication can become more clear, how eye contact for communication facilitates different ways of relating with others, how touch can have meanings, how seeing things creates visual environmental awareness, how the use of signed languages enhances meanings, how people connect with each other in communities, and how all these contribute to human diversity. When you think about people such as architects, visual artists, and surgeons, you can see how the concept of vision gain makes sense as conveyed through the term *Deaf gain*.

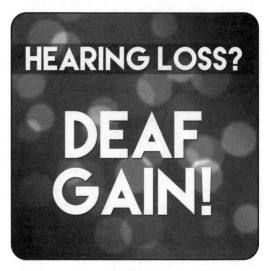

Figure 1–16. Image credit to Alexander Wilkins. Used with permission.

a gain. For them, on a fundamental level, the use of touch is viewed as a means of connection and communication. Touch has the power to unite people on a social level. Using the tactile modality, Deaf-Blind individuals have developed Protactile American Sign Language as a means of bringing their community together as well as reaching out to those who are not DeafBlind.

Brandon once worked as a surveillance system administrator. His job was to monitor surveillance cameras at truck stops all over the United States and report on incidents. His supervisor raved over his visual and memory skills and stated that he thought not being able to hear was a strong advantage for this job (Communication Service for the Deaf, 2019).

There is also what could be labeled as DeafBlind gain. How so? DeafBlind people have developed tactile expertise (McAlpine, 2017) that can be perceived as

Deaf Ethnicity

There have been arguments about whether Deaf people are an ethnic group. In support of a Deaf ethnicity, the argument is that Deaf people have a collective name (Deaf), a shared language (ASL or a signed language), feelings of community, behavior norms, distinct values, culture knowledge and customs, social/organization structures, the arts, history, and kinship (Lane, Pillard, & Hedberg, 2011). Kinship does not mean having to be in the same place geographically, but rather from a sense of human connection. Kinship here also means solidarity related to the use of visual communication. Kinship shows strong group solidarity.

Others argue that ethnicity involves biology, mostly in terms of race (Davis, 2008). Ethnicity can have all the criteria listed in the above paragraph, but many also will add biological differences between groups, often related to race. People tend to be born into ethnic groups. But most deaf people are not born into Deaf culture as they have hearing parents. Biologically, their ears are not functional. If the opportunity comes up, they may be enculturated into Deaf culture. Interestingly, Lane et al. (2011) argue that because there are genetic factors that cause people to be deaf, this is part of the biological argument for ethnicity.

Carrying this discussion further, Eckert (2010) supports the concept of Deafnicity. This is based on the ancient Greek concept of ethnos, meaning community of origin, community of language, and community of religion. Community of origin does not have to mean a biological relationship. Rather, it can mean that Deaf people are identifiable by education and culture, not necessarily a blood relationship. Community of language covers the signing community, that is, whoever uses a signed language. And finally, community of religion does not mean religion as we know it. Based on ancient Greek meanings, religion has to do with a collective consciousness of a Deaf worldview. We leave it to you to decide whether Deaf people are an ethnic group or not.

People of the Eye

This term goes all the way back to 1912 when George Veditz, at that time president of the National Association of the Deaf, wrote in his President's Message,

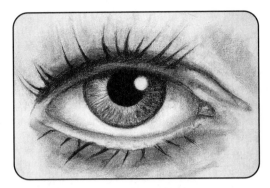

Figure 1–17. Image credit to Neil Tackaberry. Used with permission.

"The deaf are . . . first, last, and all the time the people of the eye" (Lane et al., 2011, p. vii).

Bahan (2008) describes people of the eye as living in a highly visual world. They communicate using a visual language and adapt to their environment by using their eyes. The book, *The People of the Eye* by Lane et al. (2011), describes what that term means. The term *Deaf* brings attention to the fact that deaf people cannot hear. Using "people of the eye" instead shifts the focus from hearing loss to deaf people as visual beings. Deaf people do not usually describe themselves as people of the eye but will acknowledge that, yes, they are people of the eye. However, this term does not apply to DeafBlind individuals. Dialogue between the Deaf and DeafBlind communities has led to a shift from using terms such as "eyes" or "vision" to describe Deaf people and culture toward using terms such as "hands" to describe Deaf communities, thereby being inclusive of DeafBlind people and communities.

Deaf Epistemologies

Epistemology has to do with studying knowledge and what it means. It also involves the relationship between those who know and what is known (Paul & Moores, 2012). In turn, deaf epistemologies are about studying how deaf people "know." This is a very complex topic that has been studied by anthropologists, educators, sociologists, and psychologists, among others, many of whom are also Deaf scholars (A. Kusters et al., 2017b). These scholars explore the visual and tactile ways that Deaf people use to demonstrate how they are aware of their surroundings and themselves and how they "know" whatever it is they know. For example, deaf epistemology can involve the study of exactly what the widely used phrase *Deaf same* means. This might involve exploring the value of *Deaf same* and checking for understanding with other deaf people (Friedner, 2016).

CONCLUSIONS

As you can see from this brief introduction, Deaf culture is an exciting area worth exploring. It is a rich culture that strongly encourages a sense of community. The signed language of that culture is one that draws Deaf people together to form social, psychological, and language bonding. Deaf people have their unique ways of behaving, using their bodies, eyes, and facial expressions to connect with others. They have their cultural values that encourage relationships with other Deaf people. There are gatherings or organizations where Deaf people mingle comfortably. Deaf people are often members of organizations that help bring them together. Their use of vision and taction to communicate and to orient themselves to their space, their environment, is unique. It enables them to successfully adapt to what is going on around them. They have

been able to adapt technology to fit their visual and tactile needs. For example, videophones bring them together, and they utilize the Internet to communicate as well. (See Chapter 9 for information on the technology used to access information and connect with others.) Many may use auditory technology such as hearing aids or cochlear implants, but their eyes and hands are still very important for getting through life. In the following chapters, we explain more about visual as well as auditory technology, use of taction, signed languages, education, the arts, psychological adjustment, and work, all related to Deaf culture. We hope you enjoy your journey into Deaf culture through reading, reflecting, and discussing the content of these chapters.

REFERENCES

Abrams, J. (1998). *Judaism and disability*. Washington, DC: Gallaudet University Press.

American Speech-Language-Hearing Association. (2019). *Causes of hearing loss in adults.* Retrieved from https://www.asha.org/public/hearing/causes-of-hearing-loss-in-adults/

Atherton, M. (2016). *Deafness, community and culture in Britain: Leisure and cohesion, 1945–1995.* Manchester, UK: Manchester University Press.

Bahan, B. (2008). Upon the formation of a visual variety of the human race. In H.-D. Bauman (Ed.), *Open your eyes: Deaf studies talking* (pp. 83–99). Minneapolis: University of Minnesota Press.

Bailey, K., & Miner, I. (2010). Psychotherapy for people with Usher syndrome. In I. W. Leigh (Ed.), *Psychotherapy with Deaf clients from diverse groups* (pp. 136–158). Washington, DC: Gallaudet University Press.

Bauman, H.-D. (2008). On the disconstruction of (sign) language in the Western tradition: A Deaf reading of Plato's Cratylus. In H.-D.

Bauman (Ed.), *Open your eyes: Deaf studies talking* (pp. 327–336). Minneapolis: University of Minnesota Press.

Bauman, H.-D., & Murray, J. (Eds.). (2014). *Deaf gain: Raising the stakes for human diversity.* Minneapolis: University of Minnesota Press.

Berkowitz, M., & Jonas, J. (2014). *Deaf and hearing siblings in conversation.* Jefferson, NC: McFarland.

Branson, J., & Miller, D. (2002). *Damned for their difference: The cultural construction of deaf people as disabled.* Washington, DC: Gallaudet University Press.

Buchholtz, N., & Leigh, D. J. (2020). Religion and deaf identity. In I. W. Leigh & C. O'Brien (Eds.), *Deaf identities: Exploring new frontiers* (pp. 72–95). New York, NY: Oxford University Press.

Burch, S. (2002). *Signs of resistance: American Deaf cultural history, 1900 to 1942.* Chapel Hill: University of North Carolina Press.

Cawthon, S. W., Johnson, P. M., Garberoglio, C. L., & Schoffstall, S. J. (2016). Role models as facilitators of social capital for Deaf individuals: A research synthesis. *American Annals of the Deaf, 161*(2), 115–127. https://doi.org/10.1353/aad.2016.0021

Christiansen, J., & Barnartt, S. (1995). *Deaf president now!* Washington, DC: Gallaudet University Press.

Communication Service for the Deaf. (2019, February 7). *bump: Let us work—Transportation security officer.* Retrieved from https://www.youtube.com/watch?v=bWtX0GIjB2Q)

Davis, L. (2008). Postdeafness. In H.-D. Bauman (Ed.), *Open your eyes: Deaf Studies talking* (pp. 314–325). Minneapolis: University of Minnesota Press.

Druchen, B. (2014). The legacy of Deaf President Now in South Africa. *Sign Language Studies, 15*(1), 74–86. https://doi.org/10.1353/sls.2014.0020

Dunn, L. M., & Anderson, G. B. (2020). Examining the intersectionality of deaf identity, race/ethnicity, and diversity through a Black Deaf lens. In I. W. Leigh & C. O'Brien (Eds.), *Deaf identities: Exploring new frontiers*

(pp. 279–335). New York, NY: Oxford University Press.

Eagleton, T. (2013). *The idea of culture.* Hoboken, NJ: Wiley-Blackwell.

Eckert, R. (2010). Toward a theory of Deaf ethnos: Deafnicity ≈ D/deaf (Hómaemon . Homóglosson . Homóthreskon). *Journal of Deaf Studies and Deaf Education, 15,* 317–333.

Eriksson, P. (1993). *The history of deaf people.* Örebro, Sweden: SIH Läromedel.

Frey, W. (2018, September 10). *The US will become 'minority white' in 2045, census projects.* Retrieved from https://www.brookings.edu/blog/the-avenue/2018/03/14/the-us-will-become-minority-white-in-2045-census-projects/

Friedner, M. (2016). Understanding and not-understanding: What do epistemologies and ontologies do in deaf worlds? *Sign Language Studies, 16*(2), 184-203.

Gala, N. M. (2017). *Emotional display rules of deaf culture: An evaluation of emotional expression* (Doctoral dissertation). Gallaudet University, Washington, DC.

Gallaudet Research Institute. (2011, April). *Regional and national summary report from the 2009–2010 annual survey of deaf and hard of hearing children and youth.* Washington, DC: GRI, Gallaudet University.

Gulliver, M., & Lyons, W. J. (2018). Conceptualizing the place of Deaf people in ancient Israel: Suggestions from Deaf space. *Journal of Biblical Literature, 137*(3), 537–553. https://doi.org/10.15699/jbl.1373.2018.200601

Hoffmeister, R. (2008). Border crossings by hearing children of deaf parents: The lost history of Codas. In H.-D. Bauman (Ed.), *Open your eyes: Deaf Studies talking* (pp. 189–215). Minneapolis: University of Minnesota Press.

Holcomb, T. (2013). *Introduction to American Deaf culture.* New York, NY: Oxford University Press.

International Committee of Sports for the Deaf. (2019). *History.* Retrieved from https://www.deaflympics.com/icsd/history

Jassal, Y. R. (2017). Learning about Deaf culture: More accessible than previously thought. *American Annals of the Deaf, 161*(5),

583–584. https://doi.org/10.1353/aad.2017.0008

Kusters, A., & De Meulder, M. (2013). Understanding Deafhood: In search of its meanings. *American Annals of the Deaf, 158*, 428–438.

Kusters, A., De Meulder, M., & O'Brien, D. (Eds.). (2017a). *Innovations in Deaf Studies: The role of Deaf scholars.* New York, NY: Oxford University Press.

Kusters, A., De Meulder, M., & O'Brien, D. (2017b). Innovations in Deaf Studies: Critically mapping the field. In A. Kusters, M. De Meulder, & D. O'Brien (Eds.), *Innovations in Deaf Studies: The role of Deaf scholars* (pp. 1–53). New York, NY: Oxford University Press.

Kusters, M. (2017). Intergenerational responsibilities in deaf pedagogies. In A. Kusters, M. De Meulder, & D. O'Brien (Eds.), *Innovations in Deaf Studies: The role of Deaf scholars* (pp. 241–262). New York, NY: Oxford University Press.

Ladd, P. (2003). *Understanding Deaf culture: In search of Deafhood.* Clevedon, UK: Multilingual Matters.

Lane, H., Hoffmeister, R., & Bahan, B. (1996). *A journey into the Deaf-World.* San Diego, CA: DawnSign Press.

Lane, H., Pillard, R., & Hedberg, U. (2011). *The people of the eye: Deaf ethnicity and ancestry.* New York, NY: Oxford University Press.

Languageandculture.com. (2015). *The cultural iceberg.* Retrieved from https://www.languageandculture.com/cultural-iceberg

Layton, B. (2007). Darby's story. In S. Schwartz (Ed.), *Choices in deafness* (3rd ed., pp. 208–212). Bethesda, MD: Woodbine House.

Leigh, I. W. (2009). *A lens on deaf identities.* New York, NY: Oxford University Press.

Leigh, I. W., & Andrews, J. (2017). *Deaf people and society: Psychological, sociological, and educational perspectives* (2nd ed.). New York, NY: Routledge.

McAlpine, A. (2017). *Keep in touch: A comparative analysis of visual and Protactile American Sign Language* (Honors thesis). Western Oregon University. Retrieved from https://digitalcommons.wou.edu/cgi/viewcontent.cgi?article=1133&context=honors_theses

Miles, M. (2000). Signing in the seraglio: Mutes, dwarfs, and jestures at the Ottoman Court 1500–1700. *Disability and Society, 15*, 115–134.

Mitchell, R. (2005). *Can you tell me how many deaf people there are in the United States?* Retrieved from http://research.gallaudet.edu/Demographics/deaf-US.php

Mitchell, R., & Karchmer, M. (2004). Chasing the mythical ten percent: Parental hearing status of deaf and hard of hearing students in the United States. *Sign Language Studies, 4*, 138–163.

Mitchell, R., Young, T., Bachleda, B., & Karchmer, M. (2006). How many people use ASL in the United States? *Sign Language Studies, 6*, 306–335.

Mitchiner, J. (2014). Deaf parents of cochlear implanted children: Beliefs on bimodal bilingualism. *Journal of Deaf Studies and Deaf Education, 20*, 51–56.

National Institute on Deafness and Other Communication Disorders (NIDCD). (2016). *Quick statistics about hearing.* Retrieved from https://www.nidcd.nih.gov/health/statistics/quick-statistics-hearing

Olney, K. (2007). The Chicago Mission for the Deaf. In J. Van Cleve (Ed.), *The Deaf history reader* (pp. 174–208). Washington, DC: Gallaudet University Press.

Padden, C., & Humphries, T. (1988). *Deaf in America: Voices from a culture.* Cambridge, MA: Harvard University Press.

Padden, C., & Humphries, T. (2005). *Inside Deaf culture.* Cambridge, MA: Harvard University Press.

Paul, P., & Moores, D. (2012). Towards an understanding of epistemology and deafness. In P. Paul & D. Moores (Eds.), *Deaf epistemologies: Multiple perspectives on the acquisition of knowledge* (pp. 3–15). Washington, DC: Gallaudet University Press.

Rée, J. (1999). *I see a voice.* New York, NY: Metropolitan Books.

Sass-Lehrer, M. (Ed.). (2016). *Early intervention for deaf and hard-of-hearing infants, toddlers, and their families*. New York, NY: Oxford University Press.

Schein, J. D. (1989). *At home among strangers*. Washington, DC: Gallaudet University Press.

Schein, J. D., & Delk, M. (1974). *The deaf population of the United States*. Silver Spring, MD: National Association of the Deaf.

Slane, K. (2019, January 28). *Here's who's performing at Super Bowl LIII*. Retrieved from https://www.boston.com/culture/entertainment/2019/01/18/super-bowl-2019-half-time-performer

Solomon, A. (2014). Foreword: Deaf loss. In H.-D. Bauman & J. Murray (Eds.), *Deaf gain: Raising the stakes for human diversity* (pp. ix–xi). Minneapolis: University of Minnesota Press.

Stewart, D. (1991/1993). *Deaf sport*. Washington, DC: Gallaudet University Press.

Stone, A. (2015, January 26). Breaking the sound barrier. *Washington Post*, pp. C1, C5.

Torres, A. (2009). *Signing in Puerto Rican: A hearing son and his deaf family*. Washington, DC: Gallaudet University Press.

Van Cleve, J. V., & Crouch, B. (1989). *A place of their own: Creating the deaf community in America*. Washington, DC: Gallaudet University Press.

Vesey, K., & Wilson, B. (2003). Navigating the hearing classroom with a hearing loss. *Odyssey, 4*, 10–13.

Winefield, R. (1987). *Never the twain shall meet: Bell, Gallaudet, and the communications debate*. Washington, DC: Gallaudet University Press.

World Health Organization. (2019). *World Hearing Forum*. Retrieved from https://www.who.int/deafness/world-hearing-forum/en/

Yosso, T. J. (2005). Whose culture has capital? A critical race theory discussion of community cultural wealth. *Race, Ethnicity and Education, 8*, 69–91.

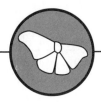

CHAPTER 2

Causes of Being Deaf and the Auditory Field

In order to understand different types of ways Deaf people are deaf, we need to understand what being "hearing" is. Deaf people call people who can hear and speak, "Hearing" or "Hearing people." Another phrase that is used for hearing people is, "Hearing world," referring to spaces populated by hearing people with speaking and hearing privileges, which is pretty much the entire world that we currently inhabit. That means that many of the services (e.g., fast-food drive-through, schools, workplaces, prisons, concert halls) and devices (e.g., doorbell intercoms in apartment buildings, loud-speakers at sporting events, automated registers) are designed *for* people who hear and speak, and *by* people who hear and speak.

People who may not hear or speak the same way hearing people do mostly identify themselves as Deaf, deaf, Deaf-Blind, DeafDisabled, hard of hearing, or late-deafened. If we meet someone from the deaf communities, how do we know which term to use to describe them? The best approach is to ask how they iden-

tify themselves. Most of the time, they'll tell you which term they identify with. But what if you want to refer to a group of people who do not hear or speak like hearing people do? You can use all those terms. Some people use this acronym, DDBDDHHLD (which represents the letters of those terms), to be inclusive of all the different identities within the Deaf communities (Council de Manos, 2019).

So, now do we know if they are DDB-DDHHLD? Often caregivers who are puzzled when an infant or a young toddler, someone recovering from an illness, or a senior citizen does not respond to sound. Those caregivers might try making a sound behind them and see if they respond and turn their heads. If they don't respond, we still don't know how much they can hear, what kind of sounds they can hear, or if it's something else. There are ways to find the answers to those questions. Keep in mind, many Deaf individuals do not tend to want answers to those questions, as they are content with being Deaf. However, during their early formative years, and even throughout their childhood and adulthood, families of Deaf children may have been exposed to conflicting information (Humphries, Kushalnagar, Mathur, Napoli, Padden, Pollard, et al., 2014; Humphries, Kushalnagar, Mathur, Napoli, Padden, & Rathmann, 2014; Humphries et al., 2019) and misinformation (Hall, 2017) from medical and audiology professionals. For example, some professionals and organizations advocate for preventing deaf children from learning sign language before implantation. It is often standard practice for them to tell parents that they need to be using spoken language only and that the use of sign language should be avoided. This is counter to the fact that there is no evidence that shows sign languages harm the child's acquisition of spoken languages. In fact, evidence points to benefits of learning speech through sign language. There is also increasing evidence that depriving a deaf child of access to sign language access has a potential negative impact on the child (Hall, 2017; Humphries, Kushalnagar, Mathur, Napoli, Padden, Pollard, et al., 2014; Humphries, Kushalnagar, Mathur, Napoli, Padden, & Rathmann, 2014;). This is not to say all audiologists are uninformed and spread misinformation (Andrews & Dionne, 2008). For a more medically focused approach to audiology testing and rehabilitative issues, please see Martin and Clark (2019).

DETERMINING ONE'S HEARING LEVEL

Audiologists and Audiograms

According to the Center for Hearing and Communication (CHC, 2020, approximately 48 million Americans have some sort of hearing challenges. This number includes those who are born deaf or are part of Deaf culture. When confronted

with the possibility of a difference in hearing, those people tend to be referred to an audiologist. An audiologist is a professional who specializes in detecting hearing levels and proposing different types of accommodations. The field an audiologist works in is called audiology. Pictured in Figure 2–1 is an audiologist working with a young client.

The purpose of an audiological evaluation is to measure the degree, type, and configuration of hearing levels by utilizing a physical examination of the ear, tests of hearing and listening, and tests of the middle ear function (Martin & Clark, 2019). An audiologist will first conduct a physical exam by looking at the outer ear for evidence of malformations. Then the audiologist uses an otoscope, which is an instrument that contains light and a magnifying glass, and inserts it into the ear to examine the ear canal and eardrum to see if there is excessive earwax or objects that could obstruct hearing. The audiologist also examines the condition of the eardrum and notes any excess fluid. A medical referral for further evaluation or treatment may be an outcome of this physical exam.

Next, the audiologist conducts tests of hearing tones or pure-tone audiometry. The individual enters a soundproof room and is fitted with earphones. Then the audiologist will leave the room and enter an adjacent room with a window through which both the client and the audiologist can see each other, as shown in Figure 2–2.

The audiologist will then proceed with turning on a machine that emits pure tones at selected pitches or frequencies to find the lowest tone that the individual responds to. The audiologist will also turn on low sounds, such as leaves rustling and water dripping, and then increase the loudness of the sounds to whispering,

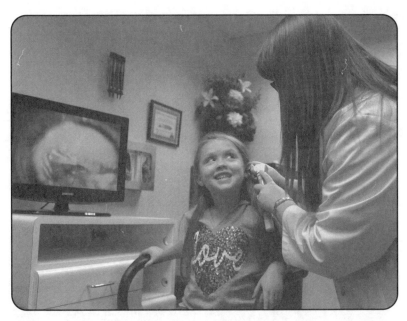

Figure 2–1. An audiologist at work. Photo courtesy of Brian Sattler. Used with permission.

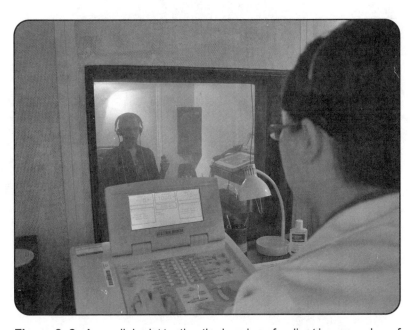

Figure 2–2. An audiologist testing the hearing of a client in a soundproof testing booth. Photo courtesy of Brian Sattler. Used with permission.

spoken language, a baby crying, a phone ringing, a dog barking, a running vacuum, a lawn mower, to a jet plane roaring by (Martin & Clark, 2019; Sheetz, 2012). The goal is to increase the sound level until the individual indicates they hear the sound by raising their hand. The audiologist varies the sounds, including the pitch level from low to high, to determine the hearing level in each ear. Figure 2–3 shows the frequencies and loudness levels of different types of sounds. Loudness is measured by decibels, which are units that measure how loud a sound is.

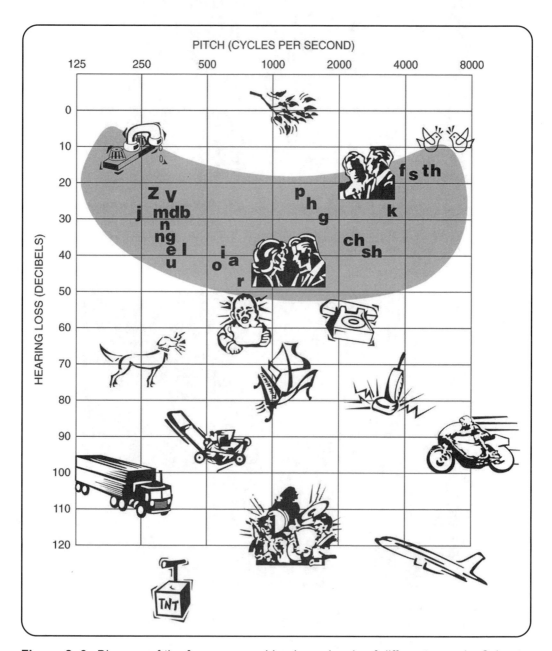

Figure 2–3. Diagram of the frequency and loudness levels of different sounds. Scheetz, Nanci A., *Deaf Education in the 21st Century: Topics and Trends.* © 2012. Printed and electronically reproduced by permission of Pearson Education, Inc., New York, NY.

The audiologist will also conduct tests to examine the "speech reception threshold," which means testing the quietest speech that can be heard. In another test, a standardized list of words is presented one at a time to the individual to assess the ability to recognize words across different loudness levels (Martin & Clark, 2019). Other tests may be administered to examine the functioning of the outer and middle ear. These are called "acoustic immittance measures" (Martin & Clark, 2019). These tests can detect blockage in the ear canal, fluid in the middle ear, or a puncture in the eardrum (Martin & Clark, 2019).

After these audiologic tests are completed, this information is then documented on an audiogram and recommendations are made for follow-up testing or medical referrals if necessary. Referrals also are made for assistive listening devices, speech and language counseling, or further audiologic rehabilitation (Martin & Clark, 2019).

The audiogram is a chart that measures sound from 0 to 120 decibels (dB) and pitch from 125 to 8,000 cycles per second (Sheetz, 2012). The hearing level of the right ear is indicated by a circle, while X is used to show the hearing level of the left ear. Here, the authors provide examples of their audiograms, as shown in Figures 2–4A–D.

Based on the information displayed in the audiograms and comparing these with Figure 2–3, we can surmise that Topher González Ávila, Raychelle Harris, and Irene Leigh (without her hearing aid) will not be able to hear a vacuum, a dog barking, a phone ringing, or a baby crying. We can surmise Jean Andrews can hear all of those, like most hearing people. However, Andrews and other hearing individuals in the late 60s age range may start to experience presbycusis, defined as changes in hearing levels, particularly in the higher frequencies, as they age.

Topher, Raychelle, and Irene will also not be able to hear spoken conversations. But they may or may not hear a lawn mower, an 18-wheeler truck, a bomb and possibly a live band, a speeding motorcycle, and a jet plane, depending on the pitch, but this is not always necessarily accurate. Intriguingly, Harris is often alerted to someone knocking on the door when her Rottweiler, Samson, barks. According to Raychelle's audiogram and Figure 2–3, Raychelle is not supposed to be able to hear a dog barking. In other words, "hearing" is not an exact science, and everyone varies in their processing of sound.

The audiologist prepares the audiogram and gives the individual a specific label that corresponds with the hearing level (dB) as indicated in the audiogram. A person with a 10- to 15-dB hearing level would be labeled as having normal or typical hearing. At the next level, 16 to 25 dB would be identified as having a *slight* hearing loss. Someone receiving a *moderate* hearing label is able to hear sounds that are 41 to 55 dB or higher. Those testing at 56 to 70 dB would be told they have a *moderately severe* hearing level. A person with a *severe* hearing label would hear a range of 71 to 90 dB or higher. People with *profound* hearing levels would only be able to hear sounds that are 91 dB or above (Martin & Clark, 2019; Sheetz, 2012). Looking at Topher, Raychelle, and Irene's audiograms, as shown above, we see that audiologists would place them in the *profound* hearing level category, or from the view of some members of Deaf communities, they would receive the designation of an ASL sign, DEAF (with puffed cheeks), which is loosely translated as "truly Deaf" or "so Deaf." Table 2–1 shows each hearing level and the labels for each.

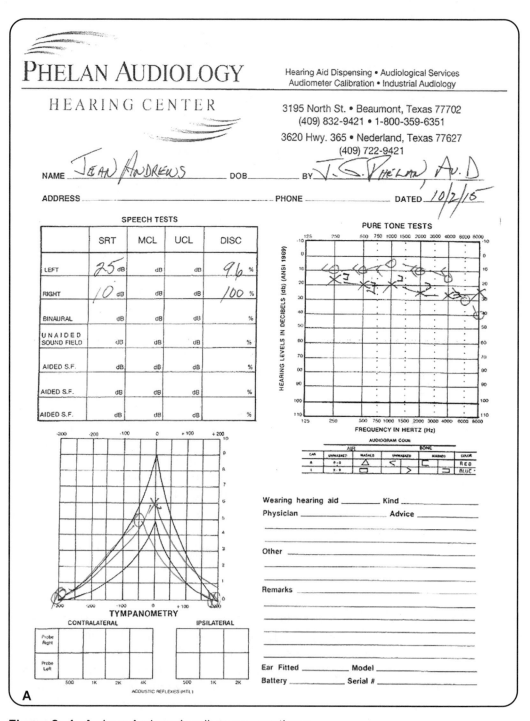

Figure 2–4. A. Jean Andrews' audiogram. *continues*

PROFESSIONAL EVALUATOR: Licensed audiologist

RESULTS (Attach audiogram and other results available)
  Otoscopic Examination   Immitance Testing

UNAIDED TESTING: ☑ Yes   ☐ No

Puretones (dBHL):	250	500	1000	2000	3000	4000	6000	8000 Hz
Right	90	100	105	100	110	115	nr110	nr110
Left, or	90	105	115	115		115	110	nr95
Soundfield								

Speech: ☑ SDT   ☐ SRT   Right: 90   Left: 85   Soundfield: _____
          Word Discrimination (Quiet)   Stimulus: _____   Presentation Level: _____
                                        Right: _____   Left: _____   Soundfield: _____

ADDITIONAL TEST RESULTS:

Auditory Brainstem Response (ABR): _____

Other, specify: _____

Type and severity of hearing loss: profound bilateral sensorineural hearing loss

☑   ☐   Need for amplification? (If yes, complete the AMPLIFICATION section.)
Yes   No

AIDED TESTING: ☐ Yes   ☑ No

Puretones (dBHL):	250	500	1000	2000	3000	4000	6000 Hz
Right							
Left, or							
Soundfield							

Speech: ☐ SDT   ☐ SRT   Right: _____   Left: _____   Binaural: _____
          Word Discrimination (Quiet)   Stimulus: _____   Presentation: _____
                                        Right: _____   Left: _____   Binaural: _____
          Word Discrimination (Noise)   Stimulus: _____   Presentation: _____   S/N Ratio: _____
B   Right: _____   Left: _____   Binaural: _____

Figure 2–4. *continued* **B.** Topher González Ávila's audiogram. *continues*

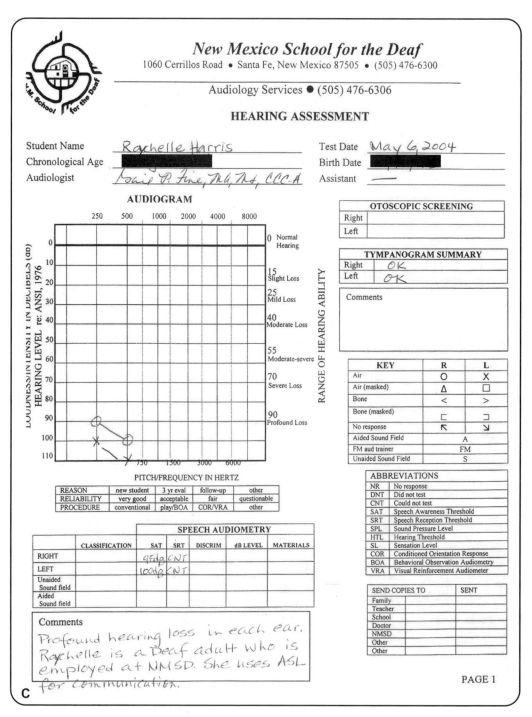

Figure 2–4. *continued* **C.** Raychelle Harris' audiogram. *continues*

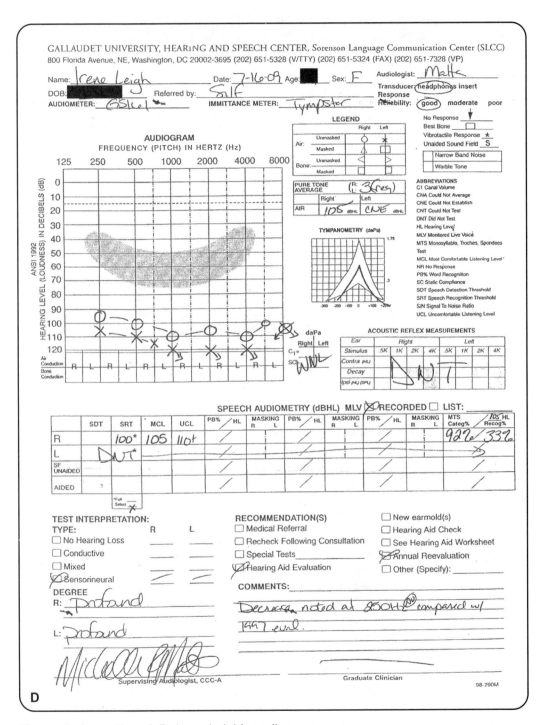

Figure 2–4. *continued* **D.** Irene Leigh's audiogram.

Table 2–1. Hearing Levels, Labels, and Examples

Hearing Level	Label	Implications in the Hearing World
−10 to 15 dB	Normal	Can participate seamlessly in spoken conversations
16 to 25 dB	Slight	Can converse in quiet environments; noisy environments can be difficult
26 to 40 dB	Mild	May be able to follow conversation if in quiet environment and topic is familiar
41 to 55 dB	Moderate	Quiet environment and conversations will need to be within 3–5 feet, may benefit from using an hearing aid
56 to 70 dB	Moderately severe	Will not be able to participate in conversations unless loud; will benefit from the above accommodations
71 to 90 dB	Severe	May identify environmental noises and loud sounds; may have difficulty producing intelligible speech
91+ dB	Profound	Does not usually rely on hearing or speech

Source: Adapted with permission of Scheetz (2012, p. 65).

Hearing people may have never seen an audiologist and may have never received an audiogram until their senior years when their family complains that they are not listening or responding only to very loud talking. On the other hand, Deaf people often grow up seeing countless audiologists and have stacks of audiograms from when they were younger. The audiogram is often used for different reasons, such as qualifying for the Deaflympics, which is similar to the Olympics, but for Deaf athletes (International Committee of Sports for the Deaf, 2018, also briefly described in Chapter 1); receiving Vocational Rehabilitation and Social Security benefits; or being eligible for admission at an educational institution or program serving deaf students.

Hearing Labels

Audiologists and speech professionals typically use the term *hearing impaired* to describe all people with different types of hearing loss. As mentioned in Chapter 1, the term *hearing impaired* is not widely embraced by Deaf people. In any case, audiologists will further categorize people with hearing loss as deaf from birth or at the age when they lost their hearing. They also categorize those who have not spoken or heard language before they became deaf as *prelingually deaf*. This applies to people who were born deaf and did not receive language input, but this does not apply to deaf infants born into language-accessible households (e.g., signing households). In contrast, those who already sign, speak, and/or hear language before they became deaf are *postlingually deaf*. People who are *postlingually deaf* usually remember what it is like to speak and hear before their hearing levels changed (Marschark & Spencer, 2016).

Another term used by audiologists, *hard of hearing*, refers to people who have a slight to moderate hearing loss. *Hard-of-hearing* people often benefit from the use of hearing aids, assistive listening devices, and other forms of amplification (Martin & Clark, 2019). Some *hard-of-hearing* people do not benefit from those devices at all. For example, a person may be able to hear only high-frequency sounds such as a whistle, a bird chirping, or a doorbell but is unable to hear speech. Sometimes a person cannot hear low-frequency sounds and is challenged in understanding mostly adult men, whose speech registers in the low-frequency range (Martin & Clark, 2019; Sheetz, 2012). Some sounds such as *b* and *d* are low frequency—if a person is unable to hear low-frequency sounds such as these, imagine how much of the conversation would be predominately guesswork? On the other hand, people unable to hear high-frequency sounds such as *th* or *s* may also struggle with understanding people whose voice registers in the high-frequency range, which is the case for most adult women. Deaf and hard-of-hearing people often receive questions and comments from naïve hearing people asking why they are able to speak but not hear (both are different skills), or why they are able to hear a dog bark but not someone who is speaking (both have different decibel levels), or why they are able to hear a man speak but not a woman speak (both speak with different frequencies) and so on (Martin & Clark, 2019; Sheetz, 2012). You may also

find hard-of-hearing people who identify as Deaf, even if they do hear.

In ASL signers within Deaf communities, there is an ASL phrase that is often transcribed as VERY-HARD-OF-HEARING (puffed cheeks). This means the opposite of what hearing people may think. That phrase is translated as the person being "almost hearing"! Similarly, LITTLE-HARD-OF-HEARING is translated as the person being able to hear just a little, but is overall, mostly Deaf. One of the classic pivotal early books on Deaf culture, titled *Deaf in America: Voices From a Culture*, goes into more detail about those terms (Padden & Humphries, 1988).

Often people are not able to separate the ability to hear from the ability to understand—for example, many Deaf people understand the spoken words for typical encounters such as, "Hello, how are you?" or "What's your name?" because those words are predictable and typically used in the beginning of most conversations between strangers. When the context of the conversation changes, Deaf people tend to try different ways to communicate, such as writing back and forth, typing on their cell phones, gesturing, and/or trying to read lips, which is usually the least effective way to communicate, as many sounds in the English language look the same on the lips such as "ball" and "mall."

> Try turning off the sound on your television or your computer device as you watch people speak. Are you able to follow what they are saying?

Additionally, there are also many other external factors influencing the ability to hear, such as background noise and reverberation, which many assistive hearing devices do not succeed in blocking. This can make it very difficult to hear conversation. If you enter noisy restaurants and have difficulty hearing conversation, you can understand how much harder this would be for people with different hearing abilities.

What Causes Changes in Hearing Levels?

What causes people to have varying hearing levels? People are put in either of those two categories: deaf before/at birth (congenital) and after birth (acquired). And within those categories, there are two areas in the ear where the hearing loss might occur. Issues in the outer and middle ear are called *conductive*. Issues happening inside the ear or within the auditory nerve are called *sensorineural* (Martin & Clark, 2019).

Genetic Causes

Genes that are inherited and gene mutations are the cause of deafness in approximately more than 50% of babies born deaf (Knoors & Marschark, 2014). So far, over 400 different genes have been found to cause people to become deaf, with scientists still trying to identify more genes (Smith, Shearer, Hildebrand, & Camp, 2014). Some of those genes make the baby deaf before birth, some during the toddler or teenager years, and some later in life. As for the hundreds of different deaf genes, approximately two-thirds of those "deaf" genes are nonsyndromic, meaning that these genes only cause the person to become deaf without any other physical

changes. Connexin 26 is one example of a common nonsyndromic gene that many Deaf families may carry from generation to generation (Clark, 2003). The remaining genes are syndromic, which means that the affected person will not only be deaf but will also have additional conditions, including, for example, blindness, heart conditions, or intellectual development challenges, among other additional disabilities (Plante & Beeson, 2008). Examples of deaf (and additional disabilities) include people having Hunter syndrome (growth failure), Usher syndrome (progressive blindness), and Waardenburg syndrome (pigment abnormalities) (Scheetz, 2012; Vernon & Andrews, 1990).

Acquired

Those who are diagnosed as acquired became deaf due to external factors—not related to genetics. Those external factors that cause deafness develop during birth or after a baby is born and can happen any time during their lives. Examples include diseases such as meningitis, Ménière disease, premature births, fetal alcohol syndrome, or simply becoming elderly (Knoors & Marschark, 2014). For example, in the 1960s, there was a sudden, large increase of deaf children due to rubella, widely known as German measles. In 1969, a rubella vaccine was developed, and after that, the number of children contracting rubella was significantly reduced. The most common cause for hearing loss in adulthood is usually due to damage to the hearing mechanism. Such damage to the hearing mechanism can be the result of prolonged exposure to acute loud noise, the taking of drugs, the aging process, accidents that cause trauma to the hearing mechanism, and diseases that attack and damage the hearing mechanism (Martin & Clark, 2019; Sheetz, 2012).

Conductive

For those diagnosed as conductive, that term specifies challenges within the outer and middle ear. Examples include ears that are not fully open, earwax in the ear, ear infections, and physical injuries to the ear (such as a Q-tip puncturing an eardrum). Often external and middle ear issues can be fixed with medicine or surgery. Surgeries include removing excessive buildup of fluid, adding a tube, removing a blockage, repairing by adding a skin graft, or reconstruction of the damaged parts inside the ear. Conductive losses tend to be temporary (Martin & Clark, 2019; Sheetz, 2012). Figure 2–5 shows the external, middle, and internal sections of the ear.

Sensorineural

Sensorineural issues are limited to the cochlea inside the inner ear and the connecting auditory nerve. The cochlea looks like a very small snail and is the size of a pea. The cochlea transmits sound from the middle of the ear to the auditory nerve. The transmission process includes over 20,000 hairs inside the cochlea, where sounds move through waves of hair to the auditory nerve. Damage to the cochlea can include missing hair or a disorder where sound is not carried from the cochlea to the auditory nerve (Martin & Clark, 2019). People with sensorineural challenges sometimes experience drastic changes in the sensation of loudness; for example, someone might ask you to speak louder and then, in the next minute, ask you why you are shouting. Sensorineural

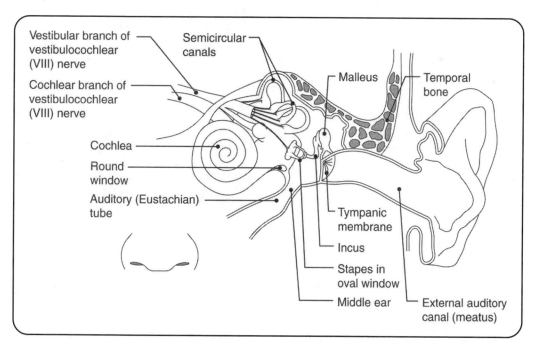

Figure 2–5. A diagram of the ear including external, middle, and internal sections. Courtesy of Marie A. Scheetz.

issues cannot be repaired by medicine or minor medical intervention (e.g., adding a tube) and is usually permanent (Sheetz, 2012).

HISTORY OF AUDITORY TECHNOLOGY

The history of the relationship between the Deaf community and auditory technology is a complicated one, fraught with heartbreaking stories of coercion, suffering, and even death in the process of trying to create the ability to "hear" (Paludneviciene & Harris, 2011). For many centuries, there was a prevailing belief that people who were disabled at birth were being punished or were manifesting demonic origins, this being predetermined by the gods. Babies with disabilities, including deaf ones, would be abandoned, killed, or imprisoned. Simultaneously, attempts to cure deaf people have existed for centuries (Davis, 2006). Many of those "cures" only aggravated the damage for the deaf person. For instance, the use of hot oil with boiled worms in the ear or an operation on the ligament of the tongue to get them to speak were excruciatingly painful treatments. Other aggressive and assault-like actions such as the repeated shaking of the head or forcing deaf people to shout so loudly that blood came out of their ears and mouths were often tried, in theory, that it would awaken their hearing (Winzer, 1993).

> Can you imagine enduring those treatments for young children in order to "cure" their being deaf?

Other miracle cures sold by get-rich-quick medicine folks included magnetic head caps, vibrating machines, artificial eardrums, blowers, inhalers, massagers, magic oils, and creams, all with promises for permanent cures (Davis, 2006). Some charlatan-healers would strike the deaf person's head hard enough to fracture it, in hopes that the blow would shake something loose. Ear infections were treated with a white-hot iron applied and poked into the area behind the ear. Those "cures" persisted well into the 20th century (Winzer, 1993). Figure 2–6 shows a pamphlet proclaiming a cure for deafness.

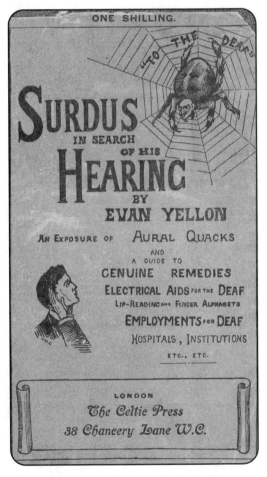

Figure 2–6. A 1906 advertisement proclaiming a cure for deafness. Courtesy of Gallaudet University Archives.

Although such cruel techniques have been abandoned in the United States, many deaf adults today remember being forced to speak English (and read lips) throughout their schooling, and if they tried to sign or gesture, they would be harshly disciplined by having their hands whipped with a ruler. Another cruel practice aimed at humiliation was to make the offending signer stand in the corner for hours (Baynton, 1996). The prohibition of deaf children from learning or using sign language still happens today, mostly without the explicit physical aspect of the punishment. However, implicitly, the punishment pervades as parents and educators may be instructed to avoid using sign language with deaf children. The thinking behind this is that if deaf children sign (or learn to sign), they will be less likely to want to learn how to speak and socialize with other deaf people. In turn, they will be more likely to successfully integrate into the hearing world (Knoors, Tang, & Marschark, 2014). However, this has not consistently proven to be the case (see Chapter 5 on Deaf education in this book).

For people with a medical perspective, utilizing auditory technology is usually the default mechanism for trying to make deaf people into hearing people. Auditory technology has evolved over time, starting with the development of ear trumpets, which were used to amplify sounds for hard-of-hearing individuals by collecting sounds and funneling them into the ear canal. The first wearable hearing aid was developed in 1936, and by the early 1950s, hearing aids could be worn on the body. See Hochheiser (2013) for more historical details.

In the 1960s through 1980s, at school, deaf children were required to wear body hearing aids upon arrival at school and to return these to the recharging station at the end of the day when going home (Conley, 2009). Body hearing aids involved a plastic case that was strapped to the chest or to the belt, with a cord attaching the case to a miniature speaker system connected to a plastic ear mold that fit in the ear canal (Welling & Ukstins, 2015). Figure 2–7 shows an old body hearing aid used in the late 1970s.

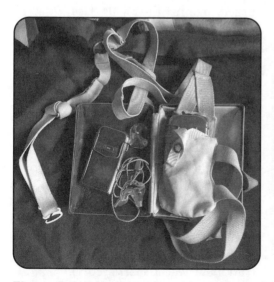
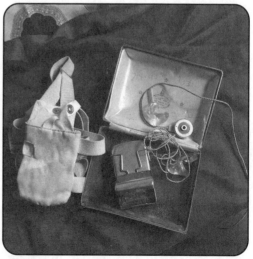

Figure 2–7. A body hearing aid used in the late 1970s. Photos courtesy of Steve Baldwin.

Deaf children were often forced to wear those types of hearing aids, which transmitted sound at very high and often painful levels that did not appropriately match their audiogram needs. Some people became used to it, but there were also many who did not (Sheetz, 2012).

Harris, one of the authors of this book, when in elementary school in the 1980s, was required by her Deaf school to wear a body hearing aid upon arrival for the full school day. Harris explained that she was receiving little or no benefit from the painful amplification of sounds—they just sounded very loud, and she had no idea what the noises were and where they were coming from. She could not concentrate in class while wearing the hearing aid. It was uncomfortable. She would often secretly disconnect or turn off the body aid, and the teachers would discipline her for turning it off once they realized what she was doing. Finally, her mother threatened the school with a lawsuit for forcing Harris to continue wearing the body hearing aid when there was no clear benefit for her. The school complied and allowed Harris to bypass wearing the body hearing aid when arriving at school. This sparked a movement for some other students at the school who felt the same way and removed their body hearing aids as well.

The U.S. Food and Drug Administration (FDA) approved cochlear implant surgery (see below for discussion about cochlear implants) in the United States for adults in 1984, then for young children ages 2 and up in 1990, and, in 2002, for children as young as 12 months old (Knoors & Marshark, 2014). Although the early cochlear implants worked for a number of deaf adults, others who underwent cochlear implant surgery in the 1980s and 1990s continue to share their traumatic stories online and post their videos online in various sites such as DeafVideo.tv or private Facebook groups. In those videos, also called vlogs (more on vlogs in Chapter 9), cochlear implant recipients would often discuss different side effects of the early cochlear implant technology, such as frequent severe and debilitating headaches and vertigo, in addition to large, visible scars from the surgery, performed when they were much younger, as seen in Figure 2–8.

In their stories, many explain that they did not fully understand why they were having surgery. Some were told that they would become hearing (in some cases, children were given a coloring book that showed them becoming a flying superhero with a cape after cochlear implant surgery) and/or forced to undergo surgery against their will (DeafVideo.tv, 2019). Those traumatic experiences by members of the Deaf community generated an atmosphere of distrust and resistance against new auditory innovations that involve surgery and extensive speech training, taking time away from educational pursuits. Some Deaf people argue that the time spent on speech training and the risk for potential side effects such as an irregular location of the ears on both sides of the face (particularly for those with one implanted ear), vertigo, headaches, and facial paralysis, while very low, are not worth the efforts to hear and speak (Paludneviciene & Harris, 2011).

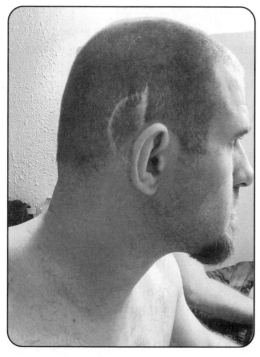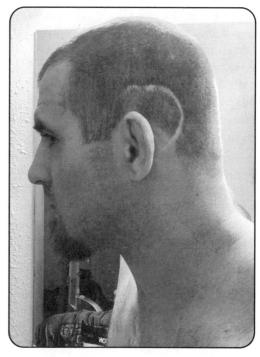

Figure 2–8. Images of a Deaf person with a large C-shaped scar on both sides of his head. Photo courtesy of Garrett Scott.

CURRENT AUDITORY INNOVATIONS AND REHABILITATION

Current auditory innovations are experiencing rapid transformation and major improvements. The medical field is expanding quickly, with fewer side effects, new experiments, updates, and releases. Audiologists, speech therapists, and teachers also work with new technology in identifying hearing differences and in developing hearing and speaking skills. This is called aural rehabilitation. There are new hearing level screening laws and organizations pushing to have hearing differences detected early in life for infants to ensure they have full access to language earlier, rather than later (Early Intervention for Infants and Toddlers,

2020), which is discussed more in detail in the next couple of chapters.

Hearing Level Screening

Some of you might ask, how do caregivers not notice an infant might be deaf until much later? Caretakers and parents may suspect something at first, for instance, when a loud noise during naptime does not wake up the baby. Then a box is dropped behind the baby and the baby is spooked. The baby looks around, not because they hear the box but because they feel the box being dropped through vibrations that travel through the floor, or maybe feel the sudden movement of the air being pushed toward the baby as the box is being dropped, or maybe the baby sees a shadow of the box being dropped, or a combination of all those signals. Likewise, when a parent arrives home, the baby looks at the door not because they hear the door opening and closing but because they see the sunlight that comes through the door as it is being opened. The baby looks up when a parent enters the bedroom not because the baby hears footsteps but because the baby smells the parent or even a slight wind blows into the room and alerts the baby. So all those signals, movements, and reactions can easily send confusing signals to caregivers.

Before early infant hearing screening laws in 1990, a child often was not identified as deaf until later in life, approximately age 2½ or 3, when caregivers realized the child wasn't responding to spoken commands or loud noises regularly (Northern & Downs, 2014). Even today, with Universal Newborn Hearing Screening (UNHS) programs, some deaf children pass the screening as they are born hearing but develop progressive losses genetically caused or from diseases, or they may not be identified until they are older because parents do not provide the necessary follow-up. These delays happen more often when children have progressive or conductive hearing loss that might respond to surgery and/or medication (Northern & Downs, 2014).

> Today, Universal Newborn Hearing Screenings (UNHS) and related public health programs are part of the Early Hearing Detection and Intervention (EHDI) system that is found in all 50 states and the District of Columbia. The National Center for Hearing Assessment and Management (NCHAM) manages these data.

Parents and caregivers are not the only ones who may miss signals that an infant who passes early hearing screening may be deaf. Most pediatricians (doctors specializing in working with infants and youth), primary care physicians (PCPs), nurses, and hospital technicians miss those signals too. They often have limited exposure to deaf babies. For one, they may have never seen a deaf child because it happens in about two to three babies per 1,000 born (NIDCD, 2016). Approximately 96% of deaf children have parents who hear (Mitchell, 2004) and those parents probably have never had exposure to deaf people or to a sign language.

Not only that, medical and audiology professionals typically do not receive training in issues related to culturally Deaf persons, the impact of early language deprivation, the use of sign language, and hearing loss in general in medical or professional schools (Andrews & Dionne, 2008; Meadow-Orlans, Mertens, & Sass-Lehrer, 2003). However, this is changing. Several major journal publications—*Journal of Clinical Ethics* (Kushalnagar et al., 2010), *Pediatrics* (Mellon et al., 2014), *Harm Reduction Journal* (Humphries et al., 2012), and *Maternal and Child Health Journal* (Hall, 2017)—printed articles discussing the importance of early identification. Not only that, a recent book publication titled *Language Deprivation and Deaf Mental Health*, edited by Glickman and Hall (2019), along with those journal publications are slowly transforming the medical field's perspective. Those publications are written by medical doctors, linguists, and educators. These Deaf scholars and their hearing colleagues explain the importance of early exposure to sign language, especially to ensure that the Deaf infant is not deprived of access to language early in life. The authors caution that if full language access is not provided early, deaf infants are at risk for cognitive, social, and academic delays as they grow older. This is discussed in detail in Chapters 4 and 5.

During early newborn hearing screening, a nurse or technician gives the infant a test using an AABR (automated auditory brainstem response), which works by recording brain activity with the baby's response to sound. If the baby does not register a response during the initial screening in either ear, the baby will be retested. If the same result is given for the second time, an audiologist will see the baby ideally within 3 weeks for a full diagnostic battery of hearing tests. The baby is then referred to an otolaryngologist (ear-nose-throat or ENT doctor) for a medical follow-up. At this point, the baby receives an otolaryngologist's clearance to see an audiologist (Northern & Downs, 2014). After the parents see the pediatrician, newborn health screener technician, and otolaryngologist, the audiologist is the parents' next professional contact (Andrews & Dionne, 2008).

Deaf involvement in the EDHI system is supported by the Best Practice Guidelines published in the journal *Pediatrics*. Goal 10 states, "Individuals who are D/HH (Deaf and Hard of Hearing) will be active participants in the development and implementation of EHDI systems at the national, state/territory, and local levels; their participation will be an expected and integral component of the EDHI system" (Muse et al., 2013, p. 1337). Is this the case in your state? Check your local and state EHDI organizations for representation of professionals who are Deaf.

Many audiologists graduated from older audiology programs, which often follow the philosophy and recommendations of the Alexander Graham Bell Association for the Deaf and Hard of Hearing, known as AG Bell. They often do not recommend sign language and Deaf culture as an option equal to auditory devices, surgery, and rehabilitation for parents of deaf infants but may do so as a last resort after all other auditory resources have been exhausted. The profit margin for the medical cochlear implant surgery as well as the device itself is high, with the burden of payment falling on the insurance companies. There are ethics involved as to the risks and to the supposed benefits for this expensive operation and device implantation. Given these considerations, some in the Deaf community, and rightly so, claim that audiologists collaborate with medical doctors and the cochlear implant industry in supplying them with patients, generating millions of dollars in profits (Durr, 2011; Ringo, 2013).

Those audiologists often recommend that parents consider Listening and Spoken Language (LSL) programs for their deaf infant (Northern & Downs, 2014). LSL programs often tell parents not to use sign language and may encourage families with deaf children to avoid contact with the Deaf community and Deaf culture. Some audiologists, speech therapists, and medical professionals recommend against the addition of sign language to the deaf child's communication opportunities (Ringo, 2013). Some require parents to sign a contract agreeing to prevent their child from being exposed to sign language (Knoors & Marschark, 2014). Santini (2015) points out that LSL is simply a rebranding of oralism and oral education (discussed further in Chapter 5), which are approaches used to exclude sign language and Deaf culture from a deaf child's life. In deconstructing the mission of LSL, Santini (2015) claims that their program design is actually a mono-modal, limited language education approach focusing solely on training the deaf child to speak and hear.

Emerging new generations of audiologists are more likely to introduce the parents to different types of early childhood programs without excluding or putting the sign language/Deaf culture option last (Andrews & Dionne, 2008). The early childhood programs include ASL/English bilingual and bimodal programs (Nussbaum, Scott, & Simms, 2012) and Total Communication programs (Bodner-Johnson & Sass-Leher, 2003). These programs promote the use of sign language(s) for all children and include the teaching of spoken English skills for deaf children who may have some residual hearing or the use of hearing aids or cochlear implants (see below) and may benefit from spoken language exposure. For children who do not benefit from access to sound, signing is the option that provides full access to language. It is important to note that children who use cochlear implants or hearing aids still do not fully hear spoken languages but may use these devices to support their spoken English development, depending on visual cues such as speechreading and signing (Byrd, Shuman, Kileny, & Kileny, 2011; Marschark, Lang, & Albertini, 2002). Those approaches embrace the multimodal (speaking, signing, and writing), multilingual (ASL, English and other sign, spoken and written languages) forms of education, as opposed to LSL, which often excludes the multimodal, multilingual approach, specifically focusing on listening, speaking, writing, and the learning of one language, English (Ringo, 2013; Santini, 2015), again discussed in detail in Chapter 5.

An increasing number of professionals support the concept of providing deaf children with opportunities to learn sign language as early as possible as the safest route to follow so the child will not suffer from language deprivation (Humphries, Kushalnagar, Mathur, Napoli, Padden, & Rathmann, 2014; Kushalnagar et al., 2010; Mellon et al., 2014). In fact, sign language has been found to support the child's learning of spoken language. In one study of 87 children with severe to profound hearing loss from 48 to 87 months of age, children who were educated in the oral-aural method combined with cochlear implants and who also learned sign language were able to learn language on the same timetable as hearing children (Yoshinaga-Itano, Baca, & Sedey, 2010). Furthermore, there is wide variability and unpredictability in outcomes for auditory devices and spoken language-only approaches (Hall, Hall, & Caselli, 2019). Moreover, being able to speak is not the same as being able to listen to a teacher and understand everything that is being said in a noisy classroom. Neither does it mean the child is progressing in the learning of language. Thus, hearing aids, cochlear implants, and listening and spoken language approaches have limitations that can be remedied by providing full access to sign language. Chapter 5 elaborates on different educational pathways for deaf children.

Hearing Aids

Hearing aids are external devices that come in many forms. The most popular ones come with a mold that is inserted in the ear and connected to a device that fits behind the ear or inside the ear. The microphone, amplifier, and speaker all are all fitted in one small plastic case worn behind the ear, as shown in Figure 2–9 (Marschark & Knoors, 2014).

Some are inserted in the frames of eyeglasses. Some simply fit in the ear canal, are barely visible, and are called in-the-canal or completely-in-the-canal, and some aids are installed inside the middle of the ear (Sheetz, 2012).

Hearing aids are used to simply amplify and channel sound into the inner ear, but lately technological advances have allowed for more sophistication in how the device processes sound for amplification. For example, hearing aid devices now can reduce environmental sounds and focus on amplifying specific types of sounds such as human voices so the listener is not distracted or confused by background sounds. Those are called *digital* hearing aids. Some features include syncing the digital hearing aid with one's smartphone wirelessly using the Bluetooth feature (Sheetz, 2012). The effectiveness of the hearing aid depends on the deaf person's residual hearing—in other words, how much hearing there is, as indicated on the audiogram. If there isn't much hearing left, the hearing aid may not be as useful. Often a profoundly

deaf person will turn the amplification much higher, and this at times may cause squealing, whistling, and severe distorting of sound, rendering the sound unintelligible if the earmold is not tightly fitted into the ear (Lane, Hoffmeister, & Bahan, 1996; Welling & Ukstins, 2015). However, there are techniques to minimize this problem.

Many members of the Deaf community wear hearing aids, which provide different types of benefits. Some individuals wearing hearing aids gain access only to environmental sounds such as sirens and someone knocking on the door. Some deaf people gain partial or full access to spoken language in specific scenarios such as a quiet room free of other noise and speaking with only one person. Some are able to manage a noisier environment with multiple people speaking (Knoors & Marschark, 2014). Some individuals simply wear hearing aids to listen to music and its rhythm and beats. Some deaf people wear their hearing aids with their hearing family members only and remove them for their daily routines. Some wear their hearing aids at work only, when communicating with hearing people. Bottom line, decisions to purchase and when to wear hearing aids greatly vary among individuals in the Deaf community. Customized digital hearing aids can range from $1,000 to $6,000 each and are often not included under most health plans (Sheetz, 2012). Sometimes people contact their local vocational rehabilitation services to help defray some of the hearing aid costs (Knoors & Marschark, 2014).

Cochlear Implants

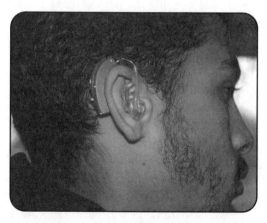

Figure 2–9. Image of a behind-the-ear hearing aid. Photo courtesy of Dezmond Moore.

For people who hear, sound travels through the ear and then finally arrives at the auditory nerve, which is connected to the inner ear. The auditory nerve then transmits the sound, now converted into electrical impulses, to the brain. The job of the brain is to interpret what you've heard. For people who have sensorineural hearing loss, the cochlea in the inner ear responsible for converting sound to electrical impulses is *not* working, so that when sound travels through the ear, the sound never arrives at the auditory nerve to be transmitted to the brain (Sheetz, 2012).

The way cochlear implants work is that there is an internal part (coil) that is surgically implanted in the cochlea (inside the inner ear) and directly attached to the auditory nerve. This implant has electrodes that allow external sounds to skip the cochlea that is not working and be converted into electrical impulses that can travel through the auditory nerve, which then sends signals to the brain—much like how people hear. In other words, the cochlear implant connects external sounds with the auditory nerve through the device that lies behind the ear. Cochlear implants do not amplify sound—instead, the sounds are transmitted directly to the auditory nerve. This device is attached to a magnet that is inserted behind the skin on the skull. The skull is slightly drilled in order to make a depression the size and depth of a quarter to fit a magnet on the side of the head. Then the external hearing aid, along with a magnetic field, is attracted to the magnet embedded under the skin behind the ear. This allows the recipient to take off or put on the device easily. Some people receive an implant for one ear, and some receive implants for both ears (Knoors & Marschark, 2014). A diagram of an implanted ear with the cochlear implant device can be seen in Figure 2–10.

Unlike hearing aids, cochlear implants also do not depend on the amount

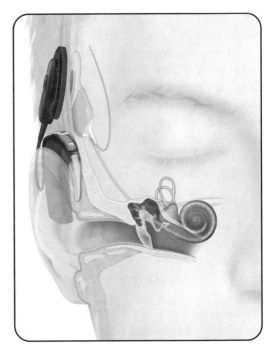

Figure 2–10. A drawing of a cochlear implant device on a human ear. Image courtesy of Cochlear Americas, ©2016.

of hearing the individual has left. Profoundly deaf people are usually better candidates for cochlear implants as long as their auditory nerve works because sometimes the surgery can wipe out the remaining hearing the person had prior to the surgery. This happens when the coil that goes through the cochlea (which is the size of a pea) is a little too rigid and damages the little hairs in the cochlea. This is why doctors usually recommend that hard-of-hearing people not receive a cochlear implant in both ears but rather in the ear that has the most hearing loss, so the other hard-of-hearing ear can work with the implanted ear (Paludneviciene & Harris, 2011).

Among medical professionals, there are a number of eligibility criteria for a successful experience with a cochlear implant. First, the infant needs to be deaf to qualify. The candidate also needs to be able to be scanned using magnetic resonance imaging (MRI). They need to have a functioning auditory nerve for the cochlear implant procedure. They need to be vaccinated against different possible infections, especially spinal meningitis. They need to be physically able to receive an implant and cleared for surgery. The caretakers need to have financial means to cover extra, unexpected costs that their insurance may not cover. The caretakers also need to have schedules that allow for, and have regular access to transportation, for frequent follow-up appointments and care. Not only that, they also need to ensure their infant will be enrolled in an educational program that includes listening and speaking practice opportunities. Of course, having realistic expectations about results and having support of family and friends also are helpful in having a successful experience (Hearing Link, 2012). For deaf adults considering implantation, in addition to the above criteria, it is better if they already have some ability to speak a language and understand a spoken language (e.g., English). If they have some benefit from using digital hearing aids, it is also important to determine whether the candidate will receive more benefit from having a cochlear implant than their digital hearing aid. The candidate needs to also socialize with hearing, nonsigning people on a regular basis to make the surgery beneficial (Cochlear Implants, 2003; Hearing Link, 2012).

For people who have heard sounds all their lives, their brain has learned to identify and interpret these sounds through repeated auditory exposure. In contrast, those individuals who have been recently implanted need to train their brains to relearn or, in other words, *map*

the impulses and the brain's interpretation of the impulses again. These impulses will be different from the sounds they are used to hearing. Adults who have had recent cochlear implantation and had some hearing before the surgery say that the sounds seem mechanical or computerized after surgery. They further commented that it takes time to make connections between the sound and the brain's interpretation of the sound so that they can recognize what the sounds mean (Chorost, 2005). Some children who receive implants pick up sounds in their brains quickly, some don't, and some are in between. Those who have just received the cochlear implant will need to attend regularly scheduled appointments with an audiologist to program the electrical impulses in the speech processor part of the cochlear implant in order to make sure the sound the person hears is at an appropriate loud level and can be interpreted by the brain. This is called "mapping" (Paludneviciene & Harris, 2011).

The American Academy of Otolaryngology-Head and Neck Surgery (2015) reports that the total cost of the cochlear implant, including evaluation, surgery, the device, and rehabilitation, can cost as much as $100,000. Some of the costs may be covered by insurance companies and Medicare, but not in every case. Those numbers do not include all of the costs associated with transportation and time off from work for multiple preoperative, postoperative surgery, and mapping appointments (Boudreault & Gertz, 2016). The devices also have an estimated shelf life of approximately 5 to 10 years, so an infant living well into his or her 70s may have to go in for multiple surgeries to replace, update, or upgrade the device. Likewise, lost or broken devices add to the overall total cost.

Aleki, a Deaf woman, had cochlear implant surgery at age 4. She used her cochlear implant until middle school when her processor broke. Her biological parents could not afford to replace her processor. When she was 17 and in foster care, the Department of Children and Families (DCF) covered the costs for a new processor. Now the current processor is 5 years old and about to die. Aleki set up a GoFundMe page to raise money for a new processor. She says her health insurance is only willing to pay up to $8,000. The total cost is $12,500. She is asking for $4,500 and so far has raised $120 in donations (Aleki, 2015).

The Cochlear Implant Controversy

With the Deaf community's past experience with medical doctors and audiologists, there understandably has been strong doubts and resistance on the part of the Deaf community toward cochlear implant technology that involves invasive surgery. In the 1980s through the early 2000s, there were reports of partial facial paralysis, painful tics caused by electrical stimulation, dizziness and vertigo, and even death as a result of obtaining a cochlear implant. The deaths were mainly caused by anesthesia before going into surgery or due to postoperative infection, particularly meningitis. Currently, patients are required to get vaccinated for meningitis before undergoing cochlear implant surgery, reducing postoperative infection leading to death (Boudreault & Gertz, 2016).

Those individuals receiving cochlear implants in the past have large scars on their head going around their ear, shaped as a big "C." Today, these scars are minor, with improved surgical techniques, and often happen behind the ear. A number of Deaf community members do not fathom putting people through an elective procedure that could potentially have serious or fatal consequences, even though the risk factors are now lower than before. This sentiment runs even stronger when involving young children due to their inability to fully understand the potential consequences (Boudreault & Gertz, 2016; Paludneviciene & Harris, 2011).

In 1993, the National Association of the Deaf (NAD) published a statement discouraging cochlear implantation in children. But since the number of children undergoing cochlear implantation continued to increase, the NAD revised its position in the year 2000 to encourage access to sign language, especially for children with cochlear implants (NAD, 2000). The Food and Drug Administration (FDA) has since then strengthened its requirements and protocol for cochlear implants, mainly to protect patients from potential harm and death. The FDA has also lowered its recommended age of surgery for children to 12 months of age, considering the procedure to be sufficiently safe (FDA, 2014).

There are many inaccurate concerns about cochlear implants that often impede the ability to open a constructive dialogue about cochlear implants among members of the Deaf community. Many common misconceptions involving cochlear implants are that they prevent children from going swimming, going on rollercoasters, or playing sports. Some say cochlear implant users cannot drive hybrid cars, go scuba diving, or walk through Travel Security Agency (TSA) metal detectors at the airport. All of those are not true. Although cochlear implant devices are water resistant, not all of them are waterproof. The device may need to be removed for showering or swimming (Cochlear, 2015). Rollercoasters, due to their speed and unpredictability, can easily dislodge cochlear implants. Extra precautions will need to be taken with sports, possibly requiring the use of helmets. Cochlear implant users can drive hybrid cars without adverse effects. There is a maximum depth limit for cochlear implant users while scuba diving (FDA, 2014). Although walking through metal detectors is not a big problem, sometimes the magnet may activate the detector alarm, and it is best to for cochlear implant recipients to carry their "Patient Emergency Identification Card" with them at all times (Cochlear, 2015).

Cochlear implant users, like people with pacemakers for their heart, may experience some lifestyle changes after receiving the implant, particularly when it comes to physical contact, water, electronics, and magnets. Boxing and other aggressive sports are discouraged for cochlear implant users.

Although water resistant, the external device cannot be submerged in water (Cochlear, 2015). Cochlear implants sometimes set off or interact awkwardly with theft detection systems, metal detectors, radio transmitters, static electricity, and more. Cochlear implant users will need to communicate with health care workers if MRIs are needed, and possibly in some situations, the magnet may need to be surgically removed (then reinserted afterward) before being scanned by an MRI (Cochlear, 2015). Users have reported some frustration after receiving an implant ranging from inability to upgrade the implant, having implant damage (from impact), unavailability of replacement parts, infection requiring removal, long-term effects, implant failure, skin irritation, dependency on batteries, and dependency on audiologists to assist with programming the settings in the device. Demagnetized implants sometimes need to be surgically replaced (Weiss, 2012). On the lighter side, some cochlear implant users rub their hand through their hair only to find discarded staples or paper clips attached to their scalp, because of the magnet underneath the skin on their head. In any case, even with all those issues, cochlear implant use continues to rise, attesting to the satisfaction some feel with their cochlear implants.

Mario (age 5) and his older brother, Antonio (age 8), both bilateral cochlear implant users, were playing as sword fighters, using sticks in place of actual swords, in their backyard. Antonio's stick accidentally struck Mario behind his ear, around the area where the magnet was located. In the next few weeks, Mario complained to his parents that he was unable to understand most of his classmates and teacher (who speak English) at his school. It was discovered later that the magnet behind his ear broke during the impact. Mario needed surgery to have his magnet replaced. Unfortunately, due to scheduling issues, Mario was not able to have surgery for another month. Fortunately, Mario and his Deaf family are fluent ASL signers and were able to communicate in ASL in the meantime.

Inspiration Porn

You may have seen (or will see) videos where deaf people or children are seen in an audiologist's office reacting to turning on of their cochlear implant device for the first time. Often those are personal video recordings of actual mapping appointments uploaded by caregivers. Those children who have been recently implanted with the devices are often crying, laughing, or smiling in slight shock. Or you've seen videos or articles of deaf children successfully speaking or hearing a word, a phrase, or a sentence.

Those types of videos tend to be uploaded to YouTube, become viral, and are often published via news outlets. Those are called "inspiration porn," a term coined by Stella Young, a disabled rights activist and writer. She argues that when disabled people are doing ordinary activities, for example, walking, driving, eating, or, in the case of Deaf people, speaking and comprehending spoken words and phrases, those uploaded pictures and videos are objectified by people who can do those things anytime, anywhere. Those people are called "abled people"; in other terms, they're not disabled.

With those uploaded materials, quotes such as, "The only disability in life is a bad attitude," "Your excuse is invalid," and "Before you quit. Try." are usually plastered on those photos or videos or written in articles about them, intended to make readers think, "Well, if that disabled person/child can do it, that means I shouldn't, ever, complain or feel bad about my life" (Pulrang, 2019; Young, 2012). Those pieces essentially make people feel good or better about their lives and feel happy about disabled people "overcoming" obstacles, essentially making those images, words, and videos "inspiration porn" for abled people (Heideman, 2015; Marcus, 2014). Marcus (2014) explains that few people actually look past those emotional moment videos, and the reality is often much more complicated and not "so shiny and perfect" as social media or media play it out to be (p. 1).

And those types of inspiration porn are actually "victim blaming" and "victim shaming" toward disabled and deaf people for not being able to walk, eat, speak, or hear like those "successful" disabled people can. If we can't walk, eat, speak, or hear like the media play them out to be, then "we didn't work hard enough like they did" (Pulrang, 2019; Young, 2012). We didn't go to speech therapy often enough, or we didn't practice hard enough, or we didn't have the right attitude. Inspiration porn is often very exploitative and only provides superficial pleasure and gratification for the reader. More often than not, the disabled person was never fully informed or asked for permission on how their image or video will be used (Pulrang, 2019).

> Now that you understand how damaging and exploitative inspiration porn is, look back on your social media and news media activity. Do you remember liking or sharing those types of posts? Do you remember reading them and feeling inspired? Now when you look at those types of posts, can you identify words and phrases that are essentially victim blaming or shaming toward Deaf people who do not hear or speak? What are the typical words and phrases? What will you do now that you know what inspiration porn is about?

Genetic Engineering

Only a few dozen of the estimated 400 genes for deafness (see earlier section on genes) have been characterized, meaning that scientists understand the characteristics of these genes. The size and complexity of these genes make testing difficult. Tests are widely available for a few common forms of genes for deafness. The most widely used test is for connexin 26, which is the name of the protein that the gene *GJB2* produces.

Whether a person is deaf because of connexin 26 depends on the genetic status of the parents. The tendency of Deaf people to marry other Deaf people who communicate using sign language (linguistic homogamy) has resulted in a significant increase in the frequency of children who are deaf due to connexin 26. However, based on the ways in which most genes for deafness (not connexin 26, but rather recessive genes) are transmitted, there is no guarantee that the children will be deaf (Nance, 2004).

There are several purposes for genetic testing. Testing can be used to determine the genetic status of a deaf child or adult (diagnostic testing), carrier testing to find out which relatives may carry genes for deafness, and prenatal testing to determine the genetic status of a fetus. Genetic testing can be used to test embryos within days of egg fertilization with in vitro fertilization in a Petri dish to allow parents to select the desired genetic outcome (Johnston, 2005; Nance, 2003; Rolland & Williams, 2006).

More and more people are participating in DNA testing through different companies such as 23andMe, AncestryDNA, FamilyTreeDNA, and many more. They include connexin 26 testing, as well as Usher syndrome and some other syndromes involving deafness. This type of voluntary testing is controversial because when you participate, you are giving up your and your entire family tree's privacy in order to learn more about yourself and where you came from. Some of the information you learn may make you or others very uncomfortable, such as a surprise sibling, or zero biological connections with people you thought were your relatives, unexpected identification of a sperm or egg donor, and even aid in police investigations of your family members (Baig, 2019). Some people use this type of testing with their partners to decide whether to have a baby (or not), inadvertently altering the futures of those not yet fertilized or unborn babies.

Diagnostic testing in deaf infants or children can be beneficial in terms of knowing genetic influences related to preventing or preparing to deal with complex medical conditions associated with syndromic deafness (see above section). Diagnostic testing for common genes for deafness in infants and children is now considered a standard of care (Pandya & Arnos, 2006). It is natural for adults to be curious about causes, and some seek diagnostic testing to understand this along with their chances of having deaf or hearing children. Others will just let nature follow its course and wait to see their babies (Arnos, 2002). Most Deaf people are resistant to genetic testing, believing it may do more harm than good (see below) (Middleton, Hewison, & Mueller, 1998; Taneja, Pandya, Foley, Nicely, & Arnos, 2004). Hearing people are more likely to consider prenatal diagnosis for genetic deafness compared to deaf people (e.g., Martinez, Linden, Schimmenti, & Palmer, 2003; Middleton, 2004). Hearing and deaf people tend to think differently, with hearing people seeing deafness as a medical issue to be prevented or cured, while culturally Deaf people feel that "deaf" is not a medical problem but a proud identity and culture (Lane, 2005; Middleton, Emery, & Turner, 2010; Scully & Burke, 2019).

> What happens when "deafness is cured"? *Zoom Focus: The End* is an award-winning movie produced by British Sign Language Broadcasting Trust (BSLBT), which commissions television programs made in British Sign Language by Deaf people for Deaf people. This movie has won over nine awards since being released in 2011. Watch and discuss among yourselves the movie's exploration of the potential impact of forced eugenics on Deaf people.

Genetic Controversy

There are social and psychological implications related to knowing more about genetic inheritance and choices about human characteristics. More and more people are thinking about this and about potential partners due to advances in genetic technology that make it possible to, for example, choose partners based on genetic makeup or to choose the sex of the child.

People will make genetic decisions depending on their cultural and/or religious perceptions and life experiences. However, more and more people will become aware of what is possible related to manipulating the genes of their future children. Much will depend on their level of comfort in choosing to go with nature as opposed to making specific reproduction choices. This knowledge, however, means that people may be passing judgment on the value of certain kinds of human lives.

The process of prenatal testing creates the opportunity to decide how acceptable it is to have babies with disabilities, babies who will develop into individuals with their own unique identities. If one accepts prenatal testing to assess chances for having a child with a disability, this challenges the typical perspective that people with disabilities, including deaf persons who see themselves as culturally Deaf, are entitled to being born just like anyone else as well as being treated by society as equal to those who are hearing (Asch, 2001; Burke, 2006; Sandel, 2007).

But when people decide on reproductive choices that are not common, others may become upset. How so? To increase the chances of having a deaf baby, a Deaf couple visited a sperm bank and were informed that potential donors were eliminated if there was a possibility the child could be deaf (Mundy, 2002). How do you

> Have you ever looked at your loved ones and appreciated the color of their eyes, height, lip shape, intelligence, or athletic ability? Research shows that people who share the same ethnic cultural background (ethnic homogamy) and/or same language background (linguistic homogamy) tend to marry each other (Stevens & Schoen, 1988).

> By screening our potential partners based on their cultural, linguistic, and genetic traits, are we practicing a form of genetic engineering as we select our partners? What about choosing the sex of your child through genetic selection? Would you want to be able to choose to have a hearing or deaf child?

think they felt? What does this say about having a deaf child? In any case, they went ahead and asked a Deaf friend (with Deaf genes) to be the donor to increase their chances of having a Deaf baby. Deaf friends asking Deaf friends with Deaf genes to be donors does happen, but we have no way of actually knowing how many babies were born deaf this way. In 2006, a survey of clinics found that 3% reported intentionally using a screening tool to select an egg with a marker for disability based on parental decision (Wordsworth, 2015).

What was society's reaction? Public opinion ranged from supportive to fiercely oppositional. Clearly, there are a lot of people who think it is an unfair burden to purposefully have a deaf child. In yet another case in Australia, during in vitro fertilization, a couple was allowed to discard embryos carrying the connexin 26 gene mutation because these were viewed as defective (Noble, 2003). Not only that, in the United Kingdom, fertility legislation enacted in 2008 required that embryo selection must be based on the grounds of avoiding disease (Emery, Middleton, & Turner, 2010). From the perspective of British legislators supporting this effort,

genes such as the connexin 26 gene mutation can easily fall into the disease category, and those who would prefer deaf children are not allowed to select embryos carrying the connexin 26 mutation. Deaf people have protested this restriction. In Russia, biologist Denis Rebrikov has started editing eggs donated by hearing women to inseminate five deaf couples so that they will give birth to hearing children. He is also working on creating gene-edited babies who are resistant to HIV (Cyranoski, 2019).

CRISPR, a gene editing kit, is available for people to purchase and use. You can order it on Amazon. It's revolutionary, cheap, effective, and easy to use. Anyone can become a genetic scientist by using that kit. Actually, professional scientists are divided on this issue—some feel this will encourage meaningful discoveries and engagement with science. Some feel this is a gateway for biohackers to accidentally create dangerous pathogens (Sneed, 2017).

Just think about the moral and ethical issues. Is it moral or ethical to discard embryos just because of the possibility of having a deaf child? What does this say about society's view of disability and of

Harris, one of the authors of this book, is Deaf because of a connexin 26 mutation, just like her father and sister. If legislation requires discarding of embryos carrying the connexin 26 gene, Harris, as well as her sister and father, would not exist. Scientists are fascinated with the connexin 26 mutation because they come with faster wound healing among other skin-related advantages. If we eradicate the connexin 26 mutation, what will happen to our ability to heal wounds? Because of the super skin-healing powers of connexin 26, she feels connexin 26 recipients should be honorary members of the X-men mutants. But let's ask the hard questions: Does removing the "bad" also come with removing the "good"? Who determines the "good" and the "bad" when it comes to genes? Why is being deaf bad if we have robust, proud Deaf communities all over the world? How do we measure goodness and badness when it comes to genes?

deaf people? Culturally Deaf people see themselves as normal and resent this perspective of society (e.g., Bova, 2008). Is society's attempt to control the number of deaf babies a form of eugenics? Eugenics is a philosophy that aims to improve the human race through different strategies, including selective breeding, forced segregation, forced sterilization, laws preventing marriage (and procreation) between less desirable people, and mass murder. Eugenics was popular in the late 1800s and throughout the early 1900s until Nazi Germany used this philosophy during the World War II years to murder people who were considered undesirable (Friedlander, 2002). Today's society can see the advances in genetic technology as either a medical triumph or as an example of cultural genocide (Nance, 2003).

Do Deaf people and Deaf communities now face cultural and linguistic genocide? Is this moral or ethical? The reality is that even if genetic testing reduces the number of deaf babies, it is still expensive and not available in most parts of the world. Also, many families are not aware of their genetic heritages, which means that the possibilities of having deaf children continue, but for how long? Let's think about why some Deaf people do not want to be Deaf. Or why some Deaf people do not want to have Deaf children. Or why people in general do not want Deaf people to exist. Now imagine if the societies of the world were all accessible, welcoming, and equal—do you think those people would think differently? Imagine if you felt welcomed and embraced for you as you are. Would you want to change yourself? Would you want to change the futures of your children? Would you want to change other people? Probably not. Why not aim for a more accessible, welcoming, and equitable society?

CONCLUSIONS

Remember the three topics you aren't supposed to discuss with your friends unless you want to get into an argument and possibly lose friends in the process? Those topics are politics, religion, and sex. Well, you can add auditory devices, surgery, rehabilitation, and genetic engineering to the list! Those topics are also difficult to discuss and can result in emotionally charged discussions. It is important for people who are not deaf to approach this topic with an open mind and listen to Deaf people, their experiences, their opinions, and their preferences. Some people have had successful experiences with auditory devices, rehabilitation, and innovations. Some love their cochlear implants, or they have to wait for additional surgery or equipment to be able to use their implants again. Some people have had traumatic experiences with audiologists and speech therapists. Some people are content and are not interested in modifying or changing their hearing levels. Some members of the Deaf community believe that Deaf babies, children, and people do not need to be fixed or cured. Some feel that if our societies were accessible, equitable, and welcoming, none of us would feel the need to fix or cure. Like the Deaf gain perspective briefly discussed in Chapter 1, Deaf people provide a unique perspective on the world and contribute to a diverse worldview. It is argued that by eliminating disability (rather than creating accessibility for all, as discussed in Chapter 9), we are interfering with the natural variations of life, biodiversity, and ecosystem that could later prove detrimental in ways we have never dreamed of. Cochlear implants, other auditory technology, and genetic advances are also seen as a significant threat to the well-being of the Deaf community. In response to that, some members of the Deaf community are trying to reach out to all parents of deaf children to educate them about the value of sign language and its benefits for all children.

REFERENCES

Aleki. (2015). *Cochlear speech processor.* Retrieved from https://www.gofundme.com/aleki

American Academy of Otolaryngology-Head and Neck Surgery. (2015). *Cochlear implants.* Retrieved from http://www.entnet.org/content/cochlearimplants

Andrews, J., & Dionne, V. (2008). Audiology and deaf education: Preparing the next generation of professionals. *ADVANCE for Speech-Language Pathologists and Audiologists, 18,* 10–13.

Arnos, K. (2002). Genetics and deafness: Impacts on the deaf community. *Sign Language Studies, 2,* 150–168.

Asch, A. (2001). Disability, bioethics, and human rights. In G. Albrecht, K. Seelman, & M. Bury (Eds.), *Handbook of disability studies* (pp. 297–326). Thousand Oaks, CA: Sage.

Baig, E. (2019). *DNA testing can share all your family secrets. Are you ready for that?* Retrieved from https://www.usatoday.com/story/tech/2019/07/04/is-23-andme-ancestry-dna-testing-worth-it/1561984001/

Baynton, D. (1996). *Forbidden signs: American culture and the campaign against sign language.* Chicago, IL: University of Chicago Press.

Bodner-Johnson, B., & Sass-Lehrer, M. (2003). *The young deaf and hard of hearing child: A family-centered approach to early education.* Baltimore, MD: Brookes.

Boudreault, P., & Gertz, G. (2016). *The SAGE deaf studies encyclopedia.* Los Angeles, CA: Sage.

Bova, M. (2008, March 17). *No to "deaf" embryos.* Retrieved March 26, 2008, from http://abcnews.go.com/print?id=4464873

Burke, T. B. (2006). Comments on "W(h)ither the Deaf community." *Sign Language Studies, 6,* 174–180.

Byrd, S., Shuman, A., Kileny, S. & Kileny, P. (2011). The right not to hear: The ethics of parental refusal of hearing rehabilitation. *Laryngoscope, 121*(8), 1800–1804.

Center for Hearing and Communication. (2020). *Statistics and facts about hearing loss.* Retrieved from http://chchearing.org/facts-about-hearing-loss/

Chorost, M. (2005). *Rebuilt: How becoming part computer made me more human.* New York, NY: Houghton Mifflin.

Clark, G. (2003). *Cochlear implants: Fundamentals & applications.* Providence, RI: Springer Verlag.

Cochlear. (2015). *Cochlear: Using a cochlear implant.* Retrieved from http://www.cochlear.com/wps/wcm/connect/au/home/support/cochlear-implant-systems/nucleus 5-system/common-questions/using-a cochlear-implant

Cochlear Implants. (2003). *Cochlear implants: Working group on cochlear implants.* Retrieved from https://www.asha.org/policy/TR 2004-00041/#sec1.5

Conley, W. (2009). *Vignettes of the deaf character and other plays.* Washington, DC: Gallaudet University Press.

Council de Manos. (2019). *Council de manos: About us.* Retrieved from https://www.councildemanos.org/about-us.html

Cyranoski, D. (2019). *Russian 'CRISPR-baby' scientist has started editing genes in human eggs with goal of altering deaf gene.* Retrieved from https://www.nature.com/articles/d4 1586-019-03018-0

Davis, L. (2006). *The disability studies reader* (2nd ed.). New York, NY: Routledge.

DeafVideo.tv. (2019). *DeafVideo.tv: Cochlear implants.* Retrieved from http://www.deaf-video.tv/?s=cochlear+implant&submit=

Durr, P. (2011). *Latest cochlear implant recall & others in the news.* Retrieved from https://hand eyes.wordpress.com/2011/09/12/latest-cochlear-implant-recall-others-inthe-news/

Early Intervention for Infants and Toddlers. (2020). *National Association of the Deaf: Resources.* Retrieved from https://www.nad.org/resources/early-intervention-for-infants-and-toddlers/

Emery, S., Middleton, A., & Turner, G. (2010). Whose deaf genes are they anyway? The Deaf community's challenge to legislation on embryo selection. *Sign Language Studies, 10,* 155–169.

Food and Drug Administration. (2014). *U.S. Food and Drug Administration: Cochlear implants.* Retrieved from http://www.fda.gov/MedicalDevices/ProductsandMedicalProcedures/ImplantsandProsthetics/CochlearImplants/default.htm

Friedlander, H. (2002). Holocaust studies and the deaf community. In D. Ryan & J. Schuchman (Eds.), *Deaf people in Hitler's Europe* (pp. 15–31). Washington, DC: Gallaudet University Press.

Glickman, N., & Hall, W. (Eds.). (2019). *Language deprivation and deaf mental health.* New York, NY: Routledge.

Hall, M., Hall, W., & Caselli, N. (2019). Deaf children need language, not (just) speech. *First Language, 39*(4), 367–395.

Hall, W. (2017). What you don't know can hurt you: The risk of language deprivation by impairing sign language development in deaf children. *Maternal and Child Health Journal, 21*(5), 961–965.

Hearing Link. (2012). *Who is eligible for a cochlear implant?* Retrieved from http://www.hearinglink.org/cochlear-implants/who-is-eligible

Heideman, E. (2015). *"Inspiration porn is not okay": Disability activists are not impressed with feel-good Super Bowl ads.* Retrieved from http://www.salon.com/2015/02/02/inspiration_porn_is_not_okay_disability_activists_are_not_impressed_with_feel_good_super_bowl_ads/

Hochheiser, S. (2013). *The history of hearing aids: Technology for the hearing impaired has come a long way.* Retrieved from http://theinstitute.ieee.org/technology-focus/technology-history/the-history-of-hearing-aids

Humphries, T., Kushalnagar, P., Mathur, G., Napoli, D. J., Padden, C., Pollard, R., & Smith, S. (2014). What medical education can do to ensure robust language development in deaf children. *Medical Science Educator, 24*(4), 409–419.

Humphries, T., Kushalnagar, P., Mathur, G., Napoli, D. J., Padden, C., & Rathmann, C. (2014). Ensuring language acquisition for deaf children: What linguists can do. *Language, 90*(2), e31–e52.

Humphries, T., Kushalnagar, P., Mathur, G., Napoli, D., Padden, C., Rathmann, C., & Smith, S. (2012). Language acquisition for deaf children: Reducing the harms of zero tolerance to the use of alternative approaches. *Harm Reduction Journal, 9,* 16. https://doi.org/10.1186/1477-7517-9-16

Humphries, T., Kushalnagar, P., Mathur, G., Napoli, D. J., Rathmann, C., & Smith, S. (2019). Support for parents of deaf children: Common questions and informed, evidence-based answers. *International Journal of Pediatric Otorhinolaryngology, 118,* 134–142.

International Committee of Sports for the Deaf. (2018). *Audiogram regulations.* Retrieved from https://www.deaflympics.com/pdf/AudiogramRegulations.pdf

Johnston, T. (2005). In one's own image: Ethics and the reproduction of deafness. *Journal of Deaf Studies and Deaf Education, 10,* 426–441.

Knoors, H., & Marschark, M. (2014). *Teaching deaf learners: Psychological and developmental foundations.* New York, NY: Oxford University Press.

Knoors, H., Tang, G., & Marschark, M. (2014). Bilingualism and bilingual deaf education: Time to take stock. In M. Marschark, G. Tang, & H. Knoors (Eds.), *Bilingualism and bilingual deaf education* (pp. 1–20). New York, NY: Oxford University Press.

Kushalnagar, P., Mathur, G., Moreland, C., Napoli, D., Osterling, W., Padden, C., & Rathmann, C. (2010). Infants and hearing loss need early language access. *Journal of Clinical Ethics, 21,* 143–154.

Lane, H. (2005). Ethnicity, ethics, and the deaf-world. *Journal of Deaf Studies and Deaf Education, 10*(3), 291–310.

Lane, H., Hoffmeister, R., & Bahan, B. (1996). *A journey into the Deaf-World.* San Diego, CA: DawnSignPress.

Marcus, L. (2014). *Why you shouldn't share those emotional 'Deaf Person Hears for the First*

Time' videos. Retrieved from http://www.thewire.com/politics/2014/03/why-you-shouldntshare-those-emotional-deaf-person-hearsfor-the-first-time-videos/359850/

Marschark, M., Lang, H., & Albertini, J. (2002). *Educating deaf students: From research to practice*. New York, NY: Oxford University Press.

Marschark, M., & Spencer, P. (2016). *The Oxford handbook of deaf studies in language*. New York, NY: Oxford University Press.

Martin, F., & Clark, J. (2019). *Introduction to audiology* (13th ed.). Boston, MA: Pearson.

Martinez, A., Linden, J., Schimmenti, L., & Palmer, C. (2003). Attitudes of the broader hearing, deaf and hard of hearing community toward genetic testing for deafness. *Genetics in Medicine, 5*, 106–112.

Meadow-Orlans, K., Mertens, D., & Sass-Lehrer, M. (2003). *Parents and their deaf children: The early years*. Washington, DC: Gallaudet University Press.

Mellon, N., Niparko, J., Rathmann, C., Mathur, G., Humphries, T., Napoli, D., . . . Lantos, J. (2014). Ethics rounds: Should all deaf children learn sign language? *Pediatrics, 1*(9), 170–176.

Middleton, A., Emery, S., & Turner, G. (2010). Views, knowledge, and beliefs about genetics and genetic counseling among deaf people. *Sign Language Studies, 10*, 170–196.

Middleton, A., Hewison, J., & Mueller, R. (1998). Attitudes of deaf adults toward genetic testing for hereditary deafness. *American Journal of Human Genetics, 63*, 1175–1180.

Mitchell, R. (2004). National profile of deaf and hard of hearing students in special education from weighted survey results. *American Annals of the Deaf, 149*, 336–344.

Mundy, L. (2002, March 31). A world of their own. *The Washington Post Magazine*, pp. 22–29, 38, 40, 42–43.

Muse, C., Harrison, J., Yoshinaga-Itano, C., Grimes, A., Brookhouser, P., Epstein, S., . . . Martin, B. (2013). Supplement to the JCIH 2007 position statement: Principles and guidelines for early intervention after confirmation that a child is deaf or hard of hearing. *Pediatrics, 131*, 1324-1349.

Nance, W. (2003). The genetics of deafness. *Mental Retardation and Developmental Disabilities Research Reviews, 9*, 109–119.

Nance, W. (2004). The epidemiology of hereditary deafness. In J. Van Cleve (Ed.), *Genetics, disability, and deafness* (pp. 94–105). Washington, DC: Gallaudet University Press.

National Association of the Deaf (NAD). (2000). *National association of the deaf position statement on cochlear implants*. Retrieved from http://nad.org/issues/technology/assistive-listening/cochlear-implants

National Institute on Deafness and Other Communication Disorders (NIDCD). (2016). *National Institute on Deafness and Other Communication Disorders: Quick statistics about hearing*. Retrieved from https://www.nidcd.nih.gov/health/statistics/quick-statistics-hearing

Noble, T. (2003). *Embryos screened for deafness: A quiet first for Australia*. Retrieved from http://www.smh.com.au/articles/2003/07/10/1057783286800.html

Northern, J., & Downs, M. (2014). *Hearing in children* (6th ed.). San Diego, CA: Plural Publishing.

Nussbaum, D., Scott, S., & Simms, L. (2012). The "why" and "how" of an ASL/English bimodal bilingual program. *Odyssey, 13*, 14–19.

Padden, C., & Humphries, T. (1988). *Deaf in America: Voices from a culture*. Cambridge, MA: Harvard University Press.

Paludneviciene, R., & Harris, R. (2011). Impact of cochlear implants on the deaf community. In R. Paludneviciene & I. Leigh (Eds.), *Cochlear implants: Evolving perspectives* (pp. 3–19). Washington, DC: Gallaudet University Press.

Pandya, A., & Arnos, K. (2006). Genetic evaluation and counseling in the context of early hearing detection and intervention. *Seminars in Hearing, 27*, 205–212.

Plante, E., & Beeson, P. (2008). *Communication and communication disorders: A clinical introduction* (3rd ed.). Boston, MA: Allyn & Bacon.

Pulrang, A. (2019). *How to avoid "inspiration porn."* Retrieved from https://www.forbes.com/sites/andrewpulrang/2019/11/29/how-to-avoid-inspiration-porn/#4c7372b95b3d

Ringo, A. (2013). *Understanding deafness: Not everyone wants to be "fixed."* Retrieved from http://www.theatlantic.com/health/archive/2013/08/understanding-deafness-not-everyone-wants-to-be-fixed/278527/

Rolland, J., & Williams, J. (2006). Toward a psychosocial model for the new era of genetics. In S. Miller, S. McDaniel, J. Rolland, & S. Feetham (Eds.), *Individuals, families, and the new era of genetics* (pp. 36–75). New York, NY: W. W. Norton.

Sandel, M. (2007). *The case against perfection.* Cambridge, MA: Harvard University Press.

Santini, J. (2015). *"Listening and spoken language": Is the rebranding of oralism a danger to students?* Retrieved from http://surdusexplores.blogspot.com/2015/08/listening-and-spoken-language-is.html

Scheetz, N. (2012). *Deaf education in the 21st century: Topics and trends.* Upper Saddle River, NJ: Pearson Education.

Sneed, A. (2017). *Mail-order CRISPR kits allow absolutely anyone to hack DNA.* Retrieved from https://www.scientificamerican.com/article/mail-order-crispr-kits-allow-absolutely-anyone-to-hack-dna/

Scully, J., & Burke, T. (2019). *Russia's CRISPR "Deaf babies": The next genome editing frontier?* Retrieved from https://www.geneticsandsociety.org/biopolitical-times/russias-crispr-deaf-babies-next-genome-editing-frontier

Smith, R., Shearer, A., Hildebrand, M., & Camp, G. (2014). *Deafness and hereditary hearing loss overview.* Bethesda, MD: National Center for Biotechnology Information.

Stevens, G., & Schoen, R. (1988). Linguistic intermarriage in the United States. *Journal of Marriage and Family, 50,* 267–279.

Taneja, P., Pandya, A., Foley, D., Nicely, L., & Arnos, K. (2004). Attitudes of deaf individuals towards genetic testing. *American Journal of Medical Genetics Part A, 130,* 17–21.

Vernon, M., & Andrews, J. (1990). *The psychology of deafness: Understanding deaf and hard of hearing people.* White Plains, NY: Allyn & Bacon.

Weiss, T. (2012). *Disabled world: Cochlear implants—Facts, benefits, and risks.* Retrieved from http://www.disabled-world.com/disability/types/hearing/communication/cochlear.php

Welling, D., & Ukstins, C. (2015). *Fundamentals of audiology for the speech-language pathologist.* Burlington, MA: Jones & Bartlett Learning.

Winzer, E. (1993). *The history of special education: From isolation to integration.* Washington, DC: Gallaudet Press.

Wordsworth, R. (2015). *Why some parents choose to have a deaf baby: Reproductive tech could threaten or preserve deaf culture.* Retrieved from https://www.vice.com/en_us/article/ypwa5j/how-reproductive-tech-could-threaten-or-preserve-deaf-culture

Yoshinago-Itano, C., Baca, R., & Sedey, A. (2010). Describing the trajectory of language development in the presence of severe-to-profound hearing loss: A closer look at children with cochlear implants versus hearing aids. *Otology & Neurotology, 31,* 1268–1274.

Young, S. (2012). *We're not here for your inspiration.* Retrieved from: https://www.abc.net.au/rampup/articles/2012/07/02/3537035.htm

PART II

Signed Languages and Learning

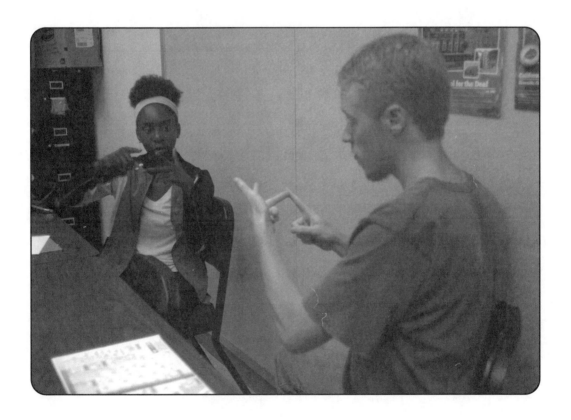

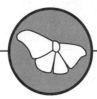

CHAPTER 3

American Sign Language

When hearing people first see American Sign Language (ASL), they recognize its expressive beauty with its flow of fingers, hands and arms, body movements, eye blinks, eye gazes, and facial grammar. ASL captivates. Is sign language universal? Is it easy to learn? How long does it take to acquire? Who uses it, besides Deaf people? These are just a few of the questions that stimulate questions about signing.

Contrary to popular belief, sign language is not universal. Each country has at least one sign language with some having more than one. Approximately 144 sign languages have been documented worldwide (Eberhard, Simons, & Fennig, 2019). And while a few words can be picked up quickly to say hello or ask "What's your name?" similar to Spanish and others languages, it takes years of practice to learn it.

In this chapter, you will learn about the history of ASL, its linguistic structure, and how it differs from English and other spoken languages. You will see how professionals worldwide use signed languages. You will also learn that despite centuries of linguistic imperialism oppression, ASL and other signed lan-

guages remain a vibrant marker of Deaf communities worldwide who cherish and celebrate its use.

BACKGROUND OF ASL AND OTHER SIGN LANGUAGES

You may wonder how sign languages were studied before we had social media and digital technology. Historical evidence documenting sign languages exists in explorers' diaries and journals (McClintock, 1910), archeological rock panel writing (McKay-Cody, 2019), and the camera and movie film footage of George Veditz in 1913 and William C. Stokoe in the 1960s (Baynton, Gannon, & Bergey, 2007). In the 21st century, scientists utilize the tools of historical and comparative linguistics (Supalla & Clark, 2015; Woodward, 2003) and computer and brain-imaging technology (see Chapter 4). One tool—lexicostatistics—enables linguists to compare the percentage of similar words between languages to determine their relationship. As such, linguists can then look for similarities across sign languages and study the roots of vocabulary. Using these tools, Woodward (2003) found that Modern Standard Thai Sign Language and ASL share 57% of their signs. This means that many Thai Sign Language signs look like ASL signs. But Woodward also found seven distinct sign languages in Thailand and neighboring Viet Nam that belong to three distinct language families, all of which are quite different from ASL (Woodward, 2003). So you can see how signed languages have complex histories.

In 1913 George Veditz, former president of the National Association for the Deaf (NAD), produced the film, *The Preservation of the Sign Language*, which was inducted into the Library of Congress National Film Registry in 2011. You can find this 14-minute film on YouTube. How do these signs compare to the signs you are learning in school?

To this end, scholars have identified four major language communities who have influenced the development of signed languages in North America: (1) Indigenous or Native, (2) African American, (3) European, and (4) American.

Indigenous Communities and "Hand-Talk"

Native American Indians (a term used by Kopper, 1986) arrived in North America about 15,000 years ago from Asia. Today, the preferred terminology is Indigenous or Native Communities (McKay-Cody, 2019). Within these communities, Indigenous Deaf people used any number of signed languages depending on where they lived geographically and in what

tribe they belonged. These signed languages are referred to as "Hand-Talk" in the wider Native communities.

Using archeology (the study of human remains; i.e., artifacts, bones, trash), linguistics (the study of languages), and art history, McKay-Cody (2019) has studied signed languages of 27 tribes using interviews, collection of lived narratives, and analyses of writing and drawings on rock panels. She has provided ancestral documentation of signed languages found in rock panel writing that predates European explorations on the continent of North America (Figure 3–1).

The term North American Indian Sign Language (NAISL) is a collective expression that designates not one

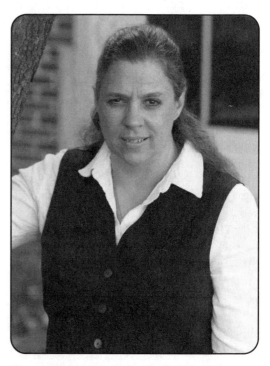

Figure 3–1. Dr. Melanie McKay-Cody, a scholar-writer who is Deaf and from the Cherokee/Choctow tribes, has investigated signed languages of Native Communities in the United States.

signed language but a specific sign language family. McKay-Cody developed the NAISL classification system, which consists of seven geographical regions with many different tribal sign languages within each area, some of which have not been formally described. For example, the Northeast Indian Sign Language region has tribal signed languages, two of which are from the Oneida and Iroquois tribes. The Southeast Indian Sign Language region also had many tribal languages, five of which are Cherokee, Creek, Seminole, Chickasaw, and Choctaw; however, these languages are now extinct. Several of the tribal signed languages of the Plains Indian Sign Language region (PISL) are Northern Cheyenne, Crow, and Kiowa. One of the many tribal signed languages of the Great Basin Indian Sign Language region is from the Ute tribe. The Southwest Indian Sign Language region also has many tribal signed languages, of which some are from the Hopi, Pueblo, and Apache tribes. Within the Northwest Indian Sign Language region is the Inuit tribal signed language, among others. And finally, there are many signed languages that were used in the West Coastal Indian Sign Language region, one of which is the tribal signed language of the Chumash tribe (McKay-Cody, 2019, p. 29). McKay-Cody (2019) points out that when early settlers and missionaries across the nation colonized the Indigenous peoples, a language genocide occurred where tribal spoken and signed languages were eradicated.

We provide such details of McKay-Cody's research to underscore the extent and complexity of the linguistic richness found in the multitude of tribal signed languages used by early Deaf Indigenous peoples prior to the coming of Europeans signed languages.

In 1886, while working for the U.S. Forest Service, William McClintock lived with the Blackfeet tribe in Montana documenting legends, religions, and signed languages. He wrote, "16 different tribes were present . . . although unable to understand each other's spoken language, they talked freely and rapidly together in gesture speech" (McClintock, 1910, p. 403). He also observed that a young deaf girl, Dives-Under-Water, used sign language with her friend and wrote, "Her busy hands moved gracefully while talking to Anatapasa" (the Chief's daughter) (McClintock, 1910, cited in Yenne, 2013).

In another case, Hovinga (2010), author of *Texas School for the Deaf Sesquicentennial: A Proud Tradition*, noted early Deaf sign and Indian sign links. In 1866, General George Custer, the infamous American army general in the Civil War who led multiple Indian massacres, visited Texas School for the Deaf. Custer purportedly wanted to meet the deaf students and "practice" sign language so he could communicate with the Indians.

Another language community—African Americans—also shares a history of early use of signed languages that predates European sign influences.

African American Communities and BASL

Under the barbaric policy of slavery, in 1619, a ship arrived near Port Comfort, Virginia. Records show that onboard were 20 to 30 Africans who were enslaved to the British to build colonies in North

America. On this account, 1619 marks the beginning of African American presence as the early builders of America. Accordingly, this date predates the 1776 (signing of the Declaration of Independence) that conventionally marks our nation's beginning ("1619 Project," 2019). There exists little (if any) documentation if any Deaf persons were on this ship. That being so, historical records do exist of British explorers engaged in the slave trade who noted that African language interpreters utilized signs and gestures to communicate among the different African tribes with their British captors. To this end, Carnes (1852) writes the following: "If no interpreter was available . . . the business is conducted in signs between parties, in the same manner that two persons deaf and dumb would act in trading with each other. Everything is done by signs and gestures of the hands and fingers." On the grounds of this, the recognition and use of signed languages can be surmised.

After the American Civil War, even though schools for Deaf students were in full operation for decades and sign language was used, Black Deaf children were segregated into separate schools. At these Black schools, formerly called Negro or Colored schools, students and faculty developed their own form of sign language. From this community, Black ASL (BASL) evolved and developed in and along the southern and border states.

See Figure 3–2 for a photo of Dr. Carolyn McCaskill, an African American linguist who has studied BASL.

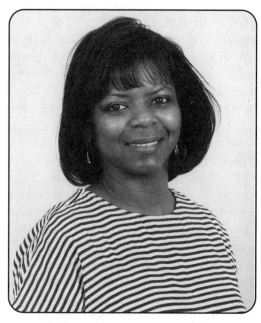

Figure 3–2. Photo of Dr. Carolyn McCaskill. Courtesy of Gallaudet University Archives.

In a study with 96 Black deaf adults from six different sites around the country, using focus groups, interviews, and storytelling, Carolyn McCaskill and her colleagues (McCaskill, Lucas, Bayley, & Hill, 2011) found that older Black signers used more two-handed signs, more forehead level signs, and a larger signing space than the younger Black deaf signers and white deaf signers. They used less mouthing and a different vocabulary or lexicon. The young Black signers showed no difference in the amount of mouthing or use of sign space, as did the white signers, but young Black signers incorporated more Black English (African American English) into their signing. You may be interested in surfing the Internet for examples of Black ASL, including STOP TRIPPING (i.e., stop imagining), DANG (i.e., darn), and slap 5 (i.e., high-five).

European Communities

The roots of ASL also run deep into the signed languages imported from Europe. Accordingly, these signed languages blended with signing already present on North American soil utilized by Native and African American communities. As such and over time, the European influences came from multiple spots on the European continent: Spain, France, Belgium, Switzerland, and Holland (Shaw & Delaporte, 2015).

In 1620, in Madrid, Spain, Juan Martin Pablo published a book describing methods of teaching deaf children, *Reducción de las letras y arte para enseñar a ablar los mudos* (Simplification of Letters and the Art of Teaching the Mute to Speak). As there were deaf children of Spanish nobility, they had to be literate in order to inherit property. For this reason, special methods of instruction were needed (Fraser, 2009). In nearby France in the 18th century, Abbe de l'Epee, a French priest, utilized Bonet's manual alphabet and also studied the natural sign language of the Parisian deaf youth freely roaming the streets. In 1760, he opened a free school, Institution Nationale des sourds-muets de Paris (now, Institut National de Jeunes Sourds de Paris [INJS] or National Institute for Deaf Children of Paris).

The innovator that he was, de l'Epee utilized the natural French signing (old LSF) but also modified it to conform to French grammar with invented signs for articles and grammatical markers. This became known as the "French Method" (Lane, 1984). Abbe de l'Epee is pictured in Figure 3–3. These methods were to make their way to America with Laurene Clerc and Thomas Hopkins Gallaudet in the early 19th century.

Not everyone thought de l'Epee's methods were forward thinking. Accord-

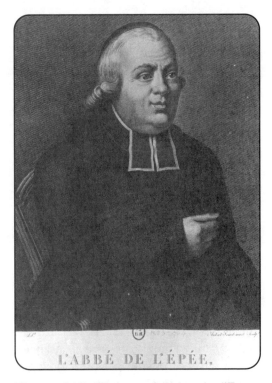

Figure 3–3. Picture of Abbe de l'Epee. Courtesy of Gallaudet University Archives.

ingly, his successor, Roch Ambroise Cucurron Sicard, in the late 18th and early 19th centuries continued to use a signed French system rather than follow the signing of the Deaf students. Debunking his teacher's methods, Roch-Ambroise Auguste Bebian criticized the French method for this reason. He considered "add-on" signs to be cumbersome and awkward. Instead, he recommended that teachers use natural sign language. Bebian's approach reflects the ongoing debate that still exists in the 21st century with some supporting the use of ASL and others supporting the use of the "methodological signs" or manual codes of English that follow English grammar (Lane, 1984).

In this direction, many Deaf students educated under de l'Epee's tutelage became teachers and were invited to lecture in Belgium, Holland, and Switzerland to share signing pedagogical practices. One of INJS's most well-known students, Laurent Clerc, was to establish the first public school for deaf students in America with Thomas Hopkins (T. H.) Gallaudet funded by a Hartford group of wealthy donors led by Mason Cogswell's family in 1817 (Lane, 1984).

Euro-American Communities

Signs and fingerspelling made their way across the Atlantic Ocean from Europe through France with some mention that the two-handed fingerspelling system came from England (Sayers, 2018). From this account, during the early 19th century, Lydia Huntley (later Sigourney) had been teaching Alice Cogswell, a young deaf girl who lived in Hartford, Connecticut. She taught Alice how to read and write using the home signs, which the young girl used with her parents. Sigourney also purportedly used the two-handed alphabet, called "the old alphabet," brought to the United States by British migrants who had settled in New England (Sayers, 2018).

While Lydia was honing her teaching skills with Alice in Hartford, a young man studying for the ministry was employed by Mason Cogswell's family to teach Alice. See Figure 3–4 for a sculpture of T. H. Gallaudet and Alice Cogswell.

Being the curious man that he was, in search of new methods, Gallaudet traveled to England to visit leaders in schools for the deaf. There he met Thomas Braidwood, who had set up schools for the deaf in Scotland and England that followed the oral approach, but T. H. Gallaudet was refused entrance to his schools. While in London, he attended an exhibition of French deaf signing students conducted

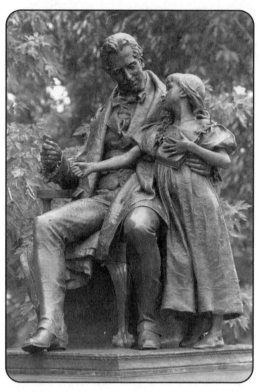

Figure 3–4. Sculpture of T. H. Gallaudet and Alice Cogswell.

by Sicard, who was then the headmaster of the Institut Royal des Sourds-Muets (now INJS) in Paris. The exhibition included two Deaf teachers, Laurent Clerc and Jean Massieu (Lane, 1984), who demonstrated how to teach. Subsequently, T. H. Gallaudet was invited to INJS, where LSF was used (Lane, 1984). T. H. Gallaudet and Clerc returned to America, where they established the first school for the deaf, the Connecticut Asylum (at Hartford) for the Education and Instruction of Deaf and Dumb Persons, now the American School for the Deaf in Hartford, Connecticut. The school used sign language as well as the methods of de l'Epee (Baynton et al., 2007).

These early forms of signing imported from Europe have provided linguists with a rich vein to examine the history of ASL from the study of old LSF. Many of the students like Clerc who were educated at INJS were invited to lecture about de l'Epee's methods and LSF in Europe and in the North, Central, and South America. In these countries, they established schools as well: Joseph Henrion in Belgium, Edouard Huet in Mexico and Brazil, Isaac Chomel in Switzerland, Brother Young in Quebec, and Henri Daniel Guyot in Holland (Shaw & Delaporte, 2015). After ASD was established in Hartford, Clerc and his students went on to establish many schools for the deaf across the United States. They used these signing methods, and their graduates further propagated these techniques as they took on teaching and administration jobs within these schools. In line with these events, the son of T. H. Gallaudet, Edward Minor Gallaudet, in 1864, went on to establish the National Deaf Mute College (now Gallaudet University) in Washington, DC, federally supported by the U.S. government beginning with Abraham Lincoln's administration (Bayton et al., 2007; Shaw & Delaporte, 2015).

their hearing families members who don't know sign language. Home signs do not have a consistent meaning-symbol relationship or formal grammar and are not passed down from generation to generation. When Deaf children meet peers and other Deaf adults as they congregate at a school for deaf students, these home signs evolve and a grammar emerges, taking two or three generations for standardization to occur (Goldin-Meadow, 2005).

> In Nicaragua, Central America, from their isolated farms and rural areas, deaf children brought their home signs and gestures to an established school and a new Nicaraguan Sign language emerged (Coppola & Senghas, 2010). This particular sign language, called Nicaraguan Sign Language (Idioma de Señas de Nicaragua), is the youngest known signed language as its historical beginnings only go back to the late 1970s (Meier, Cormier, & Quinto-Pozos, 2002).

Home Signs and Gestures

So far, we can see the Native Communities, African American, European, and Euro-American influences impacted the evolution and development of ASL. Given this, another type of signing (mentioned previously in Sigourney's work with Alice) was the use of home signs. Even before public schooling, deaf children used gesture and home signs with their hearing families to communicate. Gestures rely on body language and the labeling of objects through mime or acting out. Different from gestures, home signs are created by deaf children without adult modeling to use with

Village Sign Languages

To continue this line of thought, another form of signing influenced ASL, that is, "village sign languages." In 1694, the first deaf person arrived on the island of Martha's Vineyard from England. For more than 70 years, a large number of genetically deaf children were born and remained on the island in a community where everyone learned sign language (Groce, 1985). Other deaf-hearing signing communities emerged in two other towns: Henniker, New Hampshire, and Sandy River Valley, Maine (Lane, Pillard, & Hedberg, 2011). The numbers of deaf people significantly increased within these three towns due to a recessive hereditary trait that originated in England with subsequent intermarriage among early settlers in America. From the early 18th century to the early 1950s, to facilitate communication in the villages, both hearing and deaf persons used Martha's Vineyard Sign Language (MVSL). Precise figures of how many of these MVSL users enrolled in deaf schools are not known, nor is there any way to verify how these signs influenced the ASL signs used at the Hartford school where these signing children would have attended. See Figure 3–5 for a picture of Nora Groce, who studied MVSL.

> What would happen in the United States today if everyone learned sign language to communicate with Deaf people?

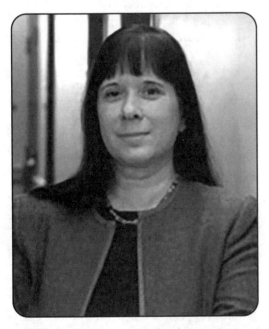

Figure 3–5. Picture of Nora Groce. Used with permission of Nora Groce.

Whether it is at school or in the marketplace, when people come together to communicate, they bring their languages or dialects to the conversation. Over time, the conversations incorporate elements from both languages. Linguists refer to this as language contact (Brentari, 2010). As European sign languages such as LSF blended with Native Communities, African American, home signs, and village sign languages, such language contact situation arose, and the result is the formation of what we now call ASL.

Researchers cherish these historical roots and work to preserve these signed languages in digital libraries where copies of historical films, illustrated dictionary entries, annotations, and written descriptions of signs are archived and analyzed. These ASL archeologists aim to trace the history of signs, as well as their changes over time, and gather evidence supporting the claim that ASL is a heritage language for Deaf people (Supalla, Limousin, & Malzkuhn, 2014).

The story of the evolution and development of ASL is not over. As what happens to all living languages, new signs in ASL are coined every day.

> Search the Internet for new ASL signs such as signs for *selfie*, *photobomb*, and *the five-second rule*.

HOW SIGN LANGUAGES ARE SPREAD

From the historical review above, we see that signed languages are found when Deaf people have regular contact with each other. With Deaf communities, when children have Deaf parents, they will learn sign language in the home and learn it as a first language. Because most deaf children have hearing parents, they typically learn to sign from a teacher at school, where there is a critical mass of other deaf children and adults. Thus, signs can be passed down from biological parent to child or from teachers, peers, or adults, particularly those with native Deaf signing parents. With the popularity of ASL, many hearing persons are taking ASL classes on college campuses and learning ASL as a second language (Rosen, 2020).

International Sign (IS) and Signed Languages Used Globally

As we pointed out, sign language is not universal; however, an international sign communication system called International Sign (IS) was developed for international meetings. IS is not a full language but rather a limited pidgin used for cross-communication, such as at the World Federation of the Deaf (WFD), the International Congress on Education of the Deaf (ICED), and Deaflympics.

This communication system has lexical items that are distinct from other sign languages and incorporates elements mostly from European sign languages (Eberhard et al., 2019) and is usually accessible only to ASL signers or European signers, despite being called "international sign." Similarly, Esperanto, a universal spoken communication system, was developed for intercommunication among first language users of other spoken languages. It is currently used by speakers in over 100 countries. (Eberhart et al., 2019). These examples show that efforts to make up a language are doomed to failure because true languages evolve within cultural communities; culture and language are inseparable.

At the 22nd International Education of the Deaf Congress held in Athens, Greece, in July 2015, with 650 scholarly presentations, 40% did not have international interpreters. Deaf professionals were excluded; they were frustrated and angry. Consequently, a resolution was drafted to provide language access to participants in international sign language and English (printed, captioned, and spoken). The proposal included guidelines for scheduling and budgeting for qualified international interpreters as well as for real-time captioning (Tucker, 2015, p. 12). This example of Deaf advocacy is and has been a sustaining characteristic present in Deaf communities for centuries.

You may think that all English-speaking countries (i.e., United States, Canada, Australia, the United Kingdom, and New Zealand) have the same sign language. This is not the case. British Sign Language (BSL), Australian Sign Language (Auslan), New Zealand Sign Language, and ASL have different histories, cultures, and structures. Likewise, Lengua de Senas Mexicana (LSM) and Lengua de Signos Espanola (LSE) are distinct sign languages with different dialects even though they are in countries where Spanish is spoken (Brentari, 2010). Canada has two sign languages—American Sign Language (ASL) and Langue des Signes Quebecois (LSQ), with each being unique (Brentari, 2010).

Signed languages are found in every country across the globe. Across the different countries, attitudes on acceptance or rejection of these sign languages differ. There are also differences in how countries utilize sign language in schools for deaf children and what government policies are set up to promote, oppress, or suppress them (Brentari, 2010).

ASL and English: Features, Content, and Structure

If we delve into the features, content, and structure of ASL, we see that it can be differentiated from spoken languages due to its use of iconicity and modality. Iconicity refers to how the form of language resembles its meaning; modality refers to how the language is expressed. These features are important because they impact how we learn language. While spoken and sign languages use different modalities, both have comparable linguistic elements, have similar acquisition timetables, and utilize both hemispheres of the brain (Mayberry, 2007). But differences exist as well. The articulators for spoken language are hidden in and around the mouth (e.g., tongue, jaws, lips, and velum). They are smaller than the articulators for signing, the hands and arms (Meier et al., 2002). Another difference is that ASL signs are made by the signer at a slower rate compared to spoken words. However, signs pack much more information in each sign/word than spoken words do. English words occur in a linear sequence, whereas ASL executes signs simultaneously. The speed or the rate of the ideas that are transmitted is about the same with both signed and spoken languages.

The iconicity of both ASL and English makes some vocabulary easier to learn. In English, the word BOW-WOW represents the sound of a barking dog. In ASL, the sign for EAT looks like a person is bringing food to the mouth with their hand. The fact that sign languages incorporate the feature of iconicity may be one reason

why deaf people may have an easier time communicating with other deaf people who use different sign languages and why babies can pick up a functional vocabulary in sign rapidly (e.g., EAT, SLEEP) (Brentari, 2010).

When looking at the features of modality, we see that when you use your voice to speak, you use the auditory modality. When you sign, you are using the visual-gestural modality. DeafBlind people use the tactile modality. They can sign into the palm of the hand or by tapping a person's shoulder or on the back. Deaf-Blind persons use touch to communicate in various ways. They can use Braille, a system of dots that enables blind persons to touch and read or write using a Braille typewriter. Or they may also make ASL handshapes into the hand. Tracing the capital letters of the alphabet into the palm of the hand is another approach. Other DeafBlind persons may prefer the use of hands-on signing where they "feel" the sign by placing their hand over the signer's hand. Some may use the Tadoma method. This uses tactile lipreading with the DeafBlind person feeling the vibration of the throat, face, and jaw positions of the speaker as he or she speaks (Reed, 1996). More recently, a new strong ASL dialect has emerged in the form of protactile (Edwards, 2015). Protactile is DeafBlind language, culture, and philosophy where DeafBlind people are always connected by touch. The protactile system has its own distinct system of classifiers (depicting verbs), specific set of signs (e.g., the ASL signs for MAN and WOMAN are essentially the same to a DeafBlind person, so in protactile, MAN is signed differently, almost like taking a cap off, to differ from the sign of WOMAN), and tactile listing or ranking (e.g., when you discuss a food shopping list in ASL, you hold up your nondominant hand and tap each finger to indicate you're going through the list, but in protactile, you hold and shake each finger) (Edwards, 2015).

In the 19th century, at age 2, Laura Dewey Bridgeman contracted scarlet fever and lost both her vision and hearing. She learned through touch, through tactile sign language, as well as the use of a technique where she touched an object, and then her teachers made the words out of raised letters on wood. Living 50 years before the well-known Helen Keller, Laura proved to the world the ability of DeafBlind students to benefit from education. See Figure 3–6 for a photo of Laura Bridgeman.

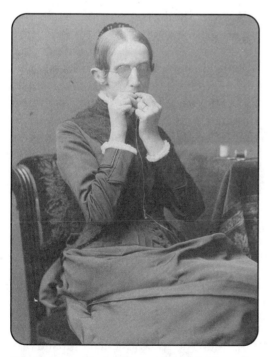

Figure 3–6. Photo of Laura Dewy Bridgeman. Courtesy of Gallaudet University Archives.

Becoming deaf and blind at age 1½ years from scarlet fever or meningitis, Helen Keller became an avid reader, writer, and international lecturer inspiring people worldwide. You may have seen the movie *The Miracle Worker* (1962) in which her teacher, Anne Sullivan, fingerspelled the word W-A-T-E-R into her hands. After this, Keller was able to learn hundreds of new words by tactile fingerspelling. See Figure 3–7 for a photo of Helen Keller.

The fourth modality is writing. English writing, a script using the Roman alphabet, is based on spoken language. Of the existing 7,111 living languages, 3,995 have a developed writing system. Around 3,116 do not have writing systems (Eberhard et al., 2019). While ASL does not have a written form used widely by Deaf people, linguists and researchers use ASL glossing notation, which allows them to analyze ASL on paper for academic publications. ASL glossing is a rudimentary system that does not fully represent ASL. It basically uses capitalized English letters. For instance, the ASL sign for cat would be designated as CAT. ASL gloss does not incorporate ASL grammar and many other important components of ASL, so it has limitations. Other than ASL glosses for research, there are a number of authors developing and promoting written systems more representative of ASL.

Search the Internet for examples of sign writing such as SignWriting, Sign Font, ASL-phabet, ASL write, and si5s. Try writing a note to a classmate in your ASL class using one of these sign writing systems.

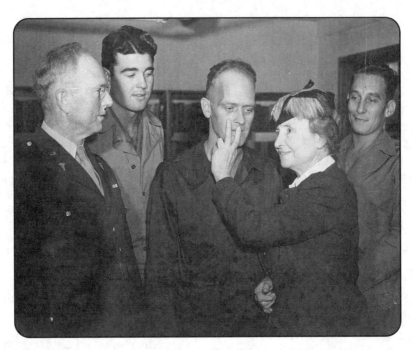

Figure 3–7. Photo of Helen Keller. Courtesy of Gallaudet University Archives.

Sometimes the four modalities can be combined and blended as in the case of hearing bilinguals, such as children of deaf parents (CODAs). These children are bimodal bilingual as they use two output channels: voice for speech and the hands for signs and two perception systems: audition and visual (Emmorey & McCullough, 2009). Bimodal bilingual persons produce unique ASL-English code blends in which ASL signs are produced at the same time with English words that are spoken (Emmorey, Borinstein, & Thompson, 2005). Deaf children also can be bimodal bilingual where they learn to separate the two languages (see Chapter 4).

ASL Content

Just like spoken languages, you can tell jokes in ASL, curse, pray, exchange news with friends, tell stories, recite poetry, or talk about philosophy or other abstract ideas. ASL has an academic technical vocabulary to convey all kinds of information, from astrophysics to zoology to theology, to concepts about early childhood to postsecondary instruction, to theater performances. Signs for computer technology, medicine, and legal terminology have been developed for instructional, medical, and legal settings.

ASL was first linguistically described and analyzed by a Deaf-hearing team: Dorothy Sueoka Casterline, Carl G. Croneberg, and William C. Stokoe (1960). They founded the first ASL linguistic laboratory as well as *Sign Language Studies*, a journal that published ASL linguistic research. After their groundbreaking research, ASL was given academic status by linguists who then set up academic linguistic programs and research laboratories worldwide. In these labs, teams of scientists and their graduate students in the fields of linguistics, psycholinguistics, cognition and learning, statistics, psychometrics, neuroscience, sociolinguistics, computer science, and engineering study various topics such as how ASL is processed in the brain, how children acquire and learn ASL, how communities use ASL and signing, how new sign languages emerge, and the role of gesture in learning. They also develop educational applications such as the ASL and English bilingual approaches and the development of electronic books that combine ASL movies with animations, illustrations, and printed texts.

> Check out the Internet of examples of bilingual children's stories books that include English text, ASL movies, animations, and illustrations.

Casterline, Croneberg, and Stokoe wrote the first ASL dictionary based on linguistic principles (DASL), first published in 1965 (Stokoe, Casterline, & Croneberg, 1965). On December 1, 2015, Gallaudet University hosted a celebration called the DASL 50th Year Anniversary. Faculty, administrators, students, and staff celebrated the linguistic breakthrough the DASL created. With a BA in English, Dorothy Sueoka Casterline was a Deaf Asian woman from Hawaii who contributed her insights and knowledge in linguistically analyzing ASL. She was also recognized for creating the tab, dez, and sig fonts, which allowed for the written notation description of ASL. Carl G. Croneberg was a Swedish Deaf man who had an MA in English and knew three other languages: Swedish, German, and ASL. During the DASL 50th year celebration at Gallaudet, Croneberg was recognized for seeing the analogies between hearing and Deaf cultures. He also wrote an early

ethnographic and sociological portrait on the Deaf communities and regional dialects. See Figure 3–8 for a photo of Dorothy Sueoka Casterline, and Figure 3–9 for a photo of Carl G. Croneberg.

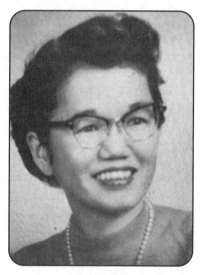

Figure 3–8. Dorothy Sueoka Casterline, a Deaf Asian woman, created the fonts for the early written notation system for the DASL.

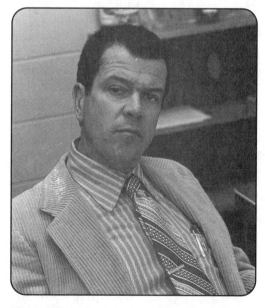

Figure 3–9. Carl G. Croneberg was a Swedish Deaf man, one of the writers of the DASL.

Since Casterline, Croneberg, and Stokoe's work on the DASL, numerous ASL dictionaries have been published cataloguing ASL signs organized by linguistic principles (Valli, 2005) and by handshape (Tennant & Brown, 2010), as well as specialized dictionaries that delve into sign histories and etymologies (word origins) (Shaw & Delaporte, 2015). Still another innovation is the TRUE-WAY ASL curriculum that has an ASL dictionary consisting of over 15,000 videos. Even with this effort, ASL dictionary-makers have barely scratched the surface of the content of the ASL lexicon (vocabulary).

ASL, like English and other languages, cannot be translated word for word. Meaning is lost. As mentioned earlier, many Deaf adults were deprived of access to language early in life, impacting their later educational abilities, and thus they face challenges even with sign language interpreters because of their lack of ASL knowledge. To make the challenge even tougher for them, many hearing interpreters do not have the ability to communicate with those Deaf adults, particularly with difficult and specialized contexts such as medical, legal, or educational situations. One way to surmount this obstacle is the use of a DI (Deaf Interpreter). The DI is a specialist who provides interpreting, translation, and transliteration services in ASL and other visual and tactual communication forms used by individuals who are Deaf, hard of hearing, and DeafBlind. The DI begins with a distinct set of formative linguistic, cultural, and life experiences that enables them to provide specialized skill and interaction in a wide range of language and communication forms influenced by region, culture, age, literacy, education, class, and physical, cognitive, and mental health. As a bilingual team, DIs work collaboratively with hearing interpreters, but with modern technology, they can also work solo with the consumer. To ensure effective communication, DIs should be provided in educational, medical, workforce, mental health, and legal settings. Unfortunately, they are limited in number because hearing interpreters, feeling offended that they cannot interpret as well as Deaf interpreters, often intentionally exclude Deaf interpreters from potential assignments and jobs.

Structure

When Casterline and Croneberg notified Stokoe of the signing around him by Deaf colleagues and students on Gallaudet campus, he was introduced to unique patterns and structures. Together they worked on describing this system based on hand positions to the body (called tabula or tab for short), configuration of the hand (called designator or dez), and movement of the hand (signifier or sig). Applying the system of structural linguistics, this Deaf-hearing team revolutionized the study of linguistics by supporting the idea that definitions of languages should include not only spoken ones but sign languages as well (Maher, 1996). See Figure 3–10 for a photo of Dr. Willian C. Stokoe.

Stokoe worked side by side with Casterline and Croneberg in observing, studying, and analyzing the structure of ASL. Deaf scholars such as Casterline and Croneberg are often overlooked in the literature discussions related to ASL linguistics, thus not getting the recognition they deserve for their work. Search the Internet. Can you find more information about Casterline and Croneberg?

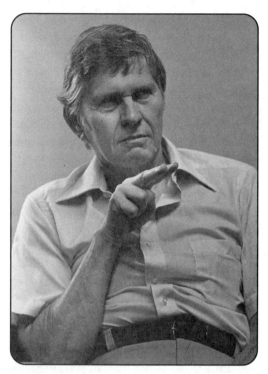

Figure 3–10. William C. Stokoe was an English professor at Gallaudet. Courtesy of Gallaudet University Archives.

For a fuller description of ASL structure, you can read your textbooks from your ASL classes. We review some key points here. Like spoken languages, ASL has a phonology, semantics or vocabulary, morphology, syntax or grammar, and discourse structures. In signed languages, its phonology consists of the following parts of signs, which are the following: (1) handshape, (2) location, (3) movement, and (4) palm orientation. A fifth parameter of nonmanual signals (NMS) such as head tilts, eyebrow raises, and facial expressions is hotly debated. To compare the phonology of English and ASL, consider the word *cat*, which can be broken down into three phonemes (*k ae t*) using the International Phonetic Alphabet (IPA). Or the word *cat* can be written as three graph-

emes or written symbols (c a t). As an ASL sign for a right-handed person, CAT can be broken down into four phonemes, the handshape (F), the palm oriented toward the cheek, the location (thumb and index finger touching the cheek), and movement (brush index finger and thumb back toward ear, twice). Nonmanual signals such as eyebrow raise (which indicates a question) could also add meaning to this sign. The sign for EXPERT is made with the same handshape as CAT with different location and movement. Refer to your ASL textbook for graphics of these examples.

Another level of ASL structure is called morphology. Defined as the study of how a language creates new words or signs, morphology shows how we can make or produce new words in our language. In English, we add *s* to the free morpheme, *cat*, to make it plural: *cats* (cat + s = cats). English can also express the concept of *more* by adding an adjective as in *more cats* or *many cats* or add numbers as in *five cats*. Like English, ASL can show plurality by adding adjectives (i.e., MORE CATS, MANY CATS) or by adding numbers, FIVE CATS, THREE CATS (Valli, Lucas, Mulrooney, & Villanueva, 2011). ASL also uses movement and facial grammar to show other meanings. Consider the sign EAT. In its basic sign stem (EAT), the signer can add movement and facial grammar to mean the cat is eating continuously, eats regularly, or eats for a prolonged period of time over and over again or eats in a hurry. Examine your ASL textbook or google this to see a graphic or movie demonstration.

In English, there are rules for forming compound words (i.e., grasshopper, meatball). Similarly, ASL has rules for forming compound words (the old sign for SISTER is a compound of two separate signs,

GIRL-SAME, which has evolved to the sign we use today for SISTER). In addition, both English and ASL can incorporate numbers and time into a word or a sign. In ASL, this would be THREE-WEEKS-AGO, which is one sign including all three concepts ("three," "weeks," and "ago") at the same time. In English, this would be a three-word sequence expressed in a linear fashion, as in "three weeks ago" (Valli et al., 2011). English has two main numerical systems, the cardinal numbers (one, two, three) and ordinal numbers (first, second, and third), while ASL has more than 20 different documented numerical systems (Humphrey, 1989).

Similar to English, ASL also uses sign order to show its relationships among words or what we call its grammar. ASL uses space and movement. For example, using the same words or signs, a person can compose two sentences with different meanings. If you change the word order, then the meaning is changed in English. When you change the movement, the meaning is changed in ASL.

When you read these two sentences, you can see how word order tells you the meaning.

1. The cat chased the dog.
2. The cat was chased by the dog.

We know that the cat chases the dog in the first sentence, and the dog chases the cat in the second sentence. Both of these have very different meanings. In ASL, the signer sets up where the cat is situated. The right-handed signer then makes a movement from one to the other: CAT (right side), DOG (left side), then with both hands moving from left to right, CAT-CHASE. The second sentence would be signed, CAT, DOG-CHASE. ASL has many grammatical processes like these that use space, movement, and direction to show relationships between signs. In contrast, English uses word order to show similar relationships.

ASL also has a complex verb system made up of special terms called classifier predicates, classifier handshapes, and locative verbs, currently called depicting verbs (Valli et al., 2011). Depicting verbs are signs that use handshapes to designate things, size, shape, or usage. For example, things shown in classifiers can be objects, people, animals, or vehicles. Shapes can include outlines, perimeters, surfaces, configurations, or gradients. Sizes can show largeness, smallness, relative size, and volume. Usage can involve movement paths, speed, and interactions (Valli et al., 2011). Please refer to your ASL textbook or online and look at different ASL signs for different shapes and sizes (e.g., The sign for FLAT).

ASL also has a genderless pronoun (he, she, it) and a determiner system (i.e., the, a, an) that are made up of similar pointing signs. The auxiliary verbs in ASL (WILL, CAN, FINISH, MUST, SHOULD) are used at the beginning and at the end of the sentence instead of internally as in English. Also, ASL does not use prepositions in the same way that English does. ASL uses depicting verbs while English uses prepositions such as in, under, on, and so on.

English uses morphemes (-s, -ing, -ed, will) to express time in a sentence. In comparison, ASL uses facial grammar along with signs to mark time (NOW, FUTURE, LONG-TIME-AGO, PAST, FINISH) and movement, which are layered in the sign sentence.

The basic order for sentences found in English, subject-verb-object, is not always found in ASL. ASL, with its more flexible sign order grammar, allows the signer to place the object before the subject. Thus, the English sentence, "The cat runs up the tree" can be signed, TREE CAT RUN-UP. Of course, English, like ASL, has many complex sentence constructions that are in different orders.

Some languages do not use the verb *to be* but instead use a different system. In ASL, for example, the sentence DOG SICK consists of a noun and a predicate that is the adjective, SICK. This ASL sentence does not include the verb *is*, but the adjective SICK functions as a predicate; it describes the dog. Verbs, nouns, and adjectives can be predicates in ASL. In English, they are predicate nominatives and predicate adjectives, but they must be accompanied by verbs such as *is, was, were*, or its various other forms (Valli et al., 2011).

ASL, like spoken language, can be used to make conversations between two or more people. The signer will use signs but also will use what linguists call discourse or conversational structures that include use of eye gazes, eye blinking, and body movement (Valli et al., 2011). As you go out and meet Deaf people and have sign conversations with them, you will notice more ASL discourse features. If you take a class in ASL, your teacher will encourage you to study videos of Deaf people signing so you can learn more about the structure of ASL conversations.

Literature is another discourse structure and can include narratives, legends, poetry, prose, and plays. In school, you may have become familiar with the rich children's literature written in English with multicultural themes and characters such as the following: Christopher Paul Curtis's *Bud, Not Buddy*, Paul Gobe's *The Girl Who Loved Wild Horses*, and Arthur Dorres's *Abuela*. Like English, ASL has a strong literary tradition. The literature of both ASL and English, interestingly enough, is based on oral language (or

sign language) stories and poems that were performed long before they were written down (Byrne, 2013). ASL has a rich reservoir of storytelling, poetry, nursery rhymes, drama, humor, and folklore, which has been passed down from generation to generation at Deaf schools and festivals and has been recorded on video, YouTube, and films (Byrne, 2013). More on ASL literacy and literature can be found in Chapter 11.

> Search the Internet and look for examples of ASL poems or stories. Can you examine them for phonology, semantics, morphology, and discourse structures? Discuss with your classmates.

THE MANUAL ALPHABET

Published charts showing fingerspelled handshapes in books came into existence as early as 1620 when Spanish monks used fingerspelling to teach deaf students reading and writing (Fraser, 2009). Fingerspelling is considered part of ASL because it uses the handshapes of ASL. However, fingerspelling also is thought of as part of English because it has 26 handshapes that correspond to the 26 letters of the English alphabet (Padden, 2011). Try this experiment in the next box.

> Find a hearing English-speaking classmate in the student center who knows no sign language. Fingerspell the word C-A-T to him and ask if he can understand what you fingerspelled. Then ask yourself: Is fingerspelling English?

Some fingerspelled letters are iconic, which means that the sign for each letter looks like their corresponding letter in English. Examples include the following iconic letters in ASL: C, O, J, L, M, N, O, U, V, W, Y, and Z (Padden, 2011). Look online and find a copy of the manual alphabet.

You can use fingerspelling for specific English words (such as book titles and names of cities and street names) and abbreviations for names, places, and objects (Valli et al., 2011). ASL uses fingerspelling. It spells out words from English, and this has resulted in a form called lexicalized signs and loan signs. As an example of lexicalized sign, BUS is a sign that is formed with a B at the beginning and an S at the end. The letter U is skillfully blended into the two handshapes B and S. There are also loan signs such as TOO BAD that is signed with a distinct movement, as TB. Lexicalized signs and loan signs provide evidence of the effects that ASL has when it meets the English language and new signs evolve.

Today fingerspelling is used in almost every deaf education classroom along with ASL to teach vocabulary, expand concepts, spell words, or identify persons, places, or things for which there are no sign equivalents yet.

As young as 13 months, Deaf children will babble using fingerspelled handshapes similar to ways hearing children babble sounds (Petitto & Marentette, 1991). Later, as hearing children match sounds to printed letters, so do deaf children match fingerspelled handshapes and letters when they learn to spell and write. Preschool children learn to fingerspell words using their own, unique, rhythmic patterns that are different from how English sequences syllables (Harris, 2010).

Adults learning ASL and fingerspelling as a second language learn letter-by-letter as they are matching them to the English alphabet (Padden, 2011). Although it takes less than an hour to learn the fingerspelling alphabet, it takes quite a bit longer to be able to read and produce fingerspelling quickly and accurately.

ASL LEARNERS AND STRATEGIES

Deaf children who attend schools for the deaf or who have Deaf families will acquire ASL as a first language through everyday conversations. We call this Social ASL, just like Social English for hearing children, their families, and schools. Through face-to-face communication, Deaf children develop shared conversation skills such as chatting with friends or just casual talk. Social ASL depends on the social situation and is highly contextual. For instance, talking to a deaf friend about plans for the evening to attend a deaf festival is an example of using Social ASL.

Deaf children also learn Academic ASL, the language of instruction in the classroom, like hearing children learn Academic English, the language of instruction in most schools in the United States. Academic ASL can include the study of ASL grammar through the use of space, classifiers, and other grammatical aspects. It can also include learning ASL poetry and literature. Classroom content in math, science, and social studies can also be expressed in Academic ASL using a specialized vocabulary for these subject areas (see Chapter 5). For example, in the science classroom, a specialized sign vocabulary is needed for terms such as photosynthesis, evolution, and global warming, to name a few.

A group of Deaf friends chatting at a coffee shop are using social ASL. When they start to talk about their upcoming test in ASL linguistics, using words such as phonology, syntax, and discourse, they switch to using Academic ASL as they are communicating and using highly complex vocabulary, grammar, and structure.

Hearing people learn ASL for many reasons. Some may simply be intrigued by it. Others learn sign to communicate and read storybooks to a deaf child. Others may meet a Deaf coworker and wish to learn to communicate with them. Or they may work in careers that involve Deaf consumers. Learning signs to have a conversation with a deaf person is one thing; however, becoming an interpreter requires years of training with developed expertise in both ASL and English, as well as knowledge of the theory and practice of interpreting, cultural competence, and knowledge of specialized signs for different content areas (Roy, Brunson, & Stone, 2019).

Against this background, ASL learners can include teachers, doctors, nurses, lawyers, social workers, interpreters, and others who work in fields that involve working with deaf consumers. Over the past 10 years, with the use of the Internet, vlogs, and videophones, ASL has spread. Additionally, the use of video relay interpreters on the videophone as well as remote interpreting through videophones and Internet videoconferencing capabilities has increased the visibility and use of ASL for hearing persons who do not know ASL and need to communicate with Deaf individuals (see Chapter 9 for details).

ASL is used in classes with all ages of deaf and hearing persons, from babies to adults. ASL signs are taught to hearing babies and children during reading instruction (Daniels, 2001). It is also utilized with hearing children with cognitive and learning disabilities, autism, Down syndrome, cerebral palsy, medical nonverbal conditions, and other communication disorders (see reviews in Leigh & Andrews, 2017). In these clinical and school settings, while ASL vocabulary is covered, the grammar of ASL grammar may not be taught.

ASL can also be taken for foreign language credit in high school, at a community college, or at a university (Rosen, 2020). Today, 45 states recognize ASL as a language that can be taken for foreign language credit at high schools, community colleges, and universities. Interest in learning sign language has caught on internationally, and sign languages of different countries are taught as L2 or second languages in elementary schools, high schools, and universities (McKee, Rosen, & McKee, 2014). Even though countries differ on their acceptance and recognition of the sign languages of their Deaf communities, still there is a surge of sign language classes taught globally due to legislation in countries giving sign language status as a language and the "linguistic rights for deaf children," a movement supported by the National Association for the Deaf (NAD) and the World Federation of the Deaf (WFD) (Murray, 2015).

Hearing students may find the facial grammar of ASL challenging such as executing question forms and negation. Other problematic areas include learning to form handshapes, using space, understanding ASL sentence structure, reading fingerspelling, using eye contact, and codeswitching between ASL and English (see reviews in McKee & McKee, 1992). These features are not found in English; hence, they require more effort for hearing signers to learn them.

Hearing students will be exposed to different learning strategies such as the use of pictures, actions, and English translations while learning ASL (Rosen, 2020). It is best to have Deaf signers as language models, either as instructors or as a community of signers with whom to communicate. There are many examples of instructional materials to teach and learn ASL available on the Internet. Going to Deaf socials at coffee shops, city and state association for the deaf meetings, residential school for the deaf football games, and other sports events are excellent ways to meet Deaf people and use your ASL skills. See Figure 3–11 for a photo of college hearing students learning ASL.

DIALECTS AND OTHER FORMS OF SIGNED COMMUNICATION

When a language comes into contact with another language or another group of users, language changes. Then a new variation or dialect emerges. Like spoken English, ASL and other signed languages have different dialects based on geographic region. Sign language linguists have found that these variations or dialects are related to sociolinguistic factors such as how old you are, your socioeconomic class, your gender, your ethnic background, where you live, your sexual orientation, and whether you have a disability or not (Brentari, 2010; McCaskill et al., 2011).

Deaf people live in communities where English is the language spoken by the majority of the hearing culture, so it's no wonder that English has influ-

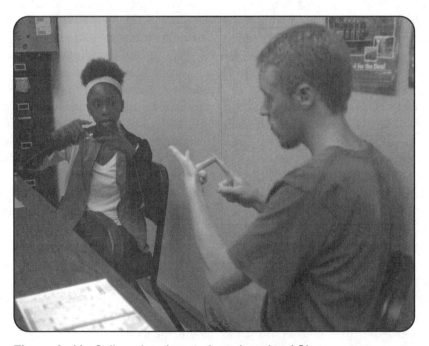

Figure 3–11. College hearing students learning ASL.

Examples of dialects in spoken and written American English include an Appalachian dialect called mountain dialect, and among Black Americans there is Black English (BE). Black English has different names such as Black English Vernacular (BEV) and Ebonics or African American Vernacular (AAVE) (MacNeil & Cran, 2005). Do you listen to rap or country western music? Can you tell the difference between Black dialect and Appalachian dialect?

enced ASL. One way is through mouthing when deaf persons silent speak words or when they read the lips of other persons (lipreading). Some Deaf people use lipreading. Some use contact signing, which is a natural blending of ASL signs with English word order (Lucas et al., 2011). Other modes of communication are not languages or dialects per se but sign codes or systems of English whose elements are derived from ASL signs but then invent signs and morphemes and place them in English word order. These include the Total Communication (TC) philosophy and English-based systems such as Manual Codes of English (MCE), Simultaneous Communication (SimCom), and Cued Speech (CS). These communication modes are used in conversational contexts as well as in the classroom. In Chapter 4, we show how signs are used in school settings to teach English.

ATTITUDES: LINGUISTIC IMPERIALISM

People have attitudes or beliefs about language in general, their language, and the language of other people. They may believe that a southern accent is less prestigious than a New England accent or that a person speaking an Appalachian dialect is less educated than a person speaking with a Midwestern accent. Taken to the extreme, these attitudes can develop into ideological beliefs that create linguistic imperialism, a concept that means some languages or dialects should be considered better and thus dominate over other languages (Phillipson, 1992).

Linguistic imperialism has been applied to the education of Deaf children, who constitute a linguistic minority. Since the international conference in Milan in 1880, signing has been considered inferior to English or other countries' spoken languages. Thus, signing was banned from schools for Deaf students in the United States and worldwide. Historically, and even today, this imperialistic attitude resulted in punishing Deaf students for signing as well as firing Deaf teachers from faculty positions.

Linguistic imperialism was also evident when spoken languages were favored over signed Native languages. This occurred when more schools for the deaf were established after the Civil War. In this context, deaf children were placed in Indian boarding schools after being forcibly removed from their Native tribal reservations for purposes of removing their Indian culture and language and assimilating them into white culture and English. Subsequently, these children were forbidden to use their Native sign languages and forced to learn ASL and English. In this same vein, as Indigenous populations were eradicated because of white European colonizers, the spread of new diseases, and forced evacuation from Indian reservations, the spoken languages and signed languages of Indigenous Communities also were stamped out and died. Today, linguists are preserving and revitalizing their Native Communities' spoken languages as well as their signed languages by preserving them in digital archives and libraries for future research (Bickford & McKay-Cody, 2018).

Linguistic imperialism also occurred against Black sign language, which Deaf children brought from their segregated Black Deaf schools when they were integrated into the white deaf schools. When Black deaf children brought their BASL, they soon dropped it to use more ASL. Fortunately, linguists are studying BASL and capturing and preserving it on videotapes for future study (McCaskill et al., 2011).

Politics and policy are not the only reasons for language genocide. Sign languages can also die of natural causes. In such a case, when the Deaf children from Martha's Vineyard attended a school for the deaf, their MVSL and other village signed languages disappeared as they became integrated into the ASL used at the school.

On the political front, many countries have not officially recognized sign language. One such example is in Ireland, where educational policies and practices for deaf students support English instruction rather than Irish Sign Language (ISL) (Rose & Conama, 2018). Still other examples are found in Taiwan and China. Here the governments primarily support one language—Mandarin Chinese—rather than the sign languages used by the Deaf communities. Within these countries, Deaf children are educated in Chinese only,

with spoken Chinese considered superior to Chinese Sign Language (CSL), Taiwanese Sign Language (TSL), and a sign-supported Chinese or Signed Chinese (SC). However, among some teachers, a sign language is utilized as compensatory tools to support spoken Chinese and for the teaching of literacy (Liu, Liu, & Andrews, 2019; Wang & Andrews, 2017).

As you can see. linguistic imperialism has infiltrated into deaf education, a practice that has persisted for centuries worldwide. Optimistically, with more open attitudes related to globalization and multilingualism, one-language instructional methodologies have receded to the sidelines with more enlightened views on bilingualism, language acquisition, and second language learning coming to the forefront (see Chapters 4 and 5).

> Hearing children of immigrant families from German-, Spanish-, Chinese-, and Japanese-speaking homes also have a long, sad history of language oppression and imperialism in American schools throughout the 19th and 20th centuries. Search the Internet for stories on how the government treated these English-language learning children.

Within this context, these language ideological beliefs, unfortunately, have carried ASL into other countries within Southeast Asia as well as countries on the African continent. For this reason, many native signed languages have been replaced with ASL and English due to the misguided efforts of missionaries and teachers who have established schools for deaf children. In Nigeria, Mali, Ghana, Gambia, Kenya, and Thailand, the use of

ASL and sign codes of English has influenced the sign languages already used there by Deaf communities (Nyst, 2010; Woodward, 2003). However, there are efforts to reverse this linguistic imperialism through language revitalization projects. For example, due to the efforts of the Save the Deaf and Endangered Languages Initiative and the Nigerian National Association of the Deaf, the indigenous and national varieties of Nigerian Sign Language (NSL) are being documented and preserved. Because there was no education or organizations for deaf people before 1960, the American-born Black Deaf missionary, Andrew Foster, introduced a sign language in the schools that was a blend of Ghana Sign Language, ASL, and English-based signs as well as local tribal signs used by deaf persons such as Hausa Sign Language, Yoruba Sign Language, and Bura Sign Language, which is today known as NSL (Ajavon, 2003; Eberhard et al., 2019).

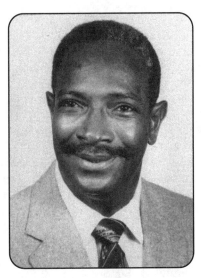

Figure 3–12. Picture of Andrew Foster. Courtesy of Gallaudet University Archives.

> Reverend Andrew Foster (1925–1987) established many mission schools in Africa between the 1950s and 1980s. He encouraged the use of signs used by the local African communities related to regional food, drinks, and ceremonial objects and rituals. See Figure 3–12 for a picture of Andrew Foster.

If you haven't yet, you can register for a beginning ASL course and start a conversation with persons who use ASL. In the next chapter, you will learn how ASL and Deaf culture are used to develop the minds and foster learning and literacy for Deaf students.

CONCLUSIONS

We hope this chapter on ASL helped you think about language and culture afresh. Studying more about ASL beyond what we described in this chapter and learning to sign are activities that you can enjoy.

REFERENCES

1619 Project. (2019, August 14). *New York Times*.

Ajavon, P. (2003). *The incorporation of Nigerian signs in deaf education in Nigeria: A pilot study. Part 1.* Frankfurt, Germany: Peter Language Publishers.

Baynton, D., Gannon, J., & Bergey, J. (2007). *Through deaf eyes: A photographic history of an American community.* Washington, DC: Gallaudet University Press.

Bickford, J. A., & McKay-Cody, M. (2018). Endangerment and revitalization of sign languages. In L. Hinton, L. Huss, & G. Roche (Eds.), *Routledge handbook of language revitalization*. New York, NY: Routledge.

Brentari, D. (Ed.). (2010). *Sign languages*. New York, NY: Cambridge University Press.

Byrne, A. (2013). *American sign language (ASL) literacy and ASL literature: A critical appraisal* (Unpublished doctoral dissertation). University of Toronto, Canada.

Carnes, J. A. (1852). *Journal of a voyage from Boston to the west coast of Africa: With a full description of the manner of trading with the natives on the coast.* Cleveland, OH: John P. Hewett & Co.

Coppola, M., & Senghas, A. (2010). Deixis in emerging sign language. In D. Brentari (Ed.), *Sign languages* (pp. 543–569). New York, NY: Cambridge University Press.

Daniels, M. (2001). *Dancing with words: Signing for hearing children's literacy.* Westport, CT: Bergin & Harvey.

Eberhard, D. M., Simons, G. F., & Fennig, C. D. (2019). *Ethnologue: Languages of the world* (22nd ed.). Dallas, TX: SIL International. Retrieved from http://www.ethnologue.com

Edwards, T. (2015). Bridging the gap between DeafBlind minds: Interactional and social foundations of intention attribution in the Seattle DeafBlind community. *Frontiers in Psychology, 6,* 1–13.

Emmorey, K., Borinstein, H., & Thompson, R. (2005). Bimodal bilingualism: Code-blending between spoken English and American Sign Language. In *Proceedings of the 4th International Symposium on Bilingualism* (pp. 663–673). Somerville, MA: Cascadilla Press.

Emmorey, K., & McCullough, S. (2009). The bimodal bilingual brain: Effects of sign language experience. *Brain and Language, 109,* 124–132.

Fraser, B. (2009). *Deaf history and culture in Spain: A reader of primary sources.* Washington, DC: Gallaudet University Press.

Goldin-Meadow, S. (2005). *The resilience of language: What gesture creation in deaf children can tell us about how all children learn language.* New York, NY: Psychology Press.

Groce, N. (1985). *Everyone here spoke sign language.* Cambridge, MA: Harvard University Press.

Harris, R. (2010). *A case study of extended discourse in an ASL/English bilingual preschool classroom* (Unpublished dissertation). Gallaudet University, Washington, DC.

Hovinga, S. (2010). *Texas School for the Deaf sesquicentennial: A proud tradition.* Austin, TX: Historical Publications.

Humphrey, J. K. (1989). *One, two, buckle your shoe: Numbering systems in ASL, course materials.* Retrieved from https://digitalcommons.unf.edu/asleimats/7

Kopper, P. (1986). *The Smithsonian book of North American Indians: Before the coming of the Europeans.* Washington, DC: Smithsonian Books.

Lane, H. (1984). *When the mind hears: A history of the deaf.* New York, NY: Vintage Books.

Lane, H., Pillard, R., & Hedberg, U. (2011). *The people of the eye: Deaf ethnicity and ancestry.* New York, NY: Oxford University Press.

Leigh, I. W., & Andrews, J. F. (2017). *Deaf people and society: Psychological, sociological, and educational perspectives.* New York, NY: Routledge.

Liu, H. T., Liu, C. J., & Andrews, J. F. (2019). Deaf Education in Taiwan: History, policies, practices and outcomes. In H. Knoors, M. Brons, & M. Marschark (Eds.). *Deaf education and beyond the Western world* (pp. 239–259). New York, NY: Oxford University Press.

Lucas, C., & Bayley, R. (2011). Variation in sign languages: Recent research on ASL and beyond. *Language and Linguistics Compass, 5*(9), 677–690.

MacNeil, R., & Cran, W. (2005). *Do you speak American?* New York, NY: Doubleday.

Maher, J. (1996). *Seeing language in sign—The work of William C. Stokoe.* Washington, DC: Gallaudet University Press.

Mayberry, R. (2007). When timing is everything: Age of first-language acquisition effects on second language learning. *Applied Psycholinguistics, 28,* 537–549.

McCaskill, M., Lucas, C., Bayley, R., & Hill, J. (2011). *The hidden treasure of Black ASL: Its history and structure.* Washington, DC: Gallaudet University Press.

McClintock, W. (1910). *The old north trail: Life, legends & religions of the Blackfeet Indians.* Lincoln: University of Nebraska Press.

McKay-Cody, M. (2019). *Memory comes before knowledge—North American Indigenous Deaf:*

Socio-cultural study of rock/picture writing, community, sign languages, and kinship (Unpublished doctoral dissertation). University of Oklahoma, Norman.

McKee, D., Rosen, R., & McKee, R. (Eds.). (2014). *Teaching learning signed languages: International perspectives and practices.* London, UK: Palgrave Macmillan.

McKee, R. L., & McKee, D. (1992). What's so hard about learning ASL? Students' & teachers' perceptions. *Sign Language Studies, 75*(1), 129–157.

Meier, R., Cormier, K., & Quinto-Pozos, D. (Eds.). (2002). *Modality and structure in signed and spoken languages.* New York, NY: Cambridge University Press.

Murray, J. (2015). Linguistic human rights: Discourse in deaf community activism. *Sign Language Studies, 15,* 379–410.

Nyst, V. (2010). Sign languages in West Africa. In D. Brentari (Ed.), *Sign languages* (pp. 405–432). New York, NY: Cambridge University Press.

Padden, C. (2011). Sign language geography. In G. Mathur & D. Napoli (Eds.), *Deaf around the world: The impact of language* (pp. 19–37). New York, NY: Oxford University Press.

Petitto, L. A., & Marentette, P. (1991). Babbling in the manual mode: Evidence for the ontogeny of language. *Science, 251,* 1483–1496.

Phillipson, R. (1992). *Linguistic imperialism.* Oxford, UK: Oxford University Press.

Reed, C. M. (1996, October). The implications of the Tadoma method of speechreading for spoken language processing. In *Proceeding of Fourth International Conference on Spoken Language Processing. ICSLP'96,* Vol. 3, pp. 1489–1492.

Rose, H., & Conama, J. B. (2018). Linguistic imperialism: Still a valid construct in relation to language policy for Irish sign language. *Language Policy, 17*(3), 385–404.

Rosen, R. (Ed.). (2020). *Routledge handbook of sign language pedagogy.* London, UK: Routledge.

Roy, C., Brunson, J., & Stone, C. (2019). *The academic foundations of interpreting studies.* Washington, DC: Gallaudet University Press.

Sayers, E. E. (2018). *The life and times of T.H. Gallaudet.* Lebanon, NH: ForeEdge.

Shaw, E., & Delaporte, Y. (2015). *A historical and etymological dictionary of American sign language.* Washington, DC: Gallaudet University Press.

Stokoe, W. (1960). *Sign language structure: An outline of visual communication systems of the American deaf.* Occasional Paper, Students in Linguistics, Buffalo, NY.

Stokoe, W., Casterline, D., & Croneberg, C. (1965). *Dictionary of American Sign Language.* Washington, DC: Gallaudet College Press.

Supalla, T., & Clark, P. (2015). *Sign language archeology: Understanding the historical roots of American sign language.* Washington, DC: Gallaudet University Press.

Supalla, T., Limousin, F., & Malzkuhn, M. (2014). Tracking our sign language heritage. *Deaf Studies Digital Journal, 4.* Retrieved from http://dsdj.gallaudet.edu/assets/section/section2/entry203/DSDJ_entry203.pdf

Tennant, R., & Brown, M. (2015). *The American sign language handshape dictionary.* Washington, DC: Gallaudet University Press.

Tucker, J. (2015). 2015 ICED. *The Maryland School for the Deaf Bulletin, CXXXV,* 12.

Valli, C. (Ed.). (2005). *The Gallaudet dictionary of American Sign Language.* Washington, DC: Gallaudet University Press.

Valli, C., Lucas, C., Mulrooney, K., & Villanueva, M. (2011). *Linguistics of American Sign Language: An introduction.* Washington, DC: Gallaudet University Press.

Wang, Q., & Andrews, J. F. (2017). Literacy instruction in primary level deaf education in China. *Deafness & Education International, 19*(2), 63–74.

Woodward, J. (2003). Sign languages and deaf identities in Thailand and Viet Nam. In L. Monaghan, C. Schmaling, K. Nakamura, & G. Turner (Eds.), *Many ways to be deaf: International variation in deaf communities* (pp. 283–301). Washington, DC: Gallaudet University Press.

Yenne, B. (2013). *Images of American: Going-to-the-sun road.* Charleston, SC: Arcadia Publishing.

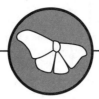

CHAPTER 4

How Deaf Children Think, Learn, and Read

Thinking, learning, and reading make us aware of our world. These mental processes help us categorize, organize, remember, and share our experiences. What if you are Deaf, Deaf multicultural, or DeafDisabled? Would you think, learn, and read in the same manner as sighted hearing people do? In this chapter, we discuss how sign language and multiculturalism, including Deaf culture and life experiences, influence intelligence and help develop cognitive abilities, world knowledge, language, and literacy. We also see how sign language and Deaf culture provide visual support for spoken language learning with cochlear implants and examine how neuroscientists have studied sign languages to better understand how Deaf people process their spoken, signed, and tactile languages.

We practice thinking skills every day. How?

Imagine that you received an unassembled computer desk. You open the box, lay out the parts, and then read the instructions. As you put the computer desk together, you discover that a board does not fit. You reread the instructions and try again. After texting a more experienced friend, who gives you several clues, you visualize your past experiences assembling furniture. After several attempts, you figure it out. During this task, how did you use thinking, memory, visual-spatial, executive functioning (planning), problem-solving, theory of mind (understanding the point of view of another person), language, reading, and writing skills? What if you were Deaf, or a Deaf student with an intellectual disability, or a DeafBlind person? Would you solve this problem in the same way?

CULTURE, LEARNING, AND INTELLIGENCE

Culture and Language

Culture impacts the way families and their Deaf children participate in deaf education, what multicultural resources they bring to school, including spoken and sign languages. As such, in order to promote thinking skills and encourage learning at school, teachers must know their students' unique cultural backgrounds and not rely on racial or ethnic stereotypes but instead rely on multiculturalism as a resource and not as a barrier (Christensen, 2017).

Cultural role modeling by families and teachers plays a pivotal role in forming how students develop thinking and learning skills. Members of ethnic communities as well as from the Deaf multicultural community, including DeafDisabled individuals, can furnish Deaf students with socially mediated learning. According to Vygotsky (1980), socially mediated learning means that children best learn how to think through interactions with an expert or more experienced others. Unfortunately, Deaf people, particularly those from multicultural backgrounds, as role models are underrepresented and their resources have only been marginally recognized in deaf education (Simms, Rusher, Andrews, & Coryell, 2008). Deaf teachers can help open the channels of language, reading, and academic learning to develop foundations of thinking, cognition, and learning using a sign language and Deaf cultural approaches (see Chapter 5 for discussion of Deaf teachers). This does not mean auditory learning objectives are not needed. Deaf teachers as experts can offer primarily visual scaffolding but also can give auditory and tactile support to Deaf students' learning. While some Deaf students may prefer to use vision, others may utilize residual hearing supported by cochlear implants or hearing aids (Marschark et al., 2015). Another group within the diverse Deaf population are students who are Deaf-Blind. As such, DeafBlind mentors can guide students and professionals on how to live and function in the DeafBlind community using visual, auditory, and tactile modes of role modeling (Bruce et al., 2016). See the next box for an example.

In a unique program offered by the DeafBlind Service Center (DBSC) in Seattle, Washington, DeafBlind individuals are trained to become mentors for sign language interpreters working with DeafBlind populations. Discuss the importance of role modeling that DeafBlind persons can provide such as what it means to live in a tactile world and use tactile communication.

IQ Tests

Intelligence cannot be fully understood outside of its cultural context. Behavior that is considered intelligent in one culture may not be thought of as intelligent in another culture (Sternberg & Grigorenko, 2004). Throughout history, using hearing norms of intelligence, psychologists have thought Deaf people were less intelligent and were mislabeled as concrete rather than abstract thinkers (Moores, 2001). Concrete thinkers experience the world through familiar objects and events while abstract thinkers find principles in recurring events and solve problems. Today, we know that intelligence is normally distributed in the Deaf population based on tests of nonverbal intelligence (Vernon, 2005). What often occurs, however, is that in early life, some Deaf children experience language delay, and this often impacts their performance on English-language-based tests (Maller & Braden, 2011). Some Deaf children and adults have even been misdiagnosed as having an intellectual disability, autism, or mental health issues and are placed in inappropriate facilities (Vernon & Andrews, 1990). Junius Wilson's tragic story is an example of such a misdiagnosis.

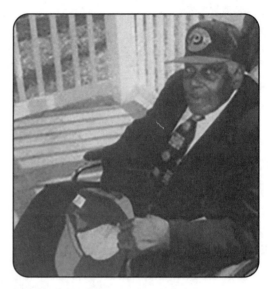

Figure 4–1. Junius Wilson. Courtesy of John Wassen.

Junius Wilson, a profoundly deaf man, lived 76 years at the Goldsboro, North Carolina, state mental hospital, 6 years of which were spent in prison. A biography of Mr. Wilson, titled *Unspeakable*, states that Mr. Wilson was never legally declared insane by a doctor, nor was he was ever found guilty of any crime. He lived in the Jim Crow South during a time when there was little understanding about being Black and Deaf. Mr. Wilson only knew a dialect of regional signs that was used in his school (Burch & Joyner, 2007). Search the Internet to find other examples of Deaf people in mental health hospitals or prisons who have not been given appropriate tests or accommodations. Junius Wilson's photo is shown in Figure 4–1.

Today we still evaluate Deaf persons using nonverbal intelligence or IQ tests to assist in planning for educational, vocational, and mental health services (Vernon & Leigh, 2007).

McCay Vernon, clinical psychologist, researcher, author, and advocate, was well known for exploring the psychosocial aspects of Deaf and DeafDisabled individuals, particularly those who are DeafBlind. He also made significant contributions in these areas: intelligence testing, mental health, education, the importance of deaf teachers and administrators, the use of sign language in schools, and legal rights (Vernon & Andrews, 1990). In 2007, the American Psychological Association awarded Vernon the Gold Medal Award for Life Achievement. See his photo in Figure 4–2.

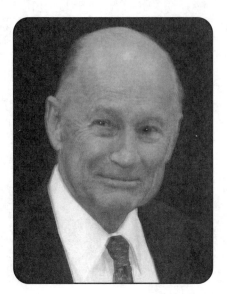

Figure 4–2. McCay Vernon. Used with permission of Marie Vernon.

Thought and Language

Since ancient times, Aristotle (384–322 BC) and other philosophers have written about the relationship between thought and language. Understanding this relationship helps us understand deaf people better because the majority have average or even above-average nonverbal intelligence even with language deprivation (Vernon, 2005). As such, this lack of access to language can create cognitive delays, mental health difficulties, lower quality of life, higher trauma, and limited health literacy (Hall, 2017).

If an early language is provided, Deaf children can develop thinking skills, label their experiences and concepts, and reorganize new patterns as they see, hear, talk about, and touch them depending on their sensory strengths and needs. Children can also use language to form new thoughts without having the experiences with real objects and events. Language is a powerful system we use to encode, organize, and remember our experiences. With language, we can translate thoughts and ideas into speech, signs, gestures, and written symbols and can share these with others (Pinker, 2007). And with language skills, children develop even more complex cognitive skills (Gleitman & Papafragou, 2005). However, some forms of cognitive organization or thinking do not need language. And interestingly enough, Deaf children who have no language are able to invent their own system of gestures to express their feelings, wants, and needs (Goldin-Meadow, 2003). All of this requires a certain level of thinking.

Do you see how important it is for all children to have early access to language? If children do not have a language, they cannot develop thinking and social skills to their maximum potential.

> What would your life be like if you had no language? What would be the quality of your thoughts, feelings, and relationships? Ildefonso, a deaf man from Mexico, was not given language access until age 27, when he learned sign language. In Susan Schaller's book, *A Man Without Words* (1991), you can read how Ildefonso's thinking, his viewpoints, and his identity changed as he learned sign language.

COGNITIVE ABILITIES

Cognition Shaped by Culture

Cognitive abilities are shaped by our culture (Sternberg & Grigorenko, 2004). It is within our family circle that thinking and language are first developed. Like the general population, Deaf people are diverse and comprise different cultural and multicultural backgrounds. But some Deaf children cannot access their family's culture and language because they do not have early familial communication. Moreover, families and also professionals may not see the benefits of a sign language or multilingualism for Deaf children when they are exposed to the family's home spoken language. Other Deaf children may experience linguicism where English and sign language of the school are favored over the home language. The Rosario case provides such an example.

Born deaf of unknown causes into a Spanish-speaking (Mexican American) home, Rosario lost her vision in early childhood from retinal detachment, leaving her with minimal light perception. Her family used English with her even though her mother did not master English until Rosario was 9 or 10 years old. Rosario used sign language with her deaf friends but used English writing, speaking, and listening with her family. She attended a public school, used a sign language interpreter, and received vision and hearing services (Ingraham & Andrews, 2010). What if Rosario's family and teachers included Spanish at home and school? How would multilingualism help Rosario develop thinking skills?

Combined with cultural beliefs, the type and extent of sensory input impacts cognitive abilities, thinking, and language skills. As such, Deaf individuals vary on their access to the quantity and quality of sensory input from vision, audition, and tactile-kinesthetic or touch and movement.

Vision and hearing are considered distant senses while the tactile-kinesthetic senses enable children with sensory input in close proximity to them. We use both distance (i.e., hearing and sight) and close (i.e., tactile-kinesthetic) input for learning. Tactile-kinesthetic skills are related to cognitive abilities, but they are different from visual learning as they involve learning about the "feel" of objects such as their texture, weight, temperature, composition, shape, and material as well as the movements of these objects. DeafBlind individuals are easily able to gather tactile-kinesthetic information that is close to them. However, they are restricted in getting sensory information from distant sources depending on the extent of their remaining hearing and sight.

Another factor to consider is that kinesthetic-tactile learning takes time, and the DeafBlind child will need multiple exposures being able to touch objects in order to build up a concept for them. To this end, DeafBlind children move through a hierarchy of tactile-kinesthetic skills from the concrete, real objects to abstract tactile concepts and skills, Braille symbols and letters. But other sensory inputs can assist in learning too. For example, Deaf students with low vision can use kinesthetic-tactile information to support impressions they get visually and auditorily (Adkins, Sewell, & Cleveland, 2016). How Deaf, DeafDisabled, and DeafBlind children access information through their available sensory avenues will provide for them their own unique path in developing thinking, language, and learning skills.

Our five senses (i.e., sight, hearing, smell, taste, and touch) enable children to perceive and gather information and experiences. From these perceptions, children organize, categorize, and develop concepts. These concepts become part of the child's thinking skills, an umbrella term that encompasses other skills such as visual and tactile attention, imagery, visual-spatial skills, memory, learning, metacognition, theory of mind (ToM), executive functioning (EF), and reasoning, to name some. Deaf people, including those who are DeafDisabled, may use spoken, signed, tactile languages or a combination of these, as well as technology and other augmentative communication devices to perceive and experience their environment from which they can develop thinking, learning, and remembering. And as they interact with others, they continue to develop their cognitive abilities by acquiring world knowledge and experiential learning at home and school, particularly through incidental learning (Hamilton, 2011).

Incidental Learning

Incidental learning and world knowledge are acquired by children through conversations with others (Meeks, 2018). Culturally Deaf families are at a marked advantage as the home environment is readily set up to naturally provide ample opportunities for incidental learning and world knowledge through daily conversational exchanges in sign language (Meeks, 2018; Ocuto, 2019). However, as most Deaf children come from hearing families, communication may fall through the cracks, which can create delays in language and conceptual and world knowledge (Hall, Smith, Sutter, DeWindt, & Dye, 2018). See the box for an example of how rich incidental learning is when accessible communication is provided in the family.

Mary, a 3-year-old hearing girl, sits at the breakfast table and listens to her older brother and parents talk about a favorite baseball player. During bath time, she listens to songs on an iPad. Later she watches cartoons on TV. While driving to the grocery store, her mother talks to her about the cows in a nearby farm. At the grocery store, Mary listens to her mother talk to the butcher. Later that evening, around the dinner table, she hears her father and mother talking about family weekend plans. What if Mary is Deaf or DeafBlind? How would you change this story to make sure she had opportunities for incidental language learning?

Incidental learning impacts Deaf-Disabled individuals in profound ways. Related to DeafBlind individuals, only about 6% are completely Deaf and blind, with most having some usable residual hearing and vision that can be used for incidental learning. However, when any extent of vision and hearing is decreased, distorted, or missing altogether, a child's world may be limited to what can be touched within arm's reach (Belote & Maier, 2014). Accordingly, DeafBlind children do not "oversee" and "overhear" information in their environment as hearing children do. While sighted Deaf children can observe what is going on around them visually even if not all visual communication is accessible to them, Deaf-Blind children miss such spontaneous learning situations. Along with low vision and low hearing levels, Deaf children may also have other physical disabilities and medical conditions that impact conditions for learning. As a result of this combination of factors, for some DeafDisabled individuals, their life experiences may be reduced and altered. Teachers, then, must depend on direct teaching of information rather than setting up experiences for incidental learning in order to stimulate thinking and learning (Belote & Maier, 2014; Knoors & Vervloed, 2015).

In a different but related vein, when Deaf individuals have a physical disability such as cerebral palsy or are persons who utilize wheelchairs, they can observe their environment and learn through incidental learning in the similar ways that sighted Deaf students do with some accommodations (i.e., giving children more time to express themselves in sign language, providing ramps to classrooms, and so on) (Burke, 2014). Other DeafDisabled persons such as those with attention-deficit disorder (ADD) or attention-deficit/ hyperactivity disorder (ADHD) may learn in a similar manner as nondisabled Deaf peers, but they may need more time and frequent repetition to learn.

Joint Attention

Joint attention using vision, touch, and sometimes hearing are avenues for the Deaf child to develop language and cognitive abilities. When Deaf babies look at or touch their caregiver's' face, they use their visual, auditory, or touch attention-getting skills. The infants direct their eye gazes or attention to their caregiver and to objects. Caregivers help the child label people and objects with names through vision, touch, or hearing depending on the child's available sensory avenues. To this end, such reciprocal attention and interactions assist the child in acquiring information and bonding with their caregivers, thus supporting social interaction (Allen, 2015; Clark et al., 2015). A reliance on vision rather than audition does not always make a Deaf child solely a visual learner. They may use their spoken language and residual hearing when they are engaged in different tasks (Marschark et al., 2015).

To further build concepts, language, and early literacy, caregivers may recite nursery rhymes in spoken language or sign language (Andrews & Baker, 2019) or even use tactile storybooks if the infant or toddler is DeafDisabled. To teach academic concepts, science and math teachers may use signed explanations, visual aids, multimedia, and rotating objects (Marschark & Wauters, 2003) with other visuals as pictures, illustration, drawings, print, movies, and visual media (Kuntze, Golos, & Enns, 2014). Deaf learners who use bimodal bilingual communication approaches may also utilize their vision to support their listening and spoken language skills supported by digital hearing aids and cochlear implants in order to support memory and language learning (Marschark, Lang, & Albertini, 2001).

Deaf children who have autism, are DeafBlind, or are both DeafBlind and autistic may access and process sensory information differently from sighted Deaf children. This impacts how they develop thinking skills and learn language (Belote & Maier, 2014). For example, Deaf children and youth with intellectual disabilities will experience developmental delay across all domains of learning that will impact their functional and adaptive skills (Bruce et al., 2016). Further, Deaf students with autism may show characteristics of echolalia, repetition of movements, and lack of eye contact, which impacts their thinking and learning skills as well (Belote & Baier, 2014).

Visual Attention and Peripheral Vision

Compared to hearing people, on average, sighted Deaf persons have the same abilities in seeing sets of color and distinguishing between flashing items and visual motion. Deaf individuals do have better peripheral vision, which is what you see on the sides when you are looking ahead (Hirshorn, 2011). Peripheral vision can be a safety asset, for instance, while crossing a street or driving. Peripheral vision, however, is not always a plus. As Deaf children are easily attuned to movements in the environment, they may appear easily distracted and inattentive and may be diverted by students working next to them or sidetracked by the flicker of lights on a television screen. Large class sizes in mainstream or inclusive settings and seating in vertical rows do not provide accessible information. Small class sizes with desks in a semicircle around the teacher may be most accessible for the deaf student (Dye, Hauser, & Bavelier, 2008).

There are also disadvantages when Deaf students switch their attention to look at the signing of the interpreter (Marschark & Hauser, 2008). Experienced teachers know how to wait until the deaf students are finished with their task, such as reading or writing. They will wait until all students' eyes are on them before they begin communicating or teaching. Teachers may set up rules for class participation so that when responding to the teacher's questions, the other students are in the line of vision. Another tip is to let the students finish reading a slide projected

in front of them before starting to teach a lesson.

With DeafBlind students, classroom rules need to be set up to ensure that class information is accessible to them through tactile measures. They may need extra time for attention-getting strategies. Deaf-Disabled students will also need their own set of classroom strategies for information access, particularly those with residual hearing.

A Deaf child with cerebral palsy may have a slower rate of signing. The child may need more time to attend to different signers in the class as well as time answering questions using expressive sign language (Burke, 2014).

And still another factor that impacts thinking and learning relates to the tactile modality. For example, Deaf students with autism, or those who are DeafBlind, or DeafBlind students with autism may have a condition called tactile defensiveness or tactile selectiveness. This is an aversion to certain textures and experiences and could be brought on by the child not having reliable information about what will happen next. This condition may also due to neurological complications (Belote & Maier, 2014). Teachers need to be sensitive to this factor in order to stimulate thinking and learning in the classroom.

Visual Imagery and Spatial Memory

Signing Deaf students may be better in forming pictures in their mind (visual imagery), remembering pictures or objects in a room (visuospatial memory), and remembering moving objects compared to their hearing peers (Hamilton, 2011). Deaf people who use sign language and their vision skills perform better than hearing signers and nonsigners on certain tasks such as quickly changing their visual attention, scanning visual material, detecting motion, and recognizing faces (Dye & Bavelier, 2010; Marschark, 2003), as in the case of Leroy Colombo, a talented lifeguard.

Frequently seen scanning the sea to the front and to the side, at the turn of the 19th century was a lifeguard named Leroy Colombo. He was born hearing but became deaf at age 7 due to spinal meningitis. Shortly after his diagnosis, his mother enrolled him at the Texas School for the Deaf, where he learned ASL and Deaf culture. The 1976 Guinness Book of World Records reported that Colombo saved more than 900 swimmers in the Gulf of Mexico on Galveston beaches from 1918 to 1967. Combining his lifeguard skills of physical strength, stamina, and endurance, as well as his knowledge of the tides and currents using his visual attention and visual motion detection abilities, he was quickly able to see and rescue swimmers from drowning (Andrews, 2010, 2011). He used his visual memory of the tides bringing in rip currents and his firsthand experiences in recognizing sink holes that trap swimmers. Colombo is pictured in Figure 4–3 holding one of his many earned trophies for saving lives and winning swim races.

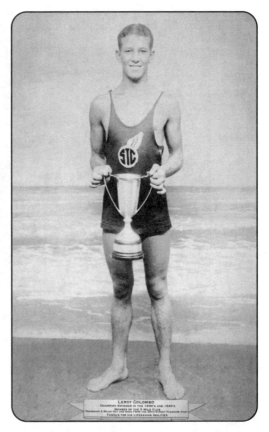

Figure 4–3. Leroy Colombo. Courtesy of Don Mize.

remember numbers, printed words, and pictures less than hearing children, but they do remember better with tasks such as recognizing unfamiliar faces and remembering paths of lights arranged in space (Hamilton, 2011). Deaf children who sign from birth show better memory than hearing children on visuospatial tasks that do not require language. Deaf children use visual imagery in place of verbal codes and spatial coding to remember information (e.g., furniture in a room) compared to hearing nonsigners (Marschark & Waulters, 2011). Figure 4–4 shows a young boy playing an action video game using visual-spatial skills.

Like Leroy, Deaf children use their visual memory to learn language, read and write, and study other school subjects (Hamilton, 2011). As expected, they

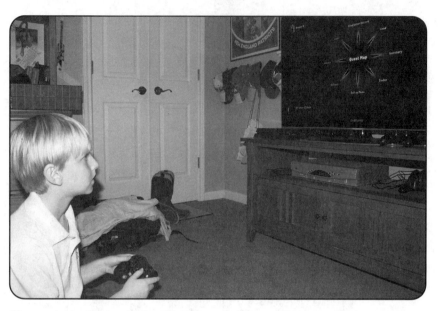

Figure 4–4. A boy playing a video game. Used with permission.

Visual memory and visual learning strategies can help deaf students remember printed words, images, and sign phrases (Hamilton, 2011). While vision may be the primary path for sighted Deaf students, other Deaf students (i.e., Deaf-Blind and DeafDisabled) may use visual, auditory, and tactile-kinesthetic memory skills for learning. As such, when reading print, they may use Braille, large print, raised print, ASL, protactile, Signed English, Tactile Signed English, or a combination of these (Edwards, 2014; Ingraham & Andrews, 2010).

Reasoning

Reasoning abilities such as logical reasoning, numerical and spatial reasoning, critical thinking, empathy, use of analogy for learning, and creativity may be challenging for Deaf students because of lack of early language access, As such, when in the upper grades, Deaf students may find it difficult to understand relationships between cause and effect of events in the learning of math, social studies, and science concepts (Marschark & Wauters, 2003). In a study with 13 Deaf students who were in middle school, researchers found that it was challenging for them to read and figure out word problems that involved a comparison of elements when they had to undertake two or more steps to correctly solve the story problem (Lee & Paul, 2019).

Metacognitive Abilities

Another cognitive ability relates to metacognition or being able to reflect on your own thinking. Both theory of mind (ToM) and executive function (EF) are metacognitive skills that help children make friends and develop relationships. Deaf teachers and peers provide modeling and conversations for deaf children so they can develop EF and ToM skills.

Theory of Mind

ToM is the ability to understand other people's feeling, intentions, and emotions. It focuses on how people get along with others and develop empathy (Siegal, 2008).

> Imagine you are interviewing for a job and tell the librarian about your experiences working in your high school library. You interpret her friendly manner to mean she will offer you the job. The next day you find out she hired someone with more library experience. You are disappointed but understand why the librarian chose the other student. That is an example of empathizing with the librarian's perspective. Can you think of a similar situation when you used your ToM skills?

Mothers' sign language proficiency and their talking to their deaf child about feelings and beliefs were factors that led to increased ToM scores for deaf children (Moeller & Schick, 2006). In another study focusing on 176 Deaf children of Deaf parents, it was found that these Deaf children had ToM skills equal to hearing children (Schick, deVilliers, deVilliers, & Hoffmeister, 2007). Deaf people who learn signing later in life often are not given access to conversations at home where they learn about other people's feelings, wants, and thoughts. Thus, they may not understand the perspectives of others, and these ToM skills may not develop until the teen years or even later (Meeks, 2018).

As ToM is associated with social and emotional development, some DeafBlind students have challenges in developing attachment, empathy, and friendships with peers and siblings. Because this environmental information is missing, some cannot see facial expressions or hear tones in voices to experience the emotions of others. Some DeafBlind individuals with other disabilities such as mood disorders may develop tantrums and aggressive behaviors so they cannot be integrated with other students in the classroom; hence, they will need their own classroom placement (Hartshorne & Schmittel, 2016).

Executive Function

Executive function (EF) refers to skills that you use to get organized, control your behavior to get things done, and problem solve. Similar to ToM, EF skills develop early from conversations with parents about everyday activities. Deaf children who did not have early language access are easily distracted in school, have difficulty completing projects, and may have difficulty with EF skills as well. Deaf children with good EF skills can control their impulses and emotions, are flexible when events don't go their way, can learn from their past mistakes, and can correct their behavior (Hauser, Lukomski, & Hillman, 2008).

EF skills are important for deaf children's schoolwork. During the preschool years, deaf children learn language and play with siblings and peers. In the elementary years, they use their EF to pay attention, apply what they learn to new situations, and control their emotions, impulses, and social behaviors. Later they use metacognitive aspects of EF for planning, reasoning and judgment, reading, and writing (Hauser et al., 2008), for example, in the writing of a term paper. Deaf teachers can provide opportunities for deaf children to learn metacognitive, ToM, and EF skills by having signed conversations with them and using stories from their own personal experiences in solving problems. Here is an example of how a Deaf teacher can support the deaf child's EF development by sharing the child's thoughts and feelings.

> A 5-year-old child used gestures to ask about a bracelet the Deaf teacher was wearing. The teacher told the child how she got the bracelet and used role-playing to show her feelings of joy in finding the bracelet (Singleton & Morgan, 2004, as cited in Hauser et al., 2008, p. 297).

As Singleton and Morgan's vignette shows, by describing everyday events and including a description of one's emotions, Deaf children can learn metacognition, ToM, and EF from Deaf adults. Deaf children who are exposed to a rich language environment in their early years are able to see and understand conversations around them, learn the language's vocabulary and grammar, and can further develop these cognitive abilities with their parents, teachers, and peers.

Since ToM and EF skills need to be learned, DeafDisabled students such as those with CHARGE syndrome or who are DeafBlind, autistic, or DeafBlind combined with autistic may not have had any or enough opportunities to learn these skills. Accordingly, these skills are refined and finally acquired with input from others' reactions and responses, which sighted Deaf and hearing persons are able to see (and hear) in another's gestures, facial expressions, vocal praise, or frustration or displeasure. Such informa-

tion is not fully available to a person with lower vision and hearing levels. Moreover, DeafDisabled individuals may not have been given ample opportunities to regulate their own behaviors and reactions based on others' responses. Hence, they may not be able to solve new problems because others with intact vision and hearing have done this for them. As the result of lack of environmental information and experiences, DeafBlind persons may not recognize a situation as being novel that they can then consider using their previously learned ToM and EF skills. For these DeafBlind students, orientation and mobility exercises are needed so they can be provided with more opportunities to interact with the environment (Belote & Maier, 2014).

Accordingly, you can see how cognitive abilities and language are related and how they interact with each other throughout the child's mental development. Cognitive skills also help build language skills, which then interact with each other to develop even more advanced cognitive and language skills.

LANGUAGE PATHWAYS

For most babies, language learning happens without effort. Language can be acquired through several pathways—the main ones being the ears and the eyes. From birth, hearing babies listen to streams of speech and can identify sounds. They hear word boundaries and learn to segment the sounds as the caregivers sing songs and nursery rhymes. They learn multiple labels or names for favorite toys. A four-legged animal toy can be a cat, dog, horse, or cow.

If the baby has Deaf parents or if the parents are hearing and use ASL, the baby will use the visual-spatial rather than the auditory-vocal modality. Instead of listening to streams of sounds, the baby will view and learn to segment streams of signs and how to identify parts of the signs, such as handshapes, movements, and positions in signed nursery rhymes just as a hearing child learns to recognize different sounds or phonemes in spoken rhymes. This pattern recognition of sounds and signs will reinforce the baby's learning of labels or names for people, objects, and events. In fact, all children have the biological capacity or innate ability to learn language (Chomsky, 1965). And if children gain input in multiple languages, they can become bilingual or even multilingual (Petitto et al., 2016). All this happens by age 4.

Early Gestures, Family Communication, and Play

Language can naturally unfold if the environment is set up so that a spoken, signed, or tactile language can be acquired. You may see a baby at the supermarket, smiling, laughing, and gurgling. Her bright eyes shine, and she may turn her face to look around, waving her hands, grabbing and pointing to objects that she wants. The caregiver smiles down at the child and gives her words or signs to label these objects (Acredolo & Goodwyn, 1994). For hearing children, early gestures turn into spoken words about 1 year of age. With constant support and scaffolding and social interaction (see Vygosky's theory above), the little girl learns words and is well on her way to develop more words, thinking, and social skills. The gestures decrease as she begins to talk. But she may still use gestures to support her spoken language (Volterra & Erting, 1994).

Nathan was born hearing to two Deaf parents who use ASL. At age 1 week, his parents saw Nathan make two natural gestures that appeared to be sign-like (i.e., the fingerspelled handshape for N on the cheek [his name sign] and the sign for LOVE on the chest). His parents knew that Nathan was too young to make these two signs linguistically, but like all new parents, they interpreted these gestures as meaningful communication. These reciprocal exchanges will later develop into linguistic communication. See Figure 4–5 for photos of Nathan and his sign-like gestures.

Both hearing and Deaf babies use gestures, vocalizations, naming of objects, and actions to build communication that assists in their development of language, thinking, and social skills.

For children born Deaf into a hearing family, the learning of signing can happen on a different schedule from early to late childhood, or even not until their teen years or young adulthood (Mayberry, 2007).

Explore the Internet and find out at what age Deaf people typically learn ASL. What do you think you will find?

Hearing families often learn ASL at the same time as their children. Even though they may not be fluent, Deaf children still benefit from their signing. Families can learn ASL at their child's school, at nearby universities, or through the community, or they can subscribe to one of the many apps for ASL instruction (see

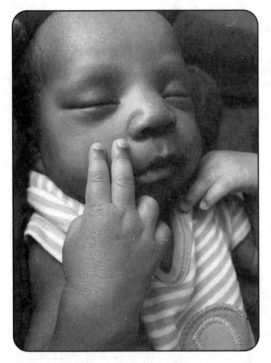
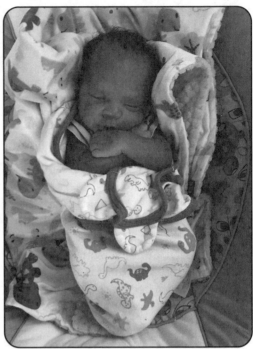

Figure 4–5. Photos of early sign-like gestures of Nathan, a hearing child of Deaf parents.

Chapter 3). Parents who have not fully learned a sign language can still communicate with their deaf children through eye gaze, joint attention, gesturing, and play (Enns & Price, 2013), as well as drawing and writing activities (Andrews, Liu, Liu, Gentry, & Smith, 2017). It is important to keep in mind that parents can bond and start communicating with their child from the first day of life.

As the infant is nurtured, play with caregivers provides the foundation for communication, language, and thinking. In a study of a 4-year-old signing Deaf girl with Deaf parents who was enrolled in a bilingual preschool, the girl's play behaviors were found to be similar to 4-year-old hearing peers. The Deaf girl's play behaviors differed depending on who she was playing with and the kind of play center she was involved in (Musyoka, 2015).

Deaf children with hearing mothers also have similar early play behaviors in the early stages of play, but when symbolic behavior or language becomes important, some Deaf children experience delays (Spencer, 2010). So you see how language is important in the development of play behaviors too. Figure 4–6 shows two sisters playing with their dolls, using their language, thinking, and creativity.

Language Milestones

In this next section, we describe the ASL milestones of culturally Deaf sighted children and the spoken and hearing milestones of sighted hearing children. Accordingly, these milestones represent what research has shown us how language is acquired from birth for these

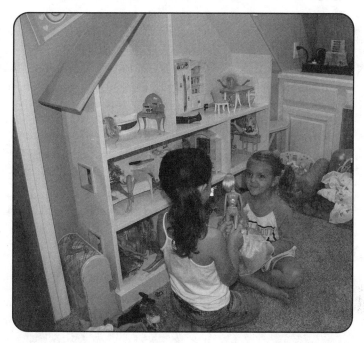

Figure 4–6. Two girls play house with their dolls. Used with permission.

two populations (Table 4–1). As such, the language developmental milestones for Deaf children of hearing families, those from multicultural families, or those who are DeafDisabled have not been fully described in the literature.

Language begins at birth. Caregivers can stimulate language by repeating words and signs, exaggerating them, and speaking and signing slower to make sure their babies understand what they are communicating. The caregivers also make words or signs on their baby's body, on objects, or near food items. As such, caregivers set up *conversational triangles* using space, pointing to a book, toy, or food item while maintaining eye contact with their child as one mother does in a book reading event. See how one father sets up the reading lesson in a similar fashion in this next box (Mather, Rodriguez, Andrews, & Rodriguez, 2006).

A Deaf father sits the child next to him on the couch and signs a picture book about the beach. He physically positions the book and the child and himself so the child can see him. He makes sure his hands are free to sign the story to the child, pausing to point to pictures and making the sign on the book or the child's body. During the storybook reading, he may expand the concept with more signs and fingerspelling and describe the child's background experiences at the beach during the family's summer vacation.

In the early stages of language development, both hearing and Deaf babies babble vocally. Deaf babies stop vocally babbling at age 6 or 7 months if they do

Table 4–1. ASL, Speech, and Hearing Developmental Milestones

Age	ASL (Deaf Children of Deaf Parents)	Speech (Hearing Children of Hearing Parents)	Hearing (Hearing Children of Hearing Parents)
Birth to 1 year	Vocal babbling, manual babbling	Vocal babbling	Eye wide, eye blink, head turn, responses to changes in tone of voice, pays attention to music, plays peek-a-boo, listens when spoken to
1–2 years	Communication gestures, sign handshape errors, baby signs, first signs	Communication gestures, word errors, baby words, first words	Turns to sounds; points to body parts when asked; follows simple commands and understands simple questions; enjoys listening to simple stories, songs, and rhymes; points to pictures in a book when named
2–3 years	Two-sign sentences, correct pronouns, Wh- questions with facial expressions, verb agreement, some classifier handshapes, fingerspelling	Two-word sentences, word parts (articles, pronouns, verbs), conversations, Wh- questions	Turns to sounds; understands difference in meaning of "go/stop," "in/on," "up/down"; follows two requests (e.g., get the book and put it on the table)
3–4 years	Topicalization and conditions, directional verbs, more fingerspelling	Consistent morphemes, irregular forms of verbs, simple sentences	Hears when someone calls from other room; hears TV or radio; understands simple questions asking who, what, when, where, why
4 years and older	Complex sentences, classifiers, more fingerspelling	Complex sentences, grammar development	Pays attention to a short story and answers simple questions about it, hears and understands most of what is said at home and in school

Source: Andrews, Logan, and Phelan (2008).

not hear sounds. They will use fingerbabbling, along with vocal babbling (Petitto & Marentette, 1991). Both produce sounds and handshapes in expected and regular sequences. Hearing babies progress to the one-word stage using a sequence of sounds that resemble words (e.g., baby talk) while deaf babies make a sequence of handshapes that are close to looking like signs (e.g., baby sign). The first spoken words and signs are made alone, but then after the babies acquire about 10 words and signs, they start to combine them into two-word sentences. These early sentences begin to expand as the now toddlers acquire the grammar of their languages. From 2 to 3 years, vocabulary continues to increase and the child begins to use pronouns. The deaf toddler learns more grammar with signs, body movements, and facial expressions. By ages 4 and 5, both deaf and hearing children have learned most of the grammar of their languages and have a vocabulary of about 8,000 signs and/or spoken words and can understand thousands more (Laurent Clerc Center, 2015).

Deaf children who acquire multiple languages, whether tactile, signed, and/ or spoken, will often naturally blend the languages, just like hearing bilingual children who naturally blend their languages. This provides them with an additional resource in learning language. With time and repeated exposure, they learn to separate the two languages with people who do not know both languages. They might continue to blend the languages with people who know both languages (Waddy-Smith, 2012).

Creating an environment where language is fully accessible is key. If parents, caregivers, and teachers open multiple pathways, deaf children can access language from birth onward. As they grow older, their languages develop in tandem.

Many Deaf children enter preschool and kindergarten without a strong foundation in any language. They often do not have the vocabulary and grammar that young children grow up having access to at home and in the community before arriving school. So, when Deaf children arrive at school, they have to learn the languages used at school and the academic information at the same time. Language-deprived deaf children may have difficulty in conversational turn-taking, asking for clarification, or communicating to the teacher what they do not know (Marschark & Wauters, 2003).

Now you can see how language can be developed through spoken language and hearing, as well as through a sign language or a tactile language. We next examine the brain's role in language development.

The Brain, Multilingualism, and Sign Languages

Neuroscientists study how we think, feel, move, remember, imagine, and experience the outside world and our bodies. Our brain, with all of its neural connections, is the hub that controls our thinking, language, literacy, and social skills processing. Neuroscience studies have provided evidence for language functions being represented in both brain hemispheres within complex and evolving neural networks that cover many different parts of the brain and are not just specific to one special region (Rutten, 2017). Neuroscientists have conducted studies in order to examine how spoken, signed, and written languages are processed in the brain

(MacSweeney, Capek, Campbell, & Woll, 2008). They have also studied how multilingualism or using three or more languages affects the structure of the brain as well as increases the brain's capacity for plasticity (Higby, Kim, & Obler, 2013; Jasinska & Petitto, 2013).

> fNIRS, or Functional Near Infrared Spectroscopy, is one of several brain-imaging technologies used to study the neural basis of language in the brain. When the neurons in the brain are active, they use up more oxygen and the blood flow is increased. Blood, rich in oxygen, absorbs light, and these lighted areas can be measured. Using this tool, neuroscientists can study movement during gesture and sign language expression with infants, children, and adults. In Figure 4–7, you can see Dr. Laura-Ann Petitto working in her Brain Language (BL2) neuroscience laboratory at Gallaudet University with her students.

Studies of fNIRS show that both spoken and signed languages stimulate the language centers of the brain. What the brain looks for are language patterns, which can occur through a spoken or a sign language (Petitto et al., 2016). Neuroscientists are also interested in studying bimodal bilingualism (two languages, with one spoken and the other signed). You can easily see that spoken language bilingualism, as in the case of Mexican American children who may know spoken Spanish and spoken English, is different from bimodal bilingualism, which uses two different modalities—signing and speaking. Bimodal bilinguals use different strategies as in the use of code-blends. Code-blend means both languages are blended together to form a communication exchange. In other words, the same information is expressed at the same time with different modalities (Emmorey, Giezen, & Gollan, 2015). In contrast, codeswitching involves the person using one language and then changing or switching to the second language within a sentence, paragraph, or longer segment of discourse.

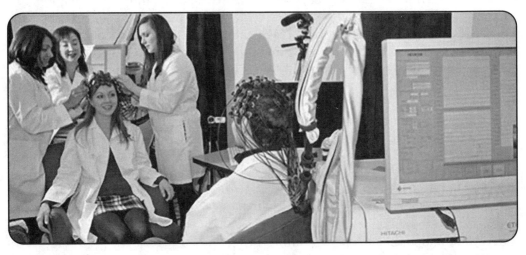

Figure 4–7. Dr. Laura-Ann Petitto, cognitive neuroscientist. Used with permission of Laura-Ann Petitto.

Deaf children of Deaf parents use both code-blending and codeswitching.

Multilingualism is ideal for Deaf babies and children from multicultural homes as they can learn the culture and identity of their families such as Black ASL, LSM, and protactile language, to name a few (see Chapter 3). The best time to receive exposure to multiple languages for children, both Deaf and hearing, is before age 5. Early bilingual or multilingual exposure, even exposure to two languages in different modalities such as speech and sign, can positively affect a person's language, culture, and cognition because it introduces them early to ways of acquiring knowledge, language, and thinking skills (Petitto et al., 2016; Rodriquez, Carrasquillo, & Lee, 2014).

Theories and Strategies

You may have a classmate or friend who speaks two or more languages. Your classmate is bilingual or even multilingual. If you are taking a sign language class, then you are on your way to becoming bilingual and join the nearly 20% or 60 million Americans or 43% of the world population who know two languages (Puerto Rico Report, 2017). In Chapter 3, we learned that the Deaf population is diverse in language and modality learning and may know two or more sign languages, spoken and tactile languages (Canon et al., 2016; Edwards, 2014).

Sign bilingualism and multilingualism is not a new concept. For hundreds of years, Deaf adults have used at least two languages in their daily lives. Since the first school for the deaf was established in 1817, Deaf children have brought their various sign languages (i.e., Native American Indian, Black ASL) into the classroom,

and teachers have been using bilingual practices with sign language and spoken and written language (see Chapter 3).

Since the 1960s, the science of bilingual/multiculturalism has provided deaf education with theories of understanding how children acquire multiple languages. One theoretical model often applied in deaf education is called the linguistic interdependence and threshold theory (LITT) (Cummins, 1981). Basically, it says that there exists in all language learners a common underlying proficiency (CUP) where the learners' first language (L1) can support the learning of their second language (L2). Cummins's LITT has been applied to studies with Deaf students around the world (see reviews in Simms & Andrews, 2020).

More recently, García (2011) proposes a dynamic model of bilingualism. In this model, García proposes that bilingual students don't build one language upon another but have a "unitary linguistic repertoire" in which they can use all of their languages as a resource. This language asset-based perspective takes into account "the total child" with all of the linguistic, cognitive, and social resources that the child brings to language learning. In other words, the languages and modalities are not bounded, but bilinguals use them together in the process of communicating.

When you learn a second or even a third language, you may use a strategy called translanguaging where you use language resources from all of your languages while communicating. If you are Deaf, this enables you to communicate with signers from different countries and languages (De Meulder, Kusters, Moriarty, & Murray, 2019). In the classroom, teachers can use translanguaging to show Deaf students how to use all of their languages as a resource to build on each language (Hoffman, Wolsey, Andrews, & Clark, 2017; Swanwick, 2016; Wolsey, Clark, & Andrews, 2018).

Besides translanguaging, there are many other bilingual and multilingual strategies used by teachers to assist students in learning other languages such as translation and codeswitching, among others. See Table 4–2 for definitions of these strategies.

Testing these bilingual strategies to determine their efficacy within bilingual program has been a challenge because students are often spread geographically across states and regions. Positive outcome data have been shown particularly among Deaf students who are educated using sign language from an early age and who are enrolled in programs that have trained bilingual teachers in sign language and written language methodologies (see Simms & Andrews, 2020, for a summary of these studies). Despite increases in inclusive education (which integrates deaf

Table 4–2. ASL/English Bilingual Strategies: Making Meaning-Based Connections

Strategies and Methods	Definition
Literal translation	Teacher reads a sentence or story then translates into ASL following the exact ideas.
Free translation	Teacher reads the sentence/story and translates into ASL with expansions.
ASL expansion	Uses more than one sign to explain a meaning of a sign or a word.
Chaining	Teacher uses sign, fingerspelling, writing, pictures, and gestures to introduce or emphasize a specific concept or term.
Sandwiching	Sandwiching is similar to using chaining; however, in this case, a purposeful and specific sequence of equivalent meaning using sign, fingerspelling, writing, pictures, and gestures, for example, sign, word, sign or sign, fingerspelling, sign, etc.
Chunking/bridging	Teacher identifies words or groups of words that represent one unit of meaning or one sign in ASL and following a discussion of appropriate translation.
Preview-view-review (PVR)	Summary of lesson presented in ASL, reading the lesson in English, followed by discussion in ASL.
Codeswitching	Teacher uses one language, then switches to another language.
ASL summary	The teacher signs a summary of a story. Then children read the print version of the story, then discuss.
Translanguaging	Teacher provides lesson in ASL, then student responds using English or vice versa.

Sources: Andrews and Rusher (2010); Ausbrooks-Rusher, Schimmel, and Edwards (2012); Gárate (2012).

children into hearing schools, with mostly monolingual students and teachers), along with the increases in cochlear implantation in the United States, and the decrease of some bilingual education programs, as a methodology, bilingualism is embraced internationally in Europe as well as in Asia (Knoors, Brons, & Marschark, 2019), with experiments in residential and coenrollment settings providing new information about positive outcomes.

LITERACY LEARNING

Importance

Reading and writing, in other words, literacy, takes on added importance for deaf people, particularly when communicating with hearing persons who do not know sign language. Smartphones are widely used by Deaf individuals for texting back and forth and have become important tools for Deaf individuals to navigate in the hearing world. The United States is heavily reliant on English in all forms of communication (e.g., school curriculum, news, traffic signs, rental agreements), so adults in the United States are exposed to different forms of English literacy every day.

Developmental Pathways

Compared to hearing children, it takes deaf children 3 or 4 years longer to learn to read because of lack of early language exposure (Hoffmeister & Caldwell-Harris, 2014). It has been often cited that Deaf students graduate from high school with an average fourth-grade reading level (Traxler, 2000). What these figures indicate is that the deaf education field has taken a deficit model approach to reporting low reading scores. The real culprit that prevents English learning is lack of early language access. Not only that, it is also statistically problematic to compare language-deprived bilinguals with privileged English monolinguals in the same data pool with a test designed for hearing English monolinguals. Can you imagine having the questions on the test signed in ASL? The majority of English monolinguals would fail. As a result, the deficit model would claim that English monolinguals graduate from high school with an average first-grade ASL level!

For all children, early home experiences related to emergent and early reading development include being read to, looking at books, turning pages and "pretend" reading of storybooks, having conversations with parents about books, reading print on signs and food vocabulary, drawing, scribbling, and writing (Andrews et al., 2017). Reading requires children to use their background and world knowledge, schema, and English structure knowledge to understand print. This is called reading comprehension. At another level, reading involves children learning vocabulary. They learn how to segment words into sounds (phonemic awareness) and then map their spoken language onto print in order to "crack the code" or learn the "alphabetic principle." This process leads them to understand the grapheme (letter) to phoneme (sound) connection. After they do this, they can read or decode any new print words that they already know in their language.

But what happens when children are Deaf? How do they learn to read? In bilingual classrooms where they have exposure to both ASL and English, deaf children are learning to read (Hoffmeister & Caldwell-Harris, 2014). Other Deaf children with residual hearing are learning to read using auditory techniques coupled with signing strategies through bilingual-bimodal methodologies (see Chapter 5). As we learn more about in the next chapter (Chapter 5), children who are DeafDisabled will learn to read and write using different methodologies and strategies than sighted Deaf students. Depending on the levels of their sensory strengths and needs, teachers will use a variety of strategies and tools including sign, spoken, and tactile languages, including braille, raised print, and enlarged print on computer screens (Ingraham & Andrews, 2010).

Two different models—the deficit and the asset models—have been proposed for Deaf students learning to read (see Andrews et al., 2017, for summary of these frameworks).

Deficit Models

In general, despite early language learning differences in access, modality, and sensory strengths and needs, some researchers follow a deficit model approach in understanding how Deaf children learn to read. They propose that learning to read for the Deaf child is the same as it is for hearing children. This means that if a deaf child receives a cochlear implant or hearing aids and goes through intensive training using oral/aural methods that include speechreading and articulation with phonologic awareness activities, then reading skills can develop similar to hearing children (Cupples, Ching, Crowe, Day, & Seeto, 2014). Another practice following the deficit model is to test deaf children in their understanding of English auditory phonology, semantics, and syntax and then design reading strategies based on their deficiencies in English (Easterbrooks et al., 2015). Alternative frameworks fol-

low an asset model. These frameworks propose that print literacy can be built upon the students' existing sign language, including fingerspelling (see Andrews et al., 2017).

Asset Model

Instead of focusing on the auditory sound system of English as hearing children do, sign-print frameworks indicate that deaf children recognize patterns in signs and print at the sign level as well as at the discourse or story level (Hoffmeister & Caldwell-Harris, 2014). This process allows deaf children to develop ASL vocabulary to bridge to English words and learn to segment printed letters when reading words. With the development of sign language phonological awareness or sign phonology, the deaf child can utilize the structure of signs and signed sentences, fingerspelling, and the orthographic patterns of letters (Pettito et al., 2016). In turn, deaf children can map these phonological units onto English print during early reading learning, particularly when learning alphabetic writing and letter shape recognition (Allen, 2015). Pattern recognition of the smallest units of language is a skill all language learners must acquire, regardless of modality. Some sounds are accessed visually (e.g., speechreading, visual phonics, cued speech, or print) or accessed through touch (e.g., protactile, tactile fingerspelling).

These frameworks presented here do not suggest deaf children will never need the sound system or phonology of English to further develop reading skills. Some skilled deaf readers use phonological coding to read. It may be that deaf readers could use these phonologic codes after they have already developed some basic English reading skills (Freel et al., 2011). Some teachers even blend these approaches as described in the following box.

Jackie is a sixth-grade teacher in a public school classroom that uses a Total Communication philosophy. She is fluent in ASL. Jackie uses spoken English, visual phonics, sign-supported speech, fingerspelling, codeswitching, chaining, and other signs to print matching strategies to teach word recognition to her deaf students. She frequently has her students read aloud or sign novels from their iPads using their preferred language. When she changes to spoken language with some students, she also will use a sign language interpreter to assist signing Deaf students in group work. She frequently directs the class to the SmartBoard where she downloads ASL and English bilingual reading programs to provide additional ASL signing models.

In using a bilingual and multilingual approach to literacy instruction, it is easy to see that sign languages are not the same as their spoken and print counterparts. Nonetheless, connecting signs with printed words, signs with spoken words using hearing aids and cochlear implant technology, and signs with visual and tactile aids (e.g., pictures, movies, tactile graphics, drawings, photos, 3-D printing) is a strategy that is practiced and seen worldwide in 15 countries or regions using 14 sign languages and 12 different spoken languages (Wang & Andrews, 2020). Future studies are needed to move past deficit models. Instead, studies are

needed that document Deaf students and DeafDisabled students *in the act of reading* while using all of their language resources to build more effective literacy strategies. As emphasized throughout this chapter and book, it is important to remember that each Deaf child is unique and will vary on the use of spoken, signed, visual, and auditory technologies throughout the life spans, and this impacts the learning of literacy. See Allie's case in the box below and her photo in Figure 4–8.

Allie was born profoundly deaf and received a cochlear implant at 2 years of age. She considers herself an ASL and English bilingual user. She uses speechreading and her cochlear implant when talking with her hearing teachers and friends. Sometimes she uses sign-supported speech, and other times, she uses ASL. Her parents learned ASL when she was a toddler. Allie attended a public school with a sign language interpreter. Her parents read to her at home, bought books for her, and frequently took her to the library. She uses captioned TV at home and chats with her deaf friends frequently on the videophone. She now attends a hearing university and is studying to become an ASL teacher for hearing students in public schools.

CONCLUSIONS

Throughout this chapter, we see that, in many ways, both Deaf and hearing individuals learn to think, learn, and read in both similar and different fashions than

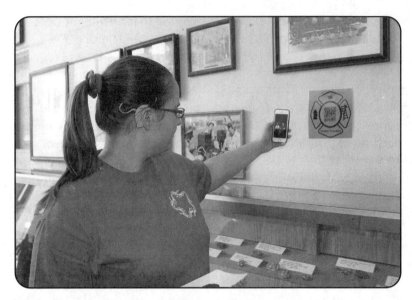

Figure 4–8. Allie using a QR code scanner and her smartphone to download information provided in ASL and spoken and written English at the Beaumont Fire Museum to enjoy the displays. Used with permission.

hearing students. Deaf students may have different life experiences at home and school with the added resources of a sign language, Deaf culture, and auditory, tactile, and visual technologies. The key to remember is that parents, educators, and professionals must provide Deaf individuals, including those who are DeafDisabled, with early access to communication and language. When such access is provided in the home, school, and community, thinking, learning, and literacy can be taught utilizing the Deaf individual's sensory strengths and needs. These skills help develop and reinforce the Deaf child's learning potential, which they can use to succeed in school.

REFERENCES

Acredolo, L., & Goodwyn, D. (1994). Sign language among hearing infants: The sponta-neous development of symbolic gestures. In V. Volterra & C. Erting (Eds.), *From gesture to language in hearing children*. Washington, DC: Gallaudet University Press.

Adkins, A., Sewell, D., & Cleveland, J. (2016). *The development of tactile skills*. Austin: TX Sense Abilities: TSBVI Outreach, Texas School for the Blind and Visually Impaired.

Allen, T. (2015). ASL skills, fingerspelling ability, home communication context and early alphabetic knowledge of preschool deaf children. *Sign Language Studies, 15*, 233–265.

Andrews, J. (2010). Leroy Colombo: The deaf lifeguard of Galveston Island, Part 1: The early years (1905–1943). *East Texas Historical Journal, XLVIII*, 85–109.

Andrews, J. (2011). Leroy Colombo: The deaf lifeguard of Galveston Island, Part II: (1943–1974). *East Texas Historical Journal, XLIX*, 9–33.

Andrews, J., Liu, H., Liu, C., Gentry, M., & Smith, Z. (2017). "Adapted little books": A shared book intervention for signing deaf children using ASL and English. *Early Child Development and Care, 187*(3–4), 583–599.

Andrews, J. F., & Baker, S. (2019). ASL nursery rhymes: Exploring a support for early language and emergent literacy skills for signing deaf children. *Sign Language Studies*, *20*(1), 5-40.

Andrews, J. F., Hamilton, B., Dunn, K. M., & Clark, M. D. (2016). Early reading for young deaf and hard of hearing children: Alternative frameworks. *Psychology*, *7*(4), 510–522.

Belote, M., & Maier, J. (2014). Why deaf-blindness and autism can look so much alike. California Deaf-Blind Services. *ReSources*, *19*(2), 1–16.

Bruce, S. M., & Parker, A. T. (2012). Young deaf-blind adults in action: Becoming self-determined change agents through advocacy. *American Annals of the Deaf*, *157*(1), 16–26.

Burch, S., & Joyner, H. (2007). *Unspeakable: The story of Junius Wilson*. Chapel Hill: University of North Carolina Press.

Burke, M. L. (2014). *Ableism in the Deaf community and the field of Deaf studies: Through the eyes of a DeafDisabled person* (MA thesis). Gallaudet University, Washington, DC.

Cannon, J. E., Guardino, C., & Gallimore, E. (2016). A new kind of heterogeneity: What we can learn from d/Deaf and hard of hearing multilingual learners. *American Annals of the Deaf*, *161*(1), 8–16.

Chomsky, N. (1965). *Aspects of syntax*. Cambridge, MA: MIT Press.

Christensen, K. (2017). *Education deaf students in a multicultural world*. San Diego, CA: DawnSignPress.

Clark, M., Galloza-Carrero, A., Keith, C., Tibbitt, J., Wolsey, J., & Zimmerman, H. (2015). Learning to look-and-looking to learn. *Advance for Speech & Hearing*. Retrieved from http://speech-language-pathology-audiology.advanceweb.com/Features/Articles/Eye-Gaze-Development-in-Infants.aspx

Cummins, J. (1981). The role of primary language development in promoting educational success for language minority students. In California State Department of Education (Ed.), *Schooling and language minority students: A theoretical framework*. Los Angeles: California State Department of Education.

Cupples, L., Ching, T., Crowe, K., Day, J., & Seeto, M. (2014). Predictors of early reading skill in 5-year-old children with hearing loss who use spoken language. *Reading Research Quarterly*, *49*, 85–104.

De Meulder, M., Kusters, A., Moriarty, E., & Murray, J. (2019) "Describe, don't prescribe. The practice and politics of translanguaging in the context of deaf signers." *Journal of Multilingual and Multicultural Development*, *17*(6), 485–496.

Dye, M., Hauser, P., & Bavelier, D. (2008). Visual attention in deaf children and adults. In M. Marschark & P. Hauser (Eds.), *Deaf cognition: Foundations and outcomes* (pp. 250–263). New York, NY: Oxford University Press.

Dye, M. W., & Bavelier, D. (2010). Differential development of visual attention skills in school-age children. *Vision Research*, *50*(4), 452–459.

Easterbrooks, S. R., Lederberg, A. R., Antia, S., Schick, B., Kushalnagar, P., Webb, M. Y., . . . Connor, C. M. (2015). Reading among diverse DHH learners: What, how, and for whom? *American Annals of the Deaf*, *159*(5), 419–432.

Edwards, T. (2014). *Language emergence in the Seattle DeafBlind community* (Unpublished doctoral dissertation). University of California, Berkeley.

Emmorey, K., Giezen, M. R., & Gollan, T. H. (2015). Psycholinguistic, cognitive, and neural implications of bimodal bilingualism. *Bilingualism: Language and Cognition*, *19*(2), 223–242.

Enns, C., & Price, L. (2013). *Family involvement in ASL acquisition* (Research Brief No. 9). Visual Language and Learning Science of Learning Center. Washington, DC: Gallaudet University Press.

Freel, B. L., Clark, M. D., Anderson, M. L., Gilbert, G. L., Musyoka, M. M., & Hauser, P. C. (2011). Deaf individuals' bilingual abilities: American Sign Language proficiency, reading skills, and family characteristics. *Psychology*, *2*(1), 18–23.

García, O. (2011). *Bilingual education in the 21st century: A global perspective*. New York, NY: John Wiley.

Gleitman, L., & Papafragou, A. (2005). Language and thought. In K. Holyoak & R. Morrison (Eds.), *Cambridge handbook of thinking and reasoning* (2nd ed., pp. 663–661). New York, NY: Cambridge University Press.

Goldin-Meadow, S. (2003). *The resilience of language: What gesture creation in deaf children can tell us about how all children learn.* New York, NY: Psychology Press.

Gruskin, D. (2003). A dual identity for hard of hearing students. *Odyssey, 4*(2), 30–35.

Hall, W. (2017). What you don't know can hurt you: The risk of language deprivation by impairing sign language development in deaf children. *Maternal Child Health Journal, 21*(5), 961–965.

Hall, W. C., Smith, S. R., Sutter, E. J., DeWindt, L. A., & Dye, T. D. (2018). Considering parental hearing status as a social determinant of deaf population health: Insights from experiences of the "dinner table syndrome." *PLoS One, 13*(9), e0202169.

Hamilton, H. (2011). Memory skills of deaf learners: Implications and applications. *American Annals of the Deaf, 156*, 402–423.

Hartshorne, T. S., & Schmittel, M. C. (2016). Social-emotional development in children and youth who are deafblind. *American Annals of the Deaf, 161*(4), 444–453.

Hauser, P., Lukomski, J., & Hillman, T. (2008). Development of deaf and hard-of-hearing students' executive function. In M. Marschark & P. Hauser (Eds.), *Deaf cognition: Foundations and outcomes* (pp. 286–308). New York, NY: Oxford University Press.

Higby, E., Kim, J., & Obler, L. K. (2013). Multilingualism and the brain. *Annual Review of Applied Linguistics, 33*, 68–101.

Hirshorn, E. (2011). *Visual attention and learning* (Research Brief No. 3). Visual Language and Visual Learning Science of Learning. Washington, DC: Gallaudet University.

Hoffman, D., Wolsey, J., Andrews, J., & Clark, D. (2017). Translanguaging supports reading with deaf adult bilinguals: A qualitative approach. *The Qualitative Report, 22*(7), 1925–1944.

Hoffmeister, R., & Caldwell-Harris, C. (2014). Acquiring English as a second language via print: The task for deaf children. *Cognition, 132*, 229–242.

Ingraham, C., & Andrews, J. (2010). The hands and reading: What DeafBlind adult readers tell us. *British Journal of Visual Impairment, 28*(2), 130–138.

Jasinska, K. K., & Petitto, L. A. (2013). How age of bilingual exposure can change the neural systems for language in the developing brain: A functional near infrared spectroscopy investigation of syntactic processing in monolingual and bilingual children. *Developmental Cognitive Neuroscience, 6*, 87–101.

Knoors, H., Brons, M., & Marschark, M. (2019). *Deaf education beyond the Western world: Context, challenges, and prospects.* New York, NY: Oxford University Press.

Knoors, H., & Vervloed, M. P. (2003). Educational programming for deaf children with multiple disabilities: Accommodating special needs. In M. Marschark & P. Spencer (Eds.). *Oxford Handbook of Deaf Studies, Language, and Education* (pp. 82–94). New York: Oxford University Press.

Kuntze, L., Golos, D., & Enns, C. (2014). Rethinking literacy: Broadening opportunities for visual learners. *Sign Language Studies, 14*, 213–224.

Laurent Clerc Center. (2015). *Setting Language in Motion: Family Supports and Early Intervention for Babies Who are Deaf or Hard of Hearing.* Retrieved from http://clerccenter.gallaudet.edu

Lee, C., & Paul, P. V. (2019). Deaf middle school students' comprehension of relational language in arithmetic compare problems. *Human: Journal for Interdisciplinary Studies, 9*(1), 4–23.

MacSweeney, M., Capek, C., Campbell, R., & Woll, B. (2008). The signing brain: The neurobiology of sign language. *Trends in Cognitive Sciences, 12*, 432–440.

Maller, S., & Braden, J. (2011). Intellectual assessment of deaf people: A critical review of core concepts. In M. Marschark & P. Spencer (Eds.), *Oxford handbook of deaf studies, language and education* (Vol. 2, pp. 473–485). New York, NY: Oxford University Press.

Marschark, M. (2003). Interactions of language and cognition in deaf learners: From research to practice. *International Journal of Audiology, 42*(Suppl. 1), S41–S48.

Marschark, M., & Hauser, P. (2008). *Deaf cognition: Foundations and outcomes*. New York, NY: Oxford University Press.

Marschark, M., Lang, H. G., & Albertini, J. A. (2001). *Educating deaf students: From research to practice*. New York, NY: Oxford University Press.

Marschark, M., Spencer, L. J., Durkin, A., Borgna, G., Convertino, C., Machmer, E., . . . Trani, A. (2015). Understanding language, hearing status, and visual-spatial skills. *Journal of Deaf Studies and Deaf Education, 20*, 310–330.

Marschark, M., & Wauters, L. (2003). Cognitive functioning in deaf adults and children. In M. Marschark & P. Spender (Eds.), *Oxford handbook of deaf studies, language and education* (Vol. 1, pp. 486–499). New York, NY: Oxford University Press.

Mather, S., Rodriguez, Y., Andrews, J., & Rodriguez, J. (2006). Sight triangles: Conversations of deaf parents and hearing toddlers in Puerto Rico. In C. Lucas (Ed.), *Multilingualism and sign languages from the Great Plains to Australia* (Vol. 12, pp. 159–187). Washington, DC: Gallaudet University Press.

Mayberry, R. I. (2007). When timing is everything: Age of first-language acquisition effects on second-language learning. *Applied Psycholinguistics, 28*, 537–549.

Meeks, D. (2018). *Experiences of family dinner conversations in the lives of deaf adults* (Unpublished doctoral dissertation). Lamar University, Beaumont, TX.

Moeller, M., & Schick, B. (2006). Relations between maternal input and theory of mind understanding in deaf children. *Child Development, 77*, 751–766.

Moores, D. (2001). *Educating the deaf: Psychology, principles and practices* (5th ed.). Boston, MA: Houghton Mifflin.

Musyoka, M. (2015). Understanding indoor play in deaf children: An analysis of play behaviors. *Psychology, 6*, 10–19.

Ocuto, O. (2019). *Chasing the why: Understanding the deaf child's home language environment* (Unpublished doctoral dissertation). Lamar University, Beaumont, TX.

Petitto, L. A., Langdon, C., Stone, A., Andriola, D., Kartheiser, G., & Cochran, C. (2016). Visual sign phonology: Insights into human reading and language from a natural soundless phonology. *Wiley Interdisciplinary Reviews: Cognitive Science, 7*(6), 366–381.

Petitto, L.-A. & Marentette, P. (1991). Babbling in the manual mode: Evidence for the ontogeny of language, *Science, 251*, 1493–1496.

Pinker, S. (2007). *The stuff of thought: Language as a window into human nature*. New York, NY: Penguin.

Puerto Rico Report. (2017). *Bilingual America*. Retrieved from https://www.puertorico report.com/bilingual-america/#.XVG7x lB7mRs

Rodriguez, D., Carrasquillo, A., & Lee, K. (2014). *The bilingual advantage: Promoting academic development, biliteracy, and native language in the classroom*. New York, NY: Teachers College Press.

Rutten, G. J. (2017). *The Broca-Wernicke Doctrine: A historical and clinical perspective on localization of language functions*. New York, NY: Springer.

Schaller, S. (1991). *A man without words*. Berkeley: University of California Press.

Schick, B., deVilliers, P., deVilliers, J., & Hoffmeister, R. (2007). Language and the theory of mind: A study of deaf children. *Child Development, 78*, 376–396.

Siegal, M. (2008). *Marvelous minds: The discovery of what children know*. New York, NY: Oxford University Press.

Simms, L., Rusher, M., Andrews, J., & Coryell, J. (2008). Apartheid in deaf education: Examining workforce diversity. *American Annals of the Deaf, 153*(4), 384–395.

Simms, L. E., & Andrews, J. F. (2020). Using L1 ASL to teach reading. In R. Rosen (Ed.),

Routledge handbook of ASL teaching (pp. 59–72). New York, NY: Routledge.

Spencer, P. (2010). Play and theory of mind: Indicators and engines of early cognitive growth. In M. Marschark & P. Spencer (Eds.), *Oxford handbook of deaf studies, language, and education* (Vol. 2, pp. 407–436). New York, NY: Oxford University Press.

Sternberg, R. J., & Grigorenko, E. L. (2004). Intelligence and culture: how culture shapes what intelligence means, and the implications for a science of well-being. *Philosophical Transactions of the Royal Society of London, Series B: Biological Sciences, 359*(1449), 1427–1434.

Swanwick, R. (2016). *Languages and languaging in deaf education: A framework for pedagogy.* New York, NY: Oxford University Press.

Traxler, C. (2000). The Stanford Achievement Test, 9th edition: National norming and performance standards for deaf and hard of hearing students. *Journal of Deaf Studies and Deaf Education, 5*, 337–348.

Vernon, M. (2005). Fifty years of research on the intelligence of deaf and hard-of-hearing children: A review of literature and discussion of implications. *Journal of Deaf Studies and Deaf Education, 10*, 225–231.

Vernon, M., & Andrews, J. (1990). *The psychology of deaf people: Understanding deaf and hard of hearing people.* Boston, MA: Allyn & Bacon.

Vernon, M., & Leigh, I. (2007). Mental health services for people who are deaf. *American Annals of the Deaf, 152*, 374–381.

Volterra, V., & Erting, C. (1994). *From gesture to language in hearing and deaf children.* Washington, DC: Gallaudet University Press.

Vygotsky, L. S. (1980). *Mind in society: The development of higher psychological processes.* Cambridge, MA: Harvard University Press.

Waddy-Smith, B. (2012). Students who are deaf and hard of hearing and use sign language: Considerations and strategies for developing spoken language and literacy skills. *Seminar in Speech and Language, 33*, 310–321.

Wang, Q., & Andrews, J. F. (2020). *Multiple paths to become literate: International perspectives in Deaf education.* Washington, DC: Gallaudet University Press.

Wolsey, J. L. A., Clark, M. D., & Andrews, J. F. (2018). ASL and English bilingual shared book reading: An exploratory intervention for signing deaf children. *Bilingual Research Journal, 41*(3), 221–237.

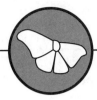

CHAPTER 5

Deaf Education, Deaf Culture, and Multiculturalism

When learning their child is deaf, hearing parents may not understand what the child's experience may be like, having never met a Deaf person. They may ask, "How will my child learn to communicate? Will my child learn to read and write? Will my child go to college?" These are some questions families ask when finding out their child is deaf.

The education of Deaf students can be impacted by many factors that influence learning and teaching. Moreover, numbers of Deaf students from multicultural and multilingual races and/or ethnicities, including DeafDisabled students, have increased in the school system, thus adding even more learner factors to consider (Cannon, Guardino, & Gallimore, 2016). Accordingly, these students are frequently underidentified and underserved, particularly those living in poverty, immigrant and refugee populations, LGBT (lesbian, gay, bisexual, and transgender) students, and DeafDisabled individuals (Burke, 2014; Christensen, 2017). We use Deaf multicultural persons as an inclusive term that refers to Deaf individuals from different heritages: Latinx,

Black (e.g., AfroLatinx, Blasian), African American, Asian/Pacific Islanders, North American Indian, and persons of multiple races and ethnic backgrounds. We use the term DeafDisabled to refer to individuals who may have cognitive, social, or sensory/physical disabilities in addition to being Deaf (Burke, 2014). In this chapter, we examine learner factors in deaf education related to Deaf culture and multiculturalism and point out disruptive dynamics as institutional and individual racism, sexism, linguicism, and audism (Christensen, 2017; Simms, Rusher, Andrews, & Coryell, 2008).

DEAF CULTURE AND MULTICULTURALISM

The field of Deaf education has historically ignored the input of the Deaf community, including Deaf multicultural individuals as well as their organizations such as the National Association of the Deaf (NAD). In this chapter and throughout this book, we view Deaf culture and multiculturalism as the cornerstone of deaf education. As such, it undergirds communication and language approaches, curriculum, pedagogy, and assessment as it includes Deaf multicultural aspects of learning (Christensen, 2017). Deaf adults are often underrepresented in teaching positions in early childhood through postsecondary programs, including at universities (O'Brien, Kuntze, & Appanah, 2015; Simms et al., 2008; Smith & Andrews, 2015), and this includes those Deaf professionals from multicultural backgrounds (Simms et al., 2008). Across this background, we discuss learning factors that impact the education of Deaf students.

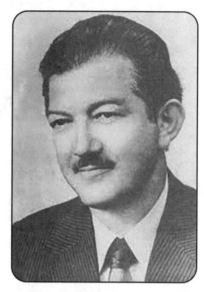

Figure 5–1. Fred Schreiber, leader and advocate for Deaf people, rebuilt the National Association for the Deaf and founded the NAD Broadcaster. Used with permission of the National Association of the Deaf.

Fred Schreiber, former Executive Director of the National Association, said, "The basic reason for becoming involved with deaf adults; we are your children grown. We can, in many instances, tell you the things your child would like to tell you, if he had the vocabulary and the experiences to put his feelings and needs into words" (Schreiber, 1980, as cited in Schein, 1981). Figure 5–1 shows a photo of Fred Schreiber.

FACTORS IMPACTING SCHOOLING

Age of Onset and Parental Hearing Status

The age of onset when a child becomes Deaf and the age of onset of additional disabilities are learner characteristics that affect type of schooling (Bruce & Borders, 2015). Accordingly, if children are born deaf (congenital) or become deaf before the age of 2, they will benefit from a strong visual language foundation. On the other hand, children who become deaf at a later age, at 5 or 6 years old, may need to recover what language they lost through speechreading instruction and auditory training (Leigh & Andrews, 2017). Those who are born with additional disabilities or are DeafDisabled individuals have communication and educational needs that are significantly different from those who acquire these disabilities in later childhood or adolescence. One such example are congenitally DeafBlind children, who will need a different communication approach and educational plan, compared to Deaf youth with Usher syndrome, who are born Deaf and learned sign language after having lost their vision later in life (Damen, Janssen, Ruijssenaars, & Schuengel, 2015). Throughout this chapter, we highlight these learning differences of DeafDisabled students.

Another learner characteristic that affects communication and schooling is parental hearing status. In this regard, about 5% of deaf children are born with

Deaf parents (Mitchell & Karchmer, 2004). These children will thrive in ASL and English bilingual school environments because of early access to both languages. The other 95% of Deaf children from hearing families may struggle with language access. At school, they may experience a variety of types of communication approaches from ASL to the Total Communication (TC) philosophy to manual codes of English (MCE) (i.e., simultaneous communication). Many of these Deaf children from hearing families are typically expected to learn both a sign language and English. And some come from homes where another signed language and/or spoken languages other than English are used, as the next section shows (Cannon et al., 2016).

Multilingualism, Multiculturalism, and Schooling

Studies show that Deaf multilingual and multicultural learners for whom neither English nor ASL is their home language are the fastest-growing groups in schools, making up 19.4% to 35% of the U.S. deaf population (Gallaudet Research Institute [GRI], 2013). After English, Spanish is the most commonly used home language, with about 19% of deaf children coming from Spanish-speaking homes (GRI, 2013). Deaf students can also come from homes where Black English is spoken and Black ASL is signed (see Chapter 3). But diversity does not stop here. Accordingly, within these ethnic groups, there is more diversity. Some Deaf Latinx students are first-generation immigrants while others are native-born citizens. Some may use spoken Spanish with hearing family members, but with their Deaf friends, they may use LSM or ASL (Baker & Scott, 2016). Other Deaf students from Asia

bring a diversity of languages and dialects, many of which are tonal languages that use pitch to signal a difference in meanings between words, which can be difficult to acquire for Deaf learners as well (Cheng & Maroonroge, 2017; Wang, Andrews, Liu, & Liu, 2016). And students from Indigenous peoples may bring any one of three tribal signed languages from the Plains Indian Sign Language region (PISL) such as Northern Cheyenne, Crow, and Kiowa (McKay-Cody, 2019). And still another example is a Deaf child who immigrated to Canada from Italy and knows Lingua dei Segni Italiana (LIS or Italian Sign Language) and spoken Italian and learns ASL and English at school (Cannon et al., 2016).

In a sample of 23,731 deaf children whose schools participated in the GRI (2013) survey, Deaf students of color made up 45.9%, of whom 28.4% were Hispanic, Latino, or Spanish origin; 15.7% Black or African American; 4.4% Asian; 1.2% American Indian or Alaskan Native; 0.6% Native Hawaiian or Pacific Islander; 2.6% other; and 0.6% unknown or cannot report.

Families from multilingual and multicultural racial and/or ethnic backgrounds have their own national language, culture, religious heritages, and beliefs, including stereotypical attitudes, which impact Deaf learners. Some multicultural families harbor myths about disabilities, and this may affect if and when they access services. Given that some view a disability as a punishment from God or is caused by evil spirits or the result of the misdeeds of ancestors, they may seek a faith healer or go on religious pilgrimages to sacred places to find a "cure" for the child rather than seek professional advice (Cheng & Maroonroge, 2017; Steinberg et al., 1997). Some in the extended family and community may stigmatize a Deaf child, causing further stress in making educational decisions. Intercultural communication may be a barrier too. In view of the foregoing, while Deaf persons use facial expressions and large gestures, in many Asian cultures, it is considered inappropriate to be overly demonstrative. As a result of this conflict, communication may be disrupted (Holcomb, Love, Nakahara, & Ostrove, 2017).

Lesbian, Gay, Bisexual, and Transgender (LGBT) Deaf Students

Another factor that may affect schooling for Deaf teens is related to gender and sexual orientation. In this regard, LGBT students represent the intersection of two oppressed minorities—being Deaf and having LGBT status. Along those lines, research shows that Deaf LGBT students at the high school and postsecondary level are vulnerable to psychological and emotional stress brought on by not only having the personal struggle of understanding their own sexual feelings but also experiencing parental rejection. At school, some become victims of physical and emotional mistreatment. As a result of this bullying, they are vulnerable to lower self-esteem, depression, negative perceptions of school climate, lower grades, and school absences, among other negative outcomes (Denniger, 2017).

DeafDisabled Students

For education purposes, the term Deaf-Disabled refers to Deaf individuals with one or more disabilities (Burke, 2014).

These can be academic/cognitive disabilities such as intellectual disabilities (IDs), including Down syndrome, attention-deficit disorder (ADD), and attention-deficit/hyperactivity disorder (ADHD). They also can have social disabilities, which include autism spectrum disorders (ASDs), emotional/behavioral disturbances (EDs) including mood disorders, depression, and so on. Finally, they can have physical/sensory disabilities, including cerebral palsy, orthopedic impairments, blindness, and low vision, as well as syndromes (i.e., CHARGE, Treacher-Collins, Waardenburg, Usher syndrome) (Wright, 2016) (see Chapter 2).

One DeafBlind community in Seattle, Washington, are primarily those who were born Deaf and lost their vision later in life from Usher syndrome. DeafBlind persons with an Usher syndrome etiology have their own culture and use a protactile language to communicate and socialize (Edwards, 2014).

The background characteristics of Individuals who exhibit each of these disabilities (or combinations of them) may vary widely on their levels of hearing, and cognitive and social functioning. Accordingly, such differences characteristics may warrant alternative communication approaches, school placement, and accommodation within the deaf education system (Cannon et al., 2016). More often than not, the deaf education system is not accessible and does not incorporate elements of universal design (UD). UD refers to the design of a setting so that it can be accessed, understood, and utilized by the largest number of individuals regardless of their age, size, ability, or disability. Related to deaf students, UD refers to providing a visual environment utilizing accommodations that include DeafSpace, Deaf teachers, and signed languages to be provided in the educational environment (Supalla, Small, & Cripps, 2013).

With this in mind, it is useful to look at demographics of this population as this affects the curriculum, evaluations, and teaching strategies established in the schools. In this regard, it has been estimated that 40% to 50% of deaf students have disabilities that can impact learning (GRI, 2013). Ranging from mild to severe, the effects of multiple disabilities interact and compound, thus creating complex secondary consequences. As a result, these Deaf learners' communication and educational needs become varied and complex (see Paul, 2015, for discussion). For example, a child with Down syndrome, a genetic cause of ID, may have a mild conductive hearing loss but can learn to talk, read, and write. A Deaf child with cerebral palsy may need more time to express herself in sign language (Burke, 2014) but can succeed with an academic curriculum. A child born Deaf who develops Usher syndrome at age 13 will have a different educational plan, including bilingualism with protactile signing (see Chapter 3).

In a sample of 23,731 deaf children enrolled in special education programs (GRI, 2013), the following programs reported 8.8% intellectual disabilities; 7.2% learning disability; 5.4% ADD/ADHD; 6.4% low vision, deafblindness, and Usher syndrome; 6.0% developmental delay; 4.1% orthopedic impairment; 2.1% emotional disturbance; 2.2% autism; 0.4% traumatic brain injury; and 14.0% other conditions and health impairments, with 12.7% not reported, for a total of 38.9% deaf with additional disabilities.

And a child born Deaf and blind with ID and autism may experience developmental differences across all domains of learning and will need still another plan that centers on functional life skills (Bruce & Borders, 2015).

COMMUNICATION AND LANGUAGE APPROACHES

History of Deaf Education

Learner factors described above drive the communication and language approaches used in deaf education with Deaf students. Accordingly, these approaches can best be understood within the context of the history deaf education. In Chapter 3, we traced the beginnings of the use of signing and English in classrooms for Deaf students during the timeframe from the 1817 setting up of the first school in Hartford to the establishment of Gallaudet College in 1864. Here we follow a chain of events that embody the *manual-oral controversy*, a historical and present friction between signers and nonsigners or oralists. As we describe these events, the 21st-century reader may recognize racism (i.e., segregated schools), audism (i.e., attitude that being hearing is better than being deaf), and linguicism (i.e., attitude that spoken languages are better than sign languages and that ASL is better than all other signed languages). On the international front, ASL is used instead of a country's own sign language of the area Deaf community, and thus the spread of ASL may be endangering these indigenous sign languages (see Chapter 3).

There is also the issue of hearing privilege and white hearing privilege or the misrepresentation of Deaf teachers, Deaf persons of color, and Deaf teachers of color in teaching positions at the early childhood through postsecondary programs. This discriminatory treatment has historically limited Deaf adult career paths as well as curtailed deaf students' language learning (Andrews & Franklin, 1997; Vernon, 1970; Vernon & Makowsky, 1969). This situation still exists today (Christensen, 2017), but the Americans With Disabilities Act (ADA) has challenged this (see Chapter 10). See Figure 5–2 for a photo of Professor Eddy Laird.

Today we have the benefit of viewing the numerous scientific revolutions from the 19th through the 21st centuries. Research in brain science, cognition, and learning; Deaf studies and sign language linguistics; computer science; and the legal protections have impacted how we view a multicultural deaf education in our modern-day world (see Chapter 10). Moreover, social movements such as bilingualism

and multilingualism, the Deaf President Now movement, the graduation of many Deaf leaders with doctorates who have assumed presidencies of universities and faculty positions, and our global economy with the recognition of the strengths and value of multicultural communities have led to more enlightened views on the education of Deaf learners. Despite these modern events, nonetheless, there is more work to be done within deaf education programs, most notably their hiring practices, to root out and replace the legacy of racism, sexism, audism, linguicism, and white privilege (Christensen, 2017; Simms et al., 2008).

While sign language spread across Europe and into the United States in schools for deaf students, at the same time, the German method or oralism was a competing classroom communication approach. Oralism had gained a stronghold due to the work of Samuel Hienicke,

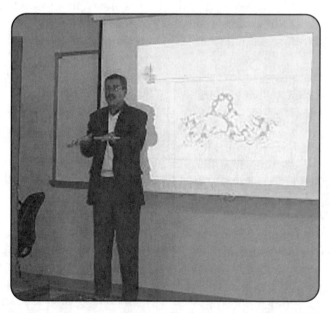

Figure 5–2. Eddy Laird, EdD professor of Deaf Education, teaches a class to Deaf and hearing teacher-trainees on bilingual-bicultural methods.

who set up the first public oral school in Germany in the 18th century. As a result of this movement, from the 18th to the latter part of the 19th century, oral schools in the United States flourished, notably the Lexington School for the Deaf in New York City (founded in 1865) and the Clarke School for the Deaf in Northampton, Massachusetts (founded in 1867). Both have lasted to this day, with the Lexington School for the Deaf now incorporating ASL along with spoken English for teaching purposes (see Leigh & Andrews, 2017, for details).

Another major historical event occurred in 1880, when members of the International Deaf Education conference convened in Milan, Italy, and voted to ban the use of sign language in the schools. Such a surprising outcome was this! Up to this point in France and Italy, sign languages were widely used in schools (see Chapter 1). E. M. Gallaudet, president of the National Deaf Mute College (now Gallaudet University), voted against this resolution. Despite this opposition, the oral or German method prevailed. Against all this, throughout Europe and the United States, there was now a profound reaction. That is, sign language was banned and oralism was adopted in schools for the deaf. Consequently, this oralism zeal and practices permeated the deaf education landscape (see Vernon & Andrews, 1990, for details).

In the latter part of the 19th century, a series of public debates ensued between E. M. Gallaudet, the son of T. H. Gallaudet and staunch advocate for sign language, and Alexander Graham Bell, a vocal supporter of spoken language for deaf students. Already we have seen that the signs versus speech debate occurred during l'Epee's time and existed throughout Europe during the 1800s to 1900s (Chapter 3). In that context, as a compromise to the oral-manual controversy, E. M. Gallaudet developed "the combined approach" that used both spoken language and signing (Winefield, 1987).

As time went on, signing was allowed in schools, primarily with older students only. But it was used more as a way to control behavior rather than as a language teaching approach. Within deaf schools, young Deaf children were segregated into manual and oral classrooms. Before the onset of medical advances and antibiotics, which reduced the occurrence of later childhood deafness, some postlingual Deaf children succeeded in the oral classes.

But as the 1950s and 1960s unfolded, the oral methods were not succeeding as more children were being born prelingually deaf. A blue-ribbon committed established by the Department of Health, Education, and Welfare (now the U.S. Department of Education) issued the Babbidge Report (1965), which was a scathing report documenting the failure of deaf education. Educators were looking for change. When sign language was recognized as a natural language in the 1960s in the United States, it crept back into the schools under the guise of Total Communication, not the signing of the Deaf World (Chapter 3). Other events promulgated by federal laws such as the Rehabilitation Act of 1973 and Education of All Handicapped Children (1975) (P.L. 94-142) (now the Individuals with Disabilities Act, 1990) moved the ball forward in improving the quality of deaf education by providing protection and support for families.

And still another historical event that impacted communication methods was the rubella epidemic from the 1960s to the 1980s. This disease resulted in the births of thousands of Deaf children, many of whom were born with disabilities such as children who are DeafBlind. As a consequence of this dramatic change in school demographics, there became a dire need for more preschools, signing teachers, and those with training for special needs children (Leigh & Andrews, 2017). Meanwhile, rather than adopting the sign language of the Deaf community, the Total Communication philosophy and Simultaneous Communication systems (speech and signing in English word order) approaches were adopted in the schools. Deaf teachers were still typically excluded from preschools and elementary schools but were allowed to teach older Deaf students. There were some exceptions, as McDaniel College (formerly Western Maryland College) and California State University at Northridge (CSUN) over a 30-year time frame did the lion's share of the work in training Deaf teachers and administrators. Despite these developments, audist hiring practices are still in existence in the 21st century and have been challenged in the legal system (see Chapter 10).

Civil unrests such as strikes and protests led up to the civil rights movement in the 1950s and 1960s. These protests shed light on the lack of power of other ethnic and culture groups, including Deaf people. As bilingual education for hearing students was gaining traction as an educational methodology, particularly for Spanish-speaking children, Deaf educators began examining its tenets for use with Deaf children (Nover, Andrews, Baker, Everhart, & Bradford, 2002).

To meet the need for language teaching change, the sociolinguist Stephen M. Nover led a language teaching and learning movement aimed at providing ASL

and English bilingual training for teachers. This in-service program began at the New Mexico School for the Deaf and included multicultural components (Parasnis, 1996). Within both the New Mexico and Texas schools for the deaf, where teachers have led bilingual training, there are large populations of Deaf students from Indigenous tribes and Mexican American families. Prior to this, as early as 1968, Judith Williams (1968), a Deaf mother of a deaf son, published a description of her son's bilingual language acquisition through the use of ASL, fingerspelling, speechreading, and auditory training that was widely read and celebrated by the Deaf community. Soon after, Stokoe wrote a proposal recommending "An Untried Experiment: Bicultural and Bilingual Education of Deaf Children" in 1972. In his proposal, he included the teaching of Deaf culture and ASL to Deaf students of all ages (Maher, 1996, pp. 125–130). Not only was Stokoe's proposal ignored, but it was not until 35 years later, in 2007, that the Board of Trustees affirmed Gallaudet's ASL and English bilingual approach by placing it in its mission statement even though since its founding in 1864, Gallaudet College (now University) already had been providing both ASL and English instruction in the classroom.

Into the 1970s and 1980s, university degree-granting sign language linguistic research programs with research labs burgeoned worldwide. This nurtured and developed sign language linguists in countries across the globe. Advanced degrees were offered in sign language linguistics, bilingualism, and interpreting, which provided training for generations of leaders to establish programs serving Deaf students that incorporated bilingual teaching and learning.

In the late 1980s and early 1990s, the bilingual-bicultural approach emerged as a teaching approach for K–12 children. Marie Jean Philip, a teacher of Deaf students from Massachusetts, introduced the term *bilingual-bicultural approach* to the field and created the sign, BI-BI, for it (Philip & Small, 1991). The same year that the Deaf President Now movement occurred (1988), the Learning Center for the Deaf in Framingham, Massachusetts, became the first private bilingual and bicultural school in the nation. Soon afterward, the Indiana School for the Deaf embraced the bilingual bicultural approach and installed Eddy Laird as the first modern-day superintendent who was Deaf (Geslin, 2007). Soon other schools for the deaf adopted this approach and began hosting workshops for parents, teachers, and staff, training them in ASL and English teaching and learning methodologies. As to be expected, this was accepted enthusiastically in the Deaf community (Gárate, 2012), particularly among Deaf scholars such as Barbara Kannapal, Stephen Nover, Laurene Simms, and others who were graduating from universities and conducting research in bilingual education for deaf students.

Ironically, bilingualism in deaf education was not a new concept. While signing and English teaching practices had been around for almost two centuries (Nover, 2000), this methodology benefited from a newfound academic credibility and was rejuvenated due to the science of bilingual theories and practices in hearing populations.

In the mid-to-late 1990s, Nover tapped into this rich resource of bilingual education for hearing children as he wrote grants to support more training in order to prepare teachers using bilingual methodologies. His programs recognized the cultural and language diversity of the Deaf experience (Parasnis, 1996).

But bilingualism still faced obstacles in deaf education. From the mid-1970s to today, another practice, called mainstreaming or educating Deaf children in public schools, dominated Deaf education. Experiments with educating Deaf children alongside hearing children had existed since Lydia Huntley Sigourney taught Alice Cogswell with hearing children in the mid-19th century (see Chapter 3). However, now mainstreaming Deaf students into public schools became a parent's right mandated by federal law (i.e., Public Law 94-142). As a result of this legislation, from the mid-1970s to the present, public schools have expanded their educational offerings when more educational sign language interpreters have become available. Now universities have begun offering sign language classes to meet this need. Interpretation training programs were established and funded by federal grant initiatives. As a result of these developments, interpreter training programs flourished.

Nover's innovative program resulted in the development of bilingual programs beyond K–12 teacher preparation. His bilingual methodologies for K–12 teachers were modified and adapted to prepare university professors at the master's and doctoral levels (Andrews, 2003; Andrews & Covell, 2006; Simms et al., 2008). As more awareness of bilingualism entered K–12 and university training, and with legislation such at the Americans With Disabilities Act, Deaf teachers began to challenge school districts who refused to hire them or who discriminated against them (see Chapter 10).

Another event that impacted communication approaches in deaf education was the development of technology. From A. G. Bell's mechanical ear tube apparatus to the telephone to the hearing aid, technology has impacted deaf education in surprising ways. After World War II, hearing aid technology improved. As a result of these advances, amplification was widely used in programs for Deaf children and youth. A new technology—the cochlear implant—came to the fore in the 1990s, when it was developed in labs in Europe and Australia (see Chapter 2). Digitization brought in digital hearing aids. Leading up to the 21st century, both digital hearing aids and cochlear implant technology have provided a new form of oralism when they are utilized without signing. However, parents and professionals found out that this technology does not always give Deaf children complete access to spoken language, and they needed sign language to support it.

The perspective of the "war against sign language," largely spearheaded by the Alexander Graham Bell Association for the Deaf and Hard of Hearing, is considered by many to be detrimental to the development of those young Deaf children who were not able to succeed with only spoken language interventions. Consequently, some Deaf children have not received early exposure to a sign language, which has resulted in cognitive and language deprivation (Hall, 2017). But, interestingly, there have been shifts in this debate. To this day, the A. G. Bell Association continues to collaborate with organizations that support ASL, such as the Joint Committee on Infant Hearing (JCIH, 2007), the Deaf and Hard of Hearing Alliance, advocates of the Language Equality and Acquisition for Deaf Kids (LEAD-K) movement, and the Council on Education of the Deaf (CED).

As a review of these historical events show, each antisigning event was distinct. Yet clear patterns emerge, including a cycle that kept repeating itself: an antisigning policy is evoked, an oral/manual debate ensues, and then Deaf community responds with calls for change.

In the 21st century, what do these communication approaches look like? We define the four approaches, which can be utilized with (or without) auditory technology (see Leigh & Andrews, 2017, for details).

Bilingual and Multilingual Approaches

The crux of the bilingual or the ASL and English approach is that ASL becomes the language of instruction and English is taught as a second language. For some Deaf students, it focuses on print (sign-print bilingualism). For others who have residual hearing, it can include spoken language instruction when appropriate. That being said, ASL and English bilingual programming must include careful language planning and explicit teaching strategies using ASL, English, and fingerspelling by teachers who have been trained in bilingual theory and practices (Gárate, 2012; Nover et al., 2002). This approach can take the form of the bimodal bilingualism, which focuses on spoken language for Deaf children who utilize cochlear implant technology and ASL. Like the bilingual approach, it requires the careful separation of spoken and sign languages (Gárate, 2011; Nussbaum, Scott, & Simms, 2012). Bilingualism is also integrated into the multilingual approach, a somewhat broader approach that includes Deaf children who come to school with multiple languages, both spoken and signed. For the most part, schools will focus on one sign language and a spoken or written language, typically ASL and English in the United States (Cannon et al., 2016). See Luis's case in the following box.

Luis was born deaf in Mexico in a home where Spanish was spoken. He never attended school in Mexico, but Luis learned Lengua de Senas Mexicana or LSM on the streets with deaf children in the neighborhood. Immigrating with his family to the United States at age 11, he enrolled in a school for the deaf. He was placed in an ASL immersion program and rapidly picked up ASL. His parents were enrolled in an ASL and Spanish and English sign language (trilingual) program offered by his school through night classes, but they had difficulty attending because they both worked two jobs. Luis's older sister attended the class and taught the family signs in the home. Luis excelled on the sports fields but struggled in school academically with his English skills.

Blended Approaches

The goal of teaching English through blended approaches includes Total Communication (TC), simultaneous communication (SimCom), contact signing, and the various manual codes of English (MCE) or cued speech (CP). See Leigh and Andrews (2017) for history, descriptions, and advantages of each. Todd's case exemplifies some features of the blended approach.

Todd was a white male who was born deaf. At age 3, he was fitted with a cochlear implant. Shortly afterward, he began intensive speech therapy. English was the language of his home, and his parents used both spoken English and ASL signs simultaneously. Todd attended a self-contained classroom with a teacher of the deaf who used Total Communication. In his class, a Deaf aide would frequently read storybooks and translate them into ASL. Todd graduated from high school and chose a hearing college with a deaf education department. Todd used an ASL interpreter in all of his college classes with hearing teachers who did not sign. With his hearing teachers in deaf education, Todd continued to speak English and try to sign ASL simultaneously, but with his Deaf classmates, he only used ASL.

At first glance, it may appear that MCE approaches are effective teaching tools to teach English grammar as they place signs in English word order. But there are challenges to learning English from them. Teachers and parents often drop the endings, resulting in incomplete and inaccurate messages. While they get MCE at school, some Deaf students do not get this modeling at home. Moreover, MCE may not make sense to Deaf students as many have not yet learned enough English to produce the English signs. There is also a lack of research on transfer of MCE to literacy skills. Another complaint about MCE systems is that they overload the child's cognitive and perceptual processes when seeing the signs (Mayberry, 2002).

There is an alternative view, though—that is, TC, SimCom, and MCE systems can be useful with Deaf students, particularly the ease it affords for hearing parents in acquiring them (see Leigh & Andrews, 2017, for review of these studies).

Monolingual Listening and Spoken Language (LSL) Approaches

Used with oral Deaf children, this monolingual approach focuses on listening and spoken English. An offshoot is the auditory-verbal approach, which utilizes visual skills such as lipreading. The goals are to give children opportunities to learn how to talk so they can be integrated into a public school classroom with hearing children. Historically, monolingual approaches were known as *pure oralism/ auditory stimulation*, the *multisensory/syllable unit method*, and the *language association-element method*, as well as the *unisensory or aural approach* (Northern & Downs, 2014). See Heather Whitestone's case.

Communication Approaches and DeafDisabled Students

These three communication and language approaches described above, along with many more, are used with DeafDisabled students (Bruce & Borders, 2015). Deaf children with learning disabilities and/ or ADD and ADHD may benefit from the same communication and language approaches used with Deaf students without disabilities, but these students may need repetition and additional time to acquire concepts and language structures. Deaf children with disabilities, such as ID, autism, and cerebral palsy, and individuals who are DeafBlind may use a sign language, protactile sign language, spoken language, or a combination of these. They also may use tangible objects, raised drawings, gestures, pictures, and augmentative and alternative communication (AAC) (Erikson & Quick, 2017). *Unaided ACC* employs graphic symbols, sign language, fingerspelling, objects, large print, and tactile communication. In comparison, *aided AAC* methods make use of electronic and nonelectronic devices (i.e., communication boards and computer displays) to send and receive messages (Light & McNaughton, 2014). Interestingly, the history of AAC methods can be traced back to the use of manual alphabets and signs recorded in Europe from the 16th century, as well as the signed languages used by North American Native Indian tribes (see Chapter 3).

Heather Whitestone, Miss America of 1995, is a white deaf female. She lost her hearing while a toddler. The family, who lived in Alabama, focused on helping her develop spoken language with the assistance of hearing aids. She attended the Central Institute for the Deaf in St. Louis, Missouri, an oral school, where she improved her listening and speaking skills. After 3 years, she caught up to hearing peers and transferred to a public high school, where she excelled. She loved ballet and learned how to follow the music and time her dancing to the music. After she won the Miss America crown, she married a hearing man, with whom she has four sons. She has supported programs to train dogs for deaf people and organizations that provide hearing aids to people in poverty.

Deaf children with emotional/behavioral disabilities and those with autism may use these three communication approaches but also may need to be taught how to socially respond to conversational partners, including making eye contact, turn-taking, and reducing highly rigid and repetitive behaviors. Parents and teachers may use a combination of voice and voice output systems (if the child wears auditory technology), sign language, pictures, and gestures for communication (Light & McNaughton, 2014). Students with physical/sensory disabilities, such as those persons who are DeafBlind, can use sign language (adapted to fit their visual field), protactile sign language, tracking, tactile fingerspelling, print on palm, Tadoma, Braille, speech, and speech reading (Edwards, 2014). Some DeafBlind teens with functional vision can use the videophone technology and computers with enlarged print (Bruce et al., 2016) (see also Chapter 2). Due to physical facial anomalies, Deaf children with Treacher Collins syndrome will need speech and language services. Those with CHARGE syndrome have a variety of physical and sensory disabilities (coloboma of the eye, heart defects, atresia of the nasal passages, retardation of physical growth, and ear abnormalities), with many having cognitive delays as well. Some may be able to use Braille and large print when they get older. Deaf children with meningitis may have learning difficulties, neuromotor disorders, seizure disorders, visual disorders, and behavioral problems, with some having cognitive delays. Deaf children with cytomegalovirus (CMV) may also have cognitive, visual, and motor delays and experience progressive decreasing of hearing levels—all of which will impact what communication approaches and type of schooling they need (Jackson, Ammerman, & Trautwein, 2015).

Keep in mind that Deaf children, including DeafDisabled individuals, from multilinguistic and multicultural homes may begin with one communication and language approach; then, as they become more comfortable and integrated into Deaf multicultural communities, they add more languages or even transition to another dominant language, as shown by the case of Nina described in the following box.

Nina was born deaf into a Mexican American family. Her family used spoken Spanish and English with her. She received a cochlear implant at age 2, then began intensive speech training. By kindergarten, she was fully mainstreamed with hearing students but frequently expressed that she was lonely at school as she was the only deaf student. At home and at school, she used spoken language—both Spanish and English. After high school graduation, she enrolled in a hearing university with a deaf education program and began to learn ASL and use ASL interpreters, because as she said, "There was so much information." She also minored in Spanish and spent a summer in Mexico, where she learned Lengua de Senas Mexicana (LSM). Nina uses spoken Spanish and English with her hearing family when she goes home. And she uses ASL daily with her Deaf friends in the United States, but uses Skype with her Mexican Deaf friends using LSM. Her goal is to become a paralegal and use her multilingual skills with clients.

These communication and language approaches can be used in all settings where Deaf students go to school, which we describe below.

SCHOOL SETTINGS

Center Schools

Center schools provide comprehensive programming, including academic, vocational, sports, and other after-school activities from parent infant programs to high school. Some provide post–high school independent living programs for Deaf youth ages 18 to 22. Most states have a state school for the deaf that is free of charge. One advantage is that they provide a critical mass of Deaf adult role models for language and cultural modeling. Another advantage is availability of a full range of extracurricular activities such as sports teams, social clubs, drama clubs, class government, and junior National Association for the Deaf clubs (Leigh & Andrews, 2017). It's a place where a Deaf girl with cerebral palsy (or other disabilities) can become a cheerleader, run for a class office, or join a debate team with Deaf peers. About 29.6% of all deaf and hard-of-hearing students attend state or center schools (GRI, 2013). Today, more Deaf children from multicultural backgrounds and those with disabilities are attending center schools because they have a broad array of trained professionals and resources. Deaf children with disabilities may be included in some classes and activities with Deaf children without disabilities. See Figure 5–3 for a picture of the Texas School for the Deaf, Austin.

Private Oral Schools

Providing intensive speech training within academic programming and dormitory living for elementary schoolchildren, these private oral schools use monolingual spo-

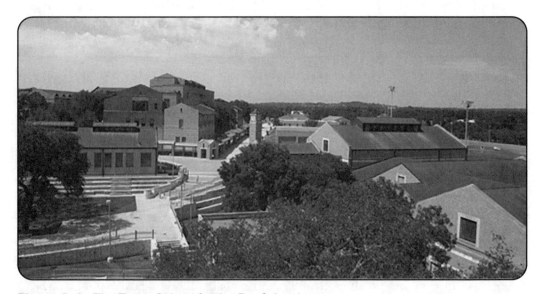

Figure 5–3. The Texas School for the Deaf, Austin.

ken language approaches only without signing. At the end of eighth grade, Deaf children are expected to have the spoken and listening skills to be mainstreamed in their neighborhood schools in high school. These schools charge tuition. There exists also oral programming in public schools that is tuition free and children live at home.

Day Schools

Day schools with separate classrooms for deaf students are found in large cities. In the past, Deaf students, including those with disabilities, were not mainstreamed with hearing students. While this was the case, in today's 21st century and with the push for inclusion, more children are integrated with hearing students. But some still are separated, particularly if they have severe disabilities. In a survey of 1,653 of special education teachers across 14 states who served children with severe IDs and hearing levels ranging from mild to profound, about 68.9% of the children were educated in separate classrooms in public schools and spent less than 40% of the day with peers without disabilities (Erikson & Quick, 2017).

Inclusion

In this placement, Deaf children and youth are placed in regular classrooms with hearing peers. Students are provided with support such as sign language interpreters or itinerant teachers to support their learning. However, there are no assurances that these services will make the curriculum accessible to Deaf students, who may be delayed because of lack of access to language at home and in school.

Mainstream, Self-Contained Resource Room

Mainstreaming can refer to total inclusion, self-contained classrooms only for deaf students, resource rooms, itinerant programs, and team teaching or coenrollment programs. Students can receive services either individually or in small groups with specialized teachers available in the resource rooms. About 13.9% of Deaf and hard-of-hearing students receive support services in resource rooms (GRI, 2013). Deaf children may attend classes with hearing children and receive extra services from an itinerant teacher who provides direct services or consultation to the school. They must be able to work with classroom teachers, administrators, speech-language pathologists, audiologists, and parents (Guardino & Cannon, 2015). Within this context, lack of socialization is a consideration. In a study of 100 Deaf children who were the only Deaf students at their public schools, the researchers reported they had difficulty in finding friends and social access. They also struggled with establishing an identity and faced challenges in obtaining qualified interpreters (Oliva & Lytle, 2014).

Coenrollment

The coenrollment model, used internationally, includes having a critical mass of Deaf students in one classroom and provides a teacher with deaf education certification. There is also a second teacher who teaches the hearing children. As a team, the two instructors teach the same on-grade level content, and hearing students take sign language classes to communicate with deaf peers (Kirchner, 2019).

The coenrollment program differs from a single deaf student or small groups of deaf students being included in a hearing school and "reverse mainstreaming," where groups of hearing children join a classroom of deaf students. While outcome research from coenrollment programs shows that deaf children still lag behind their hearing peers academically, it does provide opportunities for Deaf and hearing peer socialization. More than 10 countries, including the United States, are experimenting with this model, and more research on student outcomes should be forthcoming (Marschark, Antia, & Knoors, 2019). Figure 5–4 shows a classroom of deaf students in a public school.

Charter Schools and Home Schools

Charter schools operate under a "charter" contact between members of the charter school community and the local board of education. Some charter schools use ASL and English bilingual approaches; others use spoken language approaches. About 3.7% are home schooled (GRI, 2013). In a study of 21 families, parents reported they chose this setting so they could control the use of a specific communication approach (i.e., oral, TC, or bilingual), as well as provide academic support and religious instruction (Parks, 2009).

TECHNOLOGY, DEAFSPACE, AND CLASSROOM ACOUSTICS

Within these school settings, a variety of classroom technology is used. These include electronic devices, online instructional materials, establishing DeafSpace, and providing classroom acoustic modifications. Electronic devices that support spoken and listening skills include cochlear implants, hearing aids, and FM systems. Those devices that support visual learning (some include auditory learning as well) include online classes, ASL/Eng-

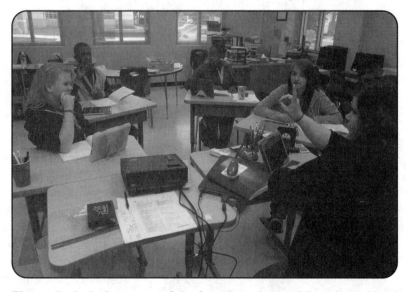

Figure 5–4. A classroom of deaf students in a public school. Used with permission. Photo courtesy of Brian Sattler.

lish bilingual e-books, whiteboards, text messaging, e-mail, multimedia materials, signing avatars, and vlogs. Other technology-oriented instructional materials and tools include ASL dictionaries and games, ASL-supported educational materials and quizzes such as supporting English text with sign and concept graphics and video in real time, and games. Lessons for Deaf students whose primary language is ASL can be developed using technologies called MAR (Mobile Augmented Reality), such as HP Reveal, which can be employed to access ASL at museums and field trips sites, and they frequently consist of inaccessible audio-based narratives and tours (Leigh & Andrews, 2017) (see Chapter 8). See Figure 5–5 for a young boy reading an ASL/English e-book.

DeafSpace refers to an aspect of universal design (UD) and aims to reduce architectural barriers for visual learning. This can include changing desk and chair arrangements to a semicircle where the teacher and students have open visual access to each other's signing. It also includes adequate room lighting.

Some Deaf students benefit from auditory technology as well as acoustically treated classrooms, which can reduce noises typically found in schools such as blaring loudspeaker announcements, banging of lockers, and the moving of desks and chairs. In this context, background noise and reverberation interfere with reception of hearing aids and cochlear implants. Schools can use special ceiling and wall tiles (called acoustic tiles), as well as rugs on the wall and on the floor to absorb these sounds. Some Deaf students may benefit from a FM system where the student wears a receiver to amplify the teacher's voice and reduce the speech-to-signal ratio. The signal-to-noise ratio (SNR) is a measure the compares the level of a signal to the level of background noise, and it is a useful index for teachers setting up an optimum environment for Deaf students to listen to spoken language (Northern & Downs, 2014).

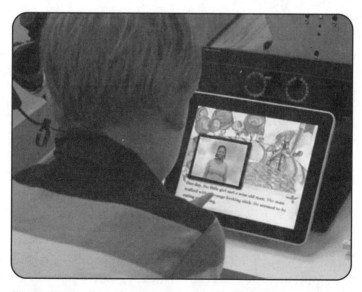

Figure 5–5. A young deaf boy reads an ASL/English bilingual e-book. Used with permission of Laura-Ann Petitto.

EDUCATIONAL PROGRAMMING

In light of the learning factors affecting schooling, communication approaches, and educational settings, we now turn to a discussion of levels of programming. In the 1980s, in an effort to improve instruction in EC to secondary education, the standards movement started. These standards were typically monolingual and provided standardized tests only in English. As such, standards-based curriculum, instruction, and assessment were developed primarily for hearing white, middle-class students, which, according to some, neither adequately addressed the needs nor measured the academic strengths and needs of students who are Deaf and Deaf multicultural individuals, including those with disabilities (Cawthon, 2011; Horn-Marsh, 2016).

Early Childhood (EC) Levels (Birth to 5 Years)

At the hospital, babies are screened for hearing loss as early as a few hours after birth. Referrals are then made to audiologists for further testing if the child does not meet the hospital's hearing-centric standards and screenings. Finding out their child is deaf often comes as a shock to hearing parents, evoking strong emotions and feelings of helplessness on where to turn to find information and services (see Chapter 2).

Curriculum and Outcomes

While the type and quantity of resources vary, every state has an early intervention system that is provided free of cost. Services are individualized based on the child's unique developmental needs.

Family-centered interventions for birth to 3 years and preschool programming grounded in best practices are recommended. These interventions can occur in the home, in a clinic, or even at an outreach program at a center school. As such, these services assist families with information and support families with communication and language approaches, use of assistive technology, and speech and hearing services. At this juncture, if the doctor suspects complications, then children are screened for other disabilities.

Education for Deaf children is protected under a series of laws enacted at the federal and the state levels. These provide families and Deaf children with early access to communication, language, and services from birth to age 21, then also into adulthood during postsecondary schooling, employment, and health care. Initiatives such as the LEAD-K campaign and Deaf Children's Bill of Rights also advocate for language access through accountability assessments, among other strategies (see Chapter 10).

Challenges in School

Challenges for Deaf children from birth to 5 years include the following: finding Deaf mentors and Deaf mentors of color to provide direction to families (Hamilton, 2017; Kite, 2014). There is also a need for family-centered interventions (FCEIs) that take a multicultural perspective and use bilingual interpreters for families (Bowen, 2016; Jackson et al., 2015).

Families who use different languages may wonder if they should use the home language with their Deaf child. Crowe and MacLeod (2014) summarize eight studies showing the benefits of teaching the Deaf child the home language in order to develop bilingual skills. Another concern is that multicultural families of Deaf children may shun services that are typically led by white professionals (Simms et al., 2008). Doctors who do not know about Deaf culture and sign language typically follow the medical-pathological perspective and prioritize spoken language as a home communication method as they may be unfamiliar with bilingual/multilingual and bimodal teaching practices.

More challenges exist for Deaf children with disabilities during the birth to age 5 span. If newborns and toddlers are medically fragile with multiple disabilities and they do not pass the newborn hearing screening, other physical disabilities will take priority over early language intervention (Erikson & Quick, 2017). Disabilities may be undiagnosed until children are older, and this delays early interven-

tion and preschool. The Joint Committee on Infant Hearing (JCIH, 2007) recommends that every family of a deaf child be offered genetic evaluation and screening for common syndromes associated with hearing loss and disabilities such as those individuals who are DeafBlind or have syndromes such as Down syndrome, Treachers Collins syndrome, CHARGE syndrome, or a combination of these. But assessment is only the beginning. Follow-up is necessary in order to find appropriate early intervention and preschool and kindergarten placements. Contacting a state center school for the Deaf is often the first step in finding information and locating appropriate services near the child's home region. Figure 5–6 shows Deaf parents playing with their two Deaf children.

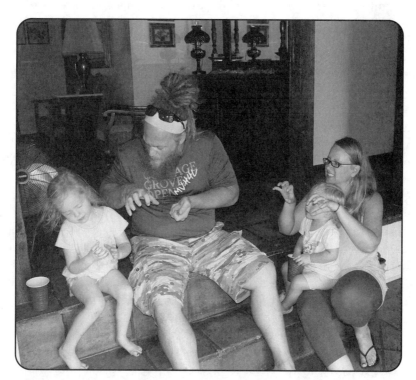

Figure 5–6. Deaf parents playing with their two Deaf children. Used with permission.

Go online and compare the services provided by the Alexander Graham Bell Association for the Deaf and Hard of Hearing, American Society for Deaf Children, Hands and Voices, and National ASL & English Bilingual Consortium for Early Childhood Education. Do you notice a difference in those organizations' stance regarding Deaf culture, multiculturalism, and sign language?

K to 12th-Grade Levels (5 to 22 Years)

Curriculum and Outcomes

The school years from kindergarten through 12th grade are vital in the Deaf students' cognitive, language, and social development. Typically, each state has its own curriculum, learning standards, and assessment measures from kindergarten to secondary levels. Even then, teachers may find it difficult to adapt, differentiate, or modify them. Related to academic achievement, some Deaf students excel and perform better than these standards. An example of such achievement is demonstrated within the Academic Bowl program sponsored by Gallaudet University (GU) (Leigh & Andrews, 2017). Every year, GU hosts four regional competitions for up to 80 teams of Deaf and hard-of-hearing high school students. Twenty teams will then advance to the national competition held at Gallaudet every year. There are also examples of many Deaf students who graduate from college, obtain advanced graduate degrees, and enter a multitude of professions in education, law, medicine, psychology, and so on (see Chapter 10).

Because of environmental language delays, inferior quality of instruction, and lack of resources, among other factors, some deaf students are often delayed in their academic skills and get further behind as they get older. On standardized, norm-referenced tests, Deaf children tend to score 3 to 4 years behind their hearing-age peers (Qi & Mitchell, 2012). And as these students move through the school system, these achievement gaps widen (Cawthon, Leppo, & Pepnet, 2013). While mathematical scores may be higher than reading scores, there is a leveling off at seventh grade in calculation skills and more difficulty with mathematical word problems (Lee & Paul, 2019). Similar delays are found in science and social studies.

In a sample of 37,700, it was reported that Deaf students completed high school at lower rates compared to hearing students. Moreover, Deaf students with disabilities are two times less likely to complete high school than Deaf students without disabilities (Garberoglio, Palmer, Cawthon, & Sales, 2019). See Chapter 10 for a series of laws that protect Deaf students at this age.

For all Deaf students, multicultural and those with disabilities, ASL, Deaf Studies, and Deaf multicultural studies can be integrated throughout the curriculum and expanded beyond a limited "Deaf Awareness Week." Information about Deaf culture is found in museums at center schools, which contain rich repositories of artifacts, memorabilia, books, old uniforms, and photographs of students. Most center schools also have published a history of their school; this provides rich, instructional curricula for Deaf students. See Figure 5–7 for a photo of the Heritage Center, the museum at the Texas School for the Deaf.

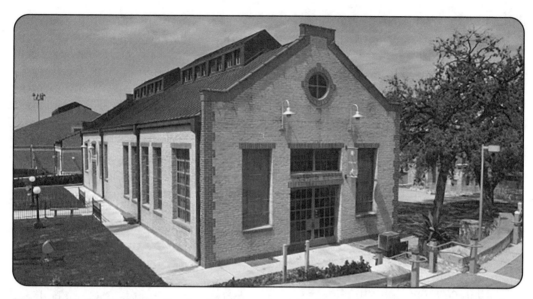

Figure 5–7. The Heritage Center, the museum at the Texas School for the Deaf. Used with permission of Texas School for the Deaf.

Search the Internet for other histori-cal museums at the Texas School, the Kentucky School, and the New Mex-ico School. What kinds of historical artifacts can you find? What do these items tell you about the role of Deaf culture in deaf education?

Support for Deaf students can be gleaned from case studies of Deaf youth and adults who make recommendations for families of Deaf multicultural students. One Latinx student reported that she used Google Translator to communicate with her parents who were Spanish speakers (Baker & Scott, 2016). Another two Asian Deaf students reported they used Skype and text messaging in Chinese to commu-nicate with their hearing families in Main-land China and Singapore (Wang et al., 2016). Denninger (2017) provides sugges-tions for middle school and high school curriculum to include information about LBGT histories and movements in order to promote tolerance and acceptance for Deaf LBGT students.

Deaf and hard-of-hearing children and youth with disabilities who now appear in the classroom are different from the children who became deaf from the rubella epidemic of the 1960s. Deaf chil-dren with disabilities in the 21st century have more complex educational needs and will require a curriculum and instruc-tional strategies that meet their unique characteristics. The possible combinations of disabilities are limitless, which impact teaching in the classroom. For instance, a child with Down syndrome and moder-ate hearing levels may learn to read and write, whereas a child born DeafBlind with intellectual disabilities and autism may require a curriculum that is based on concrete objects, signing in the hand, and a life-skills program.

For DeafDisabled children, studies of evidence-based practices are not read-ily available. That being said, a common denominator to guide instruction is using individualized approaches or a universal design that makes learning accessible and a curriculum that is based on the students' strengths and needs. Adapting and modifying practices used with hearing special needs children can be utilized as well (Borders, Bock, Probst, & Kroesch, 2017). Borders and her colleagues recommend basic special education practices that are used with non-Deaf students with disabilities, particularly those with severe to profound intellectual or multiple disabilities.

Transition and Postsecondary Educational Opportunities

What happens after the deaf student completes high school? Depending on the Deaf students' strengths and needs, after high school, they transition to post-school activities, including postsecondary education, vocational education (Chapter 10), employment (Chapter 7), continuing and adult education, adult services, independent living, or community participation (Luft, 2015). Related to postsecondary opportunities, due to legislation and increased accessibility, there are increased opportunities for Deaf students to enroll in continuing education, vocational training, universities and colleges, and other postsecondary programs (Garberoglio et al., 2019).

Curriculum and Outcomes

As part of the IEP, typically commencing at middle school or at 14 years of age, Deaf youth are required by law to have a transition plan that will assist them in their life and schooling after high school. They are eligible to receive these services up to their 22nd birthday. Luft (2015) provides

a comprehensive review of studies that describe these barriers Deaf youth face in finding appropriate transition services. These include the following: generic and superficial quality of appropriate transition training during high school, need for more time during transition training, inability to complete household chores and live independently with or without a roommate, and need for more time to complete transition training. On a positive note, Luft reports that DeafDisabled youth are provided with more social connections within the community that they did not have prior to transition services.

Academic and technical degrees and preparation are provided by four colleges that enroll many Deaf multicultural and multilingual students, as well as those with disabilities: These are Gallaudet University, Washington, DC; the National Technical Institute of the Deaf at the Rochester Institute of Technology, Rochester, New York; the California State University (CSUN) at Northridge, California; and the Southwest Collegiate Institute for the Deaf, Big Springs, Texas. These institutions provide a bilingual signing environment, with Deaf professors and hearing faculty who understand Deaf culture and are proficient in ASL. Other support services include oral and ASL interpreting, CART (computer-assisted real-time captioning), and notetaking.

Deaf students are increasingly attending community colleges and utilizing sign language interpreters. In a national sample of Deaf adults ages 18 to 64, it was reported that community colleges currently enroll 70.3% of deaf students in 2-year associate programs compared to only 61.% of hearing students (Garberoglio et al., 2019). The most popular fields of study found were business and health care, with only 26.1% of the Deaf student sample studying in the science, technology, engineer, and mathematics (STEM) fields (Garberoglio et al., 2019).

While Deaf students take longer to enroll in college (5 years) compared to hearing students (2 years), at least 51% complete at least some college. More Deaf men are enrolled in college (53.5%) compared to Deaf women (46.5%), but Deaf women have higher completing rates than Deaf men (Garberoglio et al., 2019).

Deaf college students are less racially diverse than hearing students, with those across all races and ethnicities having lower educational attainment rates than their hearing peers. Students who are Deaf Latinx, while having lower than average educational attainment, were closest to their hearing peers. Deaf Asian students were most likely to have completed their bachelor degrees, but they still showed lower achievement than their hearing peers (Garberoglio et al., 2019).

From this same sample of Deaf college students, 30.8% have learning disabilities (e.g., ADHD, ADD, or depression), 8.1% are DeafBlind, and 13.1% have ambulatory (motor) disabilities (Garberoglio et al., 2019). For DeafDisabled students with severe disabilities such as ID or autism or multiple disabilities, there are specialized transitional and vocational programs available in each state. Some DeafDisabled students will transfer from a public school to a state center school for the deaf from ages 18 to 22 to learn independent living skills (Leigh & Andrews, 2017). See Chapter 10 for education laws that support transition services.

Postsecondary Challenges

Deaf youth with disabilities face barriers in accessing work training, as well as finding and retaining employment after high school. If they are eligible for college, DeafDisabled students may need support services such as protactile interpreting, more time for testing, notetaking, writing centers, and tutoring to a greater extent than Deaf students without disabilities. Deaf multilingual students who attend college may need extra support interpreting services to meet their language needs, both spoken and signed, in the classroom.

PREPARATION OF TEACHERS AND EDUCATIONAL INTERPRETERS

Teacher-Training

There are three types of communication approaches that are taught in teacher-training in deaf education: bilingual, comprehensive (includes bilingual and blending approaches), and oral-aural. The Council for Exceptional Children (CEC) and the Council on Education of the Deaf (CED) jointly published a set of standards for teachers who work with Deaf students. Some teacher-training programs offer certification and coursework for teachers to work with Deaf students with disabilities. Some EC to 12 programs with DeafDisabled students require teachers to have dual certification in deaf education and special education.

Teachers in training can learn the bilingual-bicultural (also known as bi-bi, or the ASL and English bilingual) approach. This approach emphasizes the two languages: a native signed language and the written/spoken language used by the majority community (Gárate, 2012; Nover et al., 2002). Students receive coursework in Deaf culture, multiculturalism, ASL, and English bilingual theories, practices, and assessments (Nover et al., 2002; Simms & Thumann, 2007). Teachers develop lessons in ASL, as well as oral and written English, and learn how to administer assessments in ASL and English. They conduct their internships in schools or programs for Deaf students that use the ASL and English bilingual approach. The role of Deaf teachers, particularly those from multiethnic backgrounds, can provide important role models and mentors for the increasingly multicultural population of Deaf students (Simms et al., 2008).

The majority of teacher-training university programs follow the comprehensive approach that focuses on providing training for teachers, primarily in simultaneous communication, although they may offer select coursework in Deaf Studies and ASL. These programs teach learning pedagogy and communication practices for a wide variety of Deaf students who are enrolled in both center schools and public schools.

A few university programs provide training in monolingual oral-aural approaches to teach Deaf students. These are primarily found at private universities and may be associated with a speech-language pathology and audiology clinic. The auditory-verbal model is a habilitation and clinical model that focuses on getting Deaf children ready to be mainstreamed into the public school (Northern & Downs, 2014).

Currently, teachers in training must take teacher certification exams. These pose a barrier for Deaf people who want to become teachers because English is often their second language. The irony is that state testing does not include a test in ASL (or ASL proficiency) for those who want to teach deaf children. Whether a teacher is certified or passes a state teachers' competency exam, their certification does not ensure that the deaf child is learning. It is the quality of the communication and interaction between the student and the teacher that is most important and should be accounted for along with the coursework (Cawthon, 2011).

Search the Internet and see how the states of Texas and Oklahoma have responded to the need to increase the number of Deaf teachers by exempting them from biased English testing. Discuss how these states are combatting discrimination against Deaf teachers with these laws.

There is a need to train more teachers of DeafDisabled students as these populations are unidentified and underserved. Additional professionals, particularly teachers, are needed to provide screenings, culturally responsive evaluations, and interventions (Cawthon, 2016; Erikson & Quick, 2017).

Educational Interpreter Training

As more Deaf students are attending public schools and universities, the role of a qualified and certified educational interpreter is paramount. Educational interpreters must be qualified with specialized training for their role as the go-betweens between the hearing school setting and the deaf students. They must not only translate the English of the teachers into ASL or a manual code of English but also make sure the student is engaged in the lesson. The interpreter may also have to inform the teacher about Deaf culture and multicultural issues. Many deaf students in the lower grades are already deprived of Deaf language models in ASL and English. This interferes with their ability to understand the teacher and learn (Roberson & Shaw, 2018).

Sign language interpreters develop proficiencies in sign language and translation techniques, and they have multicultural competence, knowledge about Deaf culture and multiculturalism, and coursework in the academic areas they are interpreting. Interpreters for Deaf-Blind students must have even more skills in techniques in working with this population (i.e., protactile sign language) (Edwards, 2014; Roberson & Shaw, 2018). Figure 5–8 shows an educational interpreter working in a school setting.

Challenges for Teachers and Interpreters

When schools develop multicultural curriculum within school settings across all content areas, this is an important step in developing multicultural competence of faculty as well (Au, 2014). Deaf students of color often experience harassment or discrimination based on race, ethnicity, gender, sexual orientation, and citizenship in schools among students, teachers, and administrators and interpreters (Christensen, 2017; Denninger, 2017; Garcia-Fernandez, 2014). Deaf students of color, DeafBlind students, and Deaf-Disabled students are also often deprived of their home and natural languages, whether it be Black ASL, Plains Indian Sign Language, Lengua de Señas Mexicana, protactile, or others. Furthermore, teachers, administrators, and educational interpreters need to develop multicultural competencies as well as examine their own prejudices, stereotypes, and attitudes about cultures other than own, including attitudes of white privilege (Holcomb et al., 2017). School administrators need to examine attitudes of low expectations where Deaf students of color and those with disabilities are tracked with less frequency in academics and tracked more often into vocational and special education classes compared to their white counterparts (Simms et al., 2008).

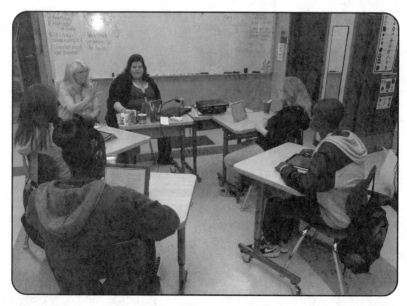

Figure 5–8. An educational interpreter working in a school setting. Used with permission. Photo courtesy of Brian Sattler.

CONCLUSIONS

Deaf children and youth from multilinguistic and multicultural backgrounds, including those who are DeafDisabled individuals, have multiple educational options and opportunities that are supported by legislation. Universal design, visual and auditory technology, and tactile language practices can provide access to spoken, sign, and tactile languages. Advances in medicine, cognitive and learning sciences, linguistics, and other sciences have improved our understanding of the learning strengths and needs of diverse populations of Deaf students. The Internet can connect teachers globally to share resources. Despite these positive directions, there is still more work to be done and obstacles to be overcome. Such barriers include meeting the shortage of trained teachers with Deaf culture and multicultural competencies, addressing the absence of teachers' and educational interpreters' sign language proficiency, and contributing to accessible on-grade content for academically oriented Deaf students. Curricula focused on independent life skills curriculum are needed for those with severe disabilities. Recognizing and removing the all too present but detrimental dynamics of racism, sexism, audism, and linguicism is also needed to foster equitable school experiences.

REFERENCES

Andrews, J., & Covell, J. (2006). Preparing future teachers and doctoral level leaders in deaf education: Meeting the challenge. *American Annals of the Deaf, 151*(6), 464–475.

Andrews, J., & Franklin, T. C. (1997). Why hire deaf teachers? *Texas Journal of Speech and Hearing (TEJAS), XXII*(1), 12013. (ERIC document: ED 425 600)

Andrews, J. F. (2003). Benefits of an Ed.D. program in deaf education: A survey. *American Annals of the Deaf, 148*(3), 259–266.

Au, W. (Ed.). (2014). *Rethinking multicultural education: Teaching for racial and cultural justice* (2nd ed.). Milwaukee, WI: Rethinking Schools.

Babbidge Report. (1965). *Education of the deaf: A report to the secretary of health, education, and welfare by his advisory committee on the education of the deaf.* Washington, DC: Department of Health, Education, and Welfare. (ERIC 011 188 EC 001 178)

Baker, S., & Scott, J. (2016). Sociocultural and academic considerations for school-aged/ Deaf and hard of hearing multilingual learners: A case study of a Deaf Latina. *American Annals of the Deaf, 161*(1), 43–55.

Borders, C. M., Bock, S. J., Probst, K. M., & Kroesch, A. M. (2017). Deaf/Hard-of-Hearing Students with Disabilities. *Preparing to teach, committing to learn: An introduction to educating children who are deaf/hard of hearing.* Retrieved from http://www.infanthearing.org/ebook-educating-children-dhh/chapters/14%20Chapter%2014%202017.pdf

Bowen, S. K. (2016). Early intervention: A multicultural perspective on d/Deaf and hard of hearing multilingual learners. *American Annals of the Deaf, 161*(1), 33–42.

Bruce, S. M., & Borders, C. (2015). Communication and language in learners who are deaf and hard of hearing with disabilities: Theories, research, and practice. *American Annals of the Deaf, 160*(4), 368–384.

Bruce, S. M., Nelson, C., Perez, A., Stutzman, B., & Barnhill, B. A. (2016). The state of research on communication and literacy in deafblindness. *American Annals of the Deaf, 161*(4), 424–443.

Burke, M. (2014). *Ableism in the Deaf community and the field of deaf students: Through the eyes of a DeafDisabled person* (Unpublished doctoral dissertation). Gallaudet University, Washington, DC.

Cannon, J. E., Guardino, C., & Gallimore, E. (2016). A new kind of heterogeneity: What we can learn from d/deaf and hard of hearing multilingual learners. *American Annals of the Deaf*, 161(1), 8–16.

Cawthon, S. (2011). *Accountability-based reforms: The impact on deaf and hard of hearing students*. Washington, DC: Gallaudet University Press.

Cawthon, S. W., Leppo, R., & Pepnet 2 Research and Evidence Synthesis Team. (2013). Accommodations quality for students who are d/Deaf or hard of hearing. *American Annals of the Deaf*, 158(4), 438–452.

Cheng, L., & Maroonroge, S. (2017). Understanding Asian deaf culture: A multicultural perspective. In K. Christensen (Ed.), *Education deaf students in a multicultural world* (pp. 97–128). San Diego, CA: DawnSignPress.

Christensen, K. (2017). *Education deaf students in a multicultural world*. San Diego, CA: DawnSignPress.

Crowe, K., & McLeod, S. (2014). A systematic review of cross-linguistic and multilingual speech and language outcomes for children with hearing loss. *International Journal of Bilingual Education and Bilingualism*, 17(3), 287–309.

Damen, S., Janssen, M. J., Ruijssenaars, W. A., & Schuengel, C. (2015). Communication between children with deafness, blindness and deafblindness and their social partners: An intersubjective developmental perspective. *International Journal of Disability, Development and Education*, 62(2), 215–243.

Denninger, M. (2017). Lesbian, gay, bisexual, and transgender deaf students: Invisible and underserved. In K. Christensen (Ed.), *Educating deaf students in a multicultural world*. San Diego, CA: DawnSignPress.

Edwards, T. (2014). *Language emergence in the Seattle DeafBlind community* (Unpublished doctoral dissertation). University of California, Berkeley.

Erickson, K., & Quick, N. (2017). The profiles of students with significant cognitive disabilities and known hearing loss. *The Journal of Deaf Studies and Deaf Education*, 22(1), 35–48.

Gallaudet Research Institute. (2013). *Regional and national summary report of data from the 2011–2012. Annual Survey of Deaf and Hard of Hearing Children and Youth*. Washington, DC: Gallaudet Research Institute, Gallaudet University.

Gárate, M. (2011). Educating children with cochlear implants in an ASL/English bilingual classroom. In R. Paludneviciene & I. W. Leigh (Eds.), *Cochlear implants: Evolving perspectives* (pp. 206–228). Washington, DC: Gallaudet University Press.

Gárate, M. (2012). *ASL/English bilingual education* (Research Brief No. 8). Washington, DC: Visual Language and Visual Learning Science of Learning Center.

Garberoglio, C. L., Palmer, J., Cawthon, S., & Sales, A. (2019). *Deaf people and educational attainment in the United States*. Washington, DC: U.S. Department of Education, Office of Special Education Programs.

García-Fernández, C. M. (2014). *Deaf-Latina/Latino critical theory in education: The lived experiences and multiple intersecting identities of deaf-Latina/o high school students* (Unpublished doctoral dissertation). University of Texas, Austin.

Geslin, J. (2010). *Deaf bilingual education: A comparison of the academic performance of deaf children of deaf parents and deaf children of hearing parents* (Unpublished doctoral dissertation). Indiana University, Bloomington.

Guardino, C., & Cannon, J. E. (2015). Theory, research, and practice for students who are deaf and hard of hearing with disabilities: Addressing the challenges from birth to postsecondary education. *American Annals of the Deaf*, 160(4), 347–355.

Hall, W. C. (2017). What you don't know can hurt you: The risk of language deprivation by impairing sign language development in deaf children. *Maternal and Child Health Journal*, 21(5), 961–965.

Individuals With Disabilities Education Act (IDEA), 34 CFR §300.34 (a). (2004).

Hamilton, B. (2017). *The Deaf Mentor Program: Benefits to families and professionals* (Unpublished doctoral dissertation). Lamar University, Beaumont, TX.

Holcomb, T., Love, A., Nakahara, C., & Ostrove, J. (2017). Preparing future American sign language/English interpreters of color: Lessons learned from an interpreter preparation program. In K. Christensen (Ed.), *Educating deaf students in a multicultural world* (pp. 175–201). San Diego, CA: DawnSign Press.

Horn-Marsh, P. (2016). Standards movement. In G. Gertz & P. Boudreault (Eds.), *The Sage deaf studies encyclopedia* (p. 941). Thousand Oaks, CA: Sage.

Individuals With Disabilities Education Act, Pub. L101-476, 20 U.S.C. & 1401 et seq. (1990).

Jackson, R. L., Ammerman, S. B., & Trautwein, B. A. (2015). Deafness and diversity: Early intervention. *American Annals of the Deaf, 160*(4), 356–367.

Joint Committee on Infant Hearing. (2007). Year 2007 position statement: Principles and guidelines for early hearing detection and intervention programs. *Pediatrics, 120*(4), 898–921.

Kirchner, C. (2019). TRIPOD: Answer to the seeds of discontent. In M. Marschark, S. Antia, & H. Knoors (Eds.), *Co-enrollment in deaf education*. New York, NY: Oxford University Press.

Kite, B. (2017). *Family language policy in American Sign Language and English bilingual families* (Unpublished doctoral dissertation). Gallaudet University, Washington, DC.

Lee, C., & Paul, P. V. (2019). Deaf middle school students' comprehension of relational language in arithmetic compare problems. *Human: Journal for Interdisciplinary Studies, 9*(1), 4–23.

Leigh, I., & Andrews, J. F. (2017). *Deaf people and society: Psychological, sociological, and educational perspectives* (2nd ed.). New York, NY: Routledge.

Light, J., & McNaughton, D. (2014). Communicative competence for individuals who require augmentative and alternative communication: A new definition for a new era of communication? *Augmentative and Alternative Communication, 30*(1), 1–18.

Luft, P. (2015). Transition services for DHH adolescents and young adults with disabilities: Challenges and theoretical frameworks. *American Annals of the Deaf, 160*(4), 395–414.

Maher, J. (1996). *Seeing language in sign: The work of William C. Stokoe*. Washington, DC: Gallaudet University Press.

Marschark, M., Antia, S., & Knoors, H. (Eds.). (2019). *Co-enrollment in deaf education*. New York, NY: Oxford University Press.

Mayberry, R. (2002). Cognitive development in deaf children: The interface of language and perception n neuropsychology. In S. J. Segalowitz & I. Rapin (Eds.), *Handbook of neuropsychology* (2nd ed., Vol 8, Part II, pp. 71–107). Amsterdam, Netherlands: Elsevier Science B.V.

McKay-Cody, M. (2019). *Memory comes before knowledge—North American Indigenous Deaf: Socio-cultural study of rock/picture writing, community, sign languages, and kinship* (Unpublished doctoral dissertation). University of Oklahoma, Norman.

Mitchell, R. E., & Karchmer, M. (2004). Chasing the mythical ten percent: Parental hearing status of deaf and hard of hearing students in the United States. *Sign Language Studies, 4*(2), 138–163.

Northern, J., & Downs, M. (2014). *Hearing in children* (6th ed.). San Diego, CA: Plural Publishing.

Nover, S., Andrews, J., Baker, S., Everhart, V., & Bradford, M. (2002). *ASL/English bilingual instruction for deaf students: Evaluation and impact study* (Final report 1997–2002). Santa Fe: New Mexico School for the Deaf.

Nover, S. M. (2000). *History of language planning in deaf education: The 19th century* (Unpublished dissertation). University of Arizona, Tuscon.

Nussbaum, D., Scott, S., & Simms, L. (2012). The "why" and "how" of an ASL/English bimodal bilingual program. *Odyssey, 13*, 14–19.

O'Brien, C., Kuntze, M., & Appanah, T. (2015). Culturally relevant leadership: A deaf education cultural approach. Book review. *American Annals of the Deaf, 159*(3), 296–301.

Olivia, G., & Lytle, L. (2014). *Turning the tide: Making life better for deaf and hard of hearing schoolchildren.* Washington, DC: Gallaudet University Press.

Parasnis, I. (1996). *Cultural and language diversity and the deaf experience.* Cambridge, UK: Cambridge University Press.

Parks, E. (2009). *Deaf and hard of hearing homeschoolers: Sociocultural motivation and approach* (Work Papers of the Summer Institute of Linguistics, University of North Dakota Session, Vol. 49). University of North Dakota. Grand Forks, ND. Retrieved from http://arts-sciences.und.edu/summer-institute-of-linguistics/work-papers/_files/docs/2009-parks.pdf

Paul, P. (2015). d/Deaf and hard of hearing with a disability or an additional disability: The need for theory, research, and practice. *American Annals of the Deaf, 160*(4), 339–343.

Philip, M. J., & Small, A. (1991). *Bilingual bicultural program development at the learning center for deaf children.* Framingham, MA: Learning Center for Deaf Children.

Qi, S., & Mitchell, R. E. (2012). Large-scale academic achievement testing of deaf and hard-of-hearing students: Past, present, and future. *Journal of Deaf Studies and Deaf Education, 17*(1), 1–18.

Roberson, L., & Shaw, S. (2018). *Signed language interpreting in the 21st century: Foundations and practice.* Gallaudet University Press: Washington, D.C.

Schein, J. (1981). *A rose for tomorrow: The biography of Frederick C. Schreiber.* Silver Spring, MD: National Association for the Deaf.

Simms, L., Rusher, M., Andrews, J. F., & Coryell, J. (2008). Apartheid in deaf education: Examining workforce diversity. *American Annals of the Deaf, 153*(4), 384–395.

Simms, L., & Thumann, H. (2007). In search of a new, linguistically and culturally sensitive paradigm in deaf education. *American Annals of the Deaf, 152*(3), 302–311.

Smith, D., & Andrews, J. (2015). Deaf and hard of hearing faculty in higher education: Enhancing access, equity, policy, and practice. *Disability & Society, 30*(10), 1521–1536.

Steinberg, A. G., Davila, J. R., Collazo Sr, J., Loew, R. C., & Fischgrund, J. E. (1997). "A little sign and a lot of love . . . ": Attitudes, perceptions, and beliefs of Hispanic families with deaf children. *Qualitative Health Research, 7*(2), 202–222.

Supalla, S. J., Small, A., & Cripps, J. S. (2013). *American Sign Language for everyone: Considerations for universal design and deaf youth identity* (Monograph Series 2). Toronto: Canadian Cultural Society of the Deaf & Knowledge Network for Applied Educational Research.

Vernon, M. (1970). The role of deaf teachers in the education of deaf children. *The Deaf American, 23,* 17–20.

Vernon, M., & Andrews, J. (1990). *The psychology of the deaf: Understanding deaf and hard of hearing people.* White Plains, NY: Longman.

Vernon, M., & Makowsky, B. (1969). Deafness and minority group dynamics. *The Deaf American, 21*(11), 3–6.

Wang, Q., Andrews, J., Liu, H. T., & Liu, C. J. (2016). Case studies of multilingual/multicultural Asian Deaf adults: Strategies for success. *American Annals of the Deaf, 161*(1), 67–88.

Williams, J. (1968). *Bilingual experiences of a deaf child* (ERIC ED030092). Retrieved from http://eric.ed.gov/?id=ED030092

Winefield, R. (1987). *Never the twain shall meet: Bell, Gallaudet, and the communications debate.* Washington, DC: Gallaudet University Press.

Wright, S. J. (2016). Diversity: Disability and deaf studies. In G. Gertz & P. Boudreault (Eds.), *The Deaf Studies encyclopedia.* Thousand Oaks, CA: Sage.

PART III

Deaf Lives, Technology, Arts, and Career Opportunities

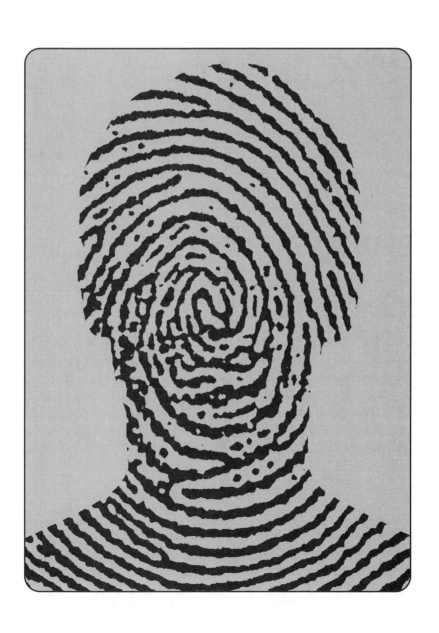

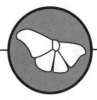

CHAPTER 6

Deaf Identities

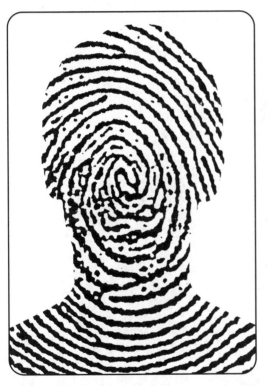

Figure 6–1. Image credit to Alexander Wilkins. Used with permission.

Identity is something we all think about, either consciously or unconsciously. It is also a very popular topic, in part because many countries have experienced an increase in diverse groups of people and in part because people outside marginalized groups are increasingly recognizing these groups. This has caused significant interest in cultural or ethnic group membership and social identity. When we ask questions about ourselves like the following, we are thinking about identity issues:

Who am I?

What is my self like?

What do I believe in?

What do I like to do?

Who do I like as my friends?

What is my personality?

In its simplest definition, identity is about how people describe themselves or how others describe them. Others may tell us we are a girl or boy, son or daughter, smart or nice, big or little, Christian, Muslim, Jewish, Hindu, or some other religion, belong to some ethnic group, and so on. We decide if these identities are true for us, and we also create our own identities. When we are in school, we can be labeled as nerds, jocks, average, basketball player, studious, academic achiever, and so on. Whether we accept these labels as our identities or not depends on how we feel about these labels. Outside of school, we may or may not identify with our family's culture, religion, or value system. When we are done with school, we may identify ourselves through our careers or occupations.

How identity develops is something that has been debated for centuries. It is well known that the self and identity have many dimensions, as shown in the tripartite model of personal identity development that lists individual, group, and universal levels (Sue & Sue, 2008) (Figure 6–2).

The individual level focuses on one's uniqueness, including genetics and experiences that are not shared, such as being treated in a certain way by a parent or play experiences in childhood. In other words, each one of us never shares the same exact experience. The group level focuses on the culture we are born into or the cultures we join. On the group level, we examine similarities and differences between ourselves and the group we are comparing ourselves to. Groups include race, sexual orientation, marital/relationship status, religion, culture, ability/disability, eth-

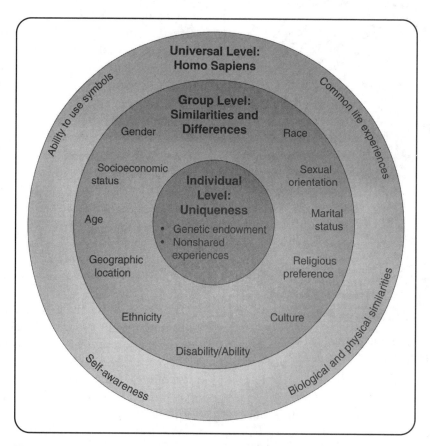

Figure 6–2. Tripartite model of personal identity development. Sue, D. W., and Sue, D. (2008). *Counseling the culturally diverse* (5th ed.). Hoboken, NJ: Wiley and Sons, p. 38. Used with permission of Wiley.

nicity, geographic location, age, socioeconomic status, gender, and language use, among others.

> Can you think of more groups? Do all the groups you can think of fit into any one of the group descriptions?

Finally, at the universal level, we are all human. Because of this, we share many similarities, including biological and physical similarities, as well as common life experiences such as birth, death, emotions, awareness about ourselves, and the ability to use symbols, especially language.

Each dimension involves a process of reflecting, accepting, and selecting identity labels based on psychological motivation, cultural knowledge, and the ability to perform appropriate roles (e.g., student, parent, worker, etc.) (Fitzgerald, 1993). It is important to understand that the meaning of each identity category will tend to change throughout life, depending on time, age, and situation. For example, what it means to be a girl at age 6 is not the same as at ages 20, 50, or 80.

DEAF IDENTITIES

When we ask a group of deaf older students or adults how they may describe themselves, very often the word *deaf* will come up. Some individuals are born deaf. They may accept or not accept calling themselves deaf or Deaf, depending on their situation or experience. This can change over time. Those individuals who identify themselves as culturally Deaf are individuals who use ASL (in the United States or Canada) or the signed language of their country or community, feel strongly that being Deaf is just fine or a gain, socialize with and get support from other culturally Deaf persons, and live a "Deaf" way of life. They feel at home with each other.

> Edmund Booth, an 1800s Deaf pioneer, became deaf from spinal meningitis at age 4. His mother taught him to read and he learned fingerspelling. He never met a deaf person until he entered the American Asylum for the Education and Instruction of Deaf and Dumb Persons, now known as the American School for the Deaf, in Hartford, Connecticut, at age 16. On his first day at school, "I was among strangers but knew I was at home" (Lang, 2004, p. 5). He is pictured in Figure 6–3.

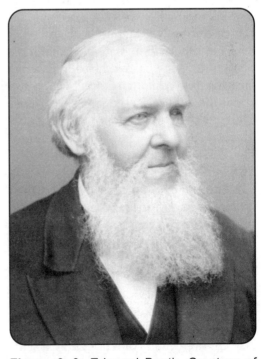

Figure 6–3. Edmund Booth. Courtesy of Gallaudet University Archives.

Could Deaf identity be called a core identity? It all depends. Corker (1996) compares core identity to personal identity. Both are identities that focus on how individuals primarily identify themselves internally and feel who they are. These are strong identities.

Personal identities start within the family of origin. The family of origin teaches the child about the family's cultural and ethnic heritages. As Irene W. Leigh (2009) explains it, a deaf child growing up in a culturally Deaf family will absorb a Deaf identity because that is the culture of the family. Therefore, it is a personal or core identity. Culturally Deaf parents do have hearing children. The hearing children's core identities may start off as culturally Deaf within their family of origin, and their first language will be ASL. As they move into the neighborhood and school, they will be increasingly exposed to English and their identities as hearing children will start to emerge. Over time, their core identities may evolve into a combination of culturally Deaf and hearing.

It is important to remember that most deaf children are born to hearing parents. Hearing parents often know very little about the cultural heritages of Deaf people. How their deaf child integrates a deaf identity depends on how the parents and the family talk about the deaf part. The deaf part starts as the sensory experience of using the eyes and hands and not so much the ears (or using the ears through hearing aids or cochlear implants) and mouths. There are also issues related to language development that differ from how hearing children develop language. Social and cultural exposures are also factors. How much exposure the child has at school or at camps where there are other deaf children, many of whom may be culturally Deaf or use ASL, may also influence how the child creates a deaf identity. That is why Deaf is not necessarily a core identity, at least not at first, for this group of deaf children whose core identities, whether consciously or unconsciously, may be ethnically or racially based.

Hilde's Norwegian family and surroundings did not reinforce being deaf as positive (Breivik, 2005). Hilde did not accept herself as deaf. Gradually, she felt something was really wrong. She was never going to be a hearing person. After meeting Deaf peers at Deaf culture events and experiencing easy communication with them, she started to feel a sense of pride in being Deaf as a strongly internalized identity and comfort as part of a culturally Deaf community.

As a deaf person in a hearing family, Tina knew she was different as a deaf person early on because of her mother being hearing, as she explained it. Tina was not really conscious about herself being Black until she entered a school for the deaf where almost everyone was white (Mauldin & Fannon, 2020).

If interactions with other deaf persons are a positive experience, and if the family is supportive of encouraging the child to be comfortable as a deaf child, it becomes easier for that child to feel a strong sense of deaf identity. If kids make fun of a child's not speaking well, it will be harder for that child to feel positive about a deaf identity. For example, Elisa Cimento (pictured in Figure 6–4) felt dif-

Categories of Deaf Identities

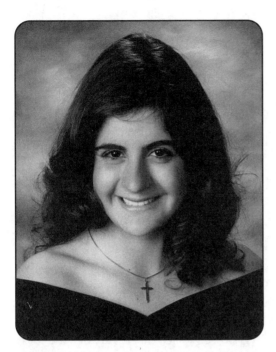

Figure 6–4. Elisa Cimento. Used with permission of Elisa Cimento.

ferent and this embarrassed her. She had worked to hide her deafness and blend in with hearing classmates at her mainstream school, where she was the only deaf student. But then one summer, she participated in a national conference that included a program track for deaf high school peers from the mainstream, most of whom were the only deaf students in their schools. At the conference, she realized that she was no longer alone and had new connections with other deaf teenagers who were fine about being deaf and having auditory aids, including hearing aids and cochlear implants. She now had the motivation to stop feeling shame as a deaf person and reveal herself as a teenager with a solid, positive, proud deaf identity. She was able to state, "I no longer feel ashamed of who I am; instead, those who treat me as less than I am are now the problem, not me" (Cimento, 2013, p. 44).

There are different deaf identities. Some may call themselves "big D" deaf, others "little d" deaf. Some will say they don't hear too well and avoid the word *deaf*. At times, they may call themselves hard of hearing, hearing impaired, or late deafened. It is not easy to know the meaning of each of these identity categories because they can be quite broad. Researchers have tried to develop theoretical frameworks that help explain specific deaf identity categories. Here, we describe a few theories that support categories of deaf identities. The theories that are listed here were developed by psychologists.

Disability Framework

One theoretical framework is that of disability. In 1986, Weinberg and Sterritt wanted to better understand how deaf persons identify themselves and how this may be associated with psychological adjustment. They used the medical model of deafness as a disability to describe possible identity categories. This model is different from the sociolinguistic model that describes deaf people as a cultural minority. The authors defined deaf children as having a disability. Their categories are as follows:

Hearing Identification = able-bodied

Deaf Identification = disabled

Dual Identification = identification with both able-bodied and disabled worlds

Weinberg and Sterritt acknowledged the potential negative impact of using their disability-related categories. They wrote that when parents do not encourage their deaf children to use sign language and minimize identifying them as deaf, their children could possibly feel inferior because they cannot be "able-bodied," especially when they see themselves as physically able.

To do their study, Weinberg and Sterritt developed the Deaf Identity Scale using items that would place deaf adolescent participants into these three identity categories. They found that most of their participants were labeled as Dual Identification. This group was also the best adjusted overall compared to those who were in the Deaf Identification and Hearing Identification categories. This may have been the first formal research study that created an identity category that covered identifying with both hearing and Deaf cultures.

Social Identity Theory

The social identity theory, developed by Tajfel (1981), suggests that group relationships and social orientations are important for identity. If the minority status individual is not comfortable with a minority group, he or she will not join that group. If the individual is able to see that minority group as empowering, that person will move to join that group. Here we explain how the theory may apply to deaf students who are introduced to Deaf peers.

If Max grew up in a mainstream school where he was the only deaf student and never met a Deaf person who communicated using ASL until he started at a high school that had a deaf program for students who lived in the area, how might he start connecting with the Deaf students in that program? Would he be uncomfortable at first, or would he just be curious?

Processes in developing a Deaf identity based on social identity theory:

1. If Max does not have a satisfactory social identity as a Deaf person, he may be uncomfortable about the Deaf students in his high school program. But after seeing how much these Deaf students interact with each other, he may become curious. This may encourage a psychological process that pushes him to connect positively with the Deaf student group, even though it is a minority or possibly stigmatized group (stigmatized by hearing students). This will help him feel better about himself.
2. Max changes his behavior to behave similarly to those within the new Deaf group by learning ASL and how to communicate with his new Deaf friends.
3. Max internalizes the social name or category of this new Deaf group as part of his identity and proudly states that he is Deaf.

Researchers have studied high school adolescents using this theory. If students are able to participate in activities with Deaf peers, feel that the activities are right for them, feel connected or related to their Deaf peers, and feel competent in communicating with their Deaf friends, they are socially oriented to Deaf groups. In one study that used the Social Activity Scale to measure social orientation using 451 high school students in mainstream schools, researchers found that the majority of the students (37.1%) were socially oriented to both hearing and deaf peers, while 30.3% were mostly oriented to deaf peers and 12.4% were oriented to hearing peers (Kluwin & Stinson, 1993). Representing the remainder, 20.2% were not oriented to either group.

> How would you feel if you did not belong to any group in high school or college?

Communication and language issues were important in this study. Those deaf students who were oriented to Deaf peers had profound hearing levels and preferred to use sign language or knew it, while those oriented to hearing peers preferred spoken language and had less severe hearing levels. The other two groups fell into the middle for how well they thought they knew sign language. Many follow-up studies have generally supported the findings from this research project. The bottom line is that language and communication competency help support relationships. If there is shared communication, and this communication is going well, whether in a signed or spoken language, whether the person has a cochlear implant or not, this will positively influence social relationships and social identity, whether hearing oriented, Deaf oriented, or both.

Racial Identity Development Framework

Theorists have studied how people in racial minority groups become aware of their racial identities (e.g., Atkinson, Morten, & Sue, 1989; Wijeyesinghe & Jackson, 2012). Their models focus on how members of oppressed racial or ethnic groups develop a positive identity in difficult situations. See Table 6–1 for an example of a racial/cultural identity development model. We explain this model and then later show how it may apply to deaf people.

As you may notice, in Stage 1, which is the Preencounter or Conformity stage, members of minority groups strongly prefer the values of the majority or dominant culture. They believe it is important to be as much like the majority culture as possible. In the United States, this means striving to assimilate white people's ways. They do not fully accept their minority culture and may feel uncomfortable at times. They may want to have white friends and join white groups.

However, if they have negative experiences with some white people, experience rejection because they are not white, or hear news about reports of discrimination against their minority group, they may experience Dissonance/Encounter. That is Stage 2. Another possibility is that they see a strong leader, a great actor, or some other famous person who is a member of their minority group. In that stage, they begin to realize that being a minority can be acceptable and that becoming as "white" as possible is never going to be possible. Then they may experience Dissonance/Encounter. Whatever their experience, their old beliefs begin to crumble. They start questioning their old beliefs and begin to think that the majority or white culture is not that superior after all. This stage is not a stage that always happens quickly. It takes time for people to enter and move through this stage.

In moving through Stage 2, minority group members start to get a greater understanding of the problems in trying so hard to be a member of the majority culture. They may start to feel guilt, shame, or anger about not recognizing the problems that come up in dealing with the majority culture. The majority culture does have

Table 6–1. Racial/Cultural Identity Development

Stages of Development	Description
Stage 1: Preencounter or Conformity	Believes that one should integrate into the majority culture. This means conforming to its values. Most often this means conforming to white culture values.
Stage 2: Dissonance/Encounter	The person experiences or hears about discrimination. There is realization that conforming to the majority culture is not going to work. The person starts the process of thinking differently about her or his racial/cultural identity.
Stage 3: Resistance and Immersion	The person supports only the minority culture and goes against the majority culture. Racism, oppression, and discrimination are important topics. Feelings are very strong.
Stage 4: Internalization/Introspection	The minority identity is internalized and appreciated. The person now feels more comfortable about reaching out to other groups.
Stage 5: Integrative Awareness	Can appreciate oneself, feels secure inside, and can appreciate other cultures. Recognizes the strengths and problems in each culture.

Sources: Adapted from Atkinson, Morten, and Sue (1989); Cross (1995); Parham and Helms (1985); Sue and Sue (2008).

its own problems. Individuals may realize that they have been brainwashed to believe in the majority culture. The feelings build up and they move into Stage 3, which involves Resistance and Immersion. They resist the majority culture and feel it is important to fully immerse into the minority culture, which "is the best." They will not criticize the minority culture at this time.

However, we know that no culture is perfect. In time, it is going to become clear that there are problems with the minority culture. The values of the minority culture may not always match the person's inner values. And sometimes, it becomes clear that there are some good things about the

majority culture. It no longer makes sense to resist the majority culture 100%. That is why this Stage 4 is called the Internalization/Introspection stage. The internalization of the minority culture has been successful, and the person now has worked through the negative emotions of guilt, shame, and anger. Now is the time for introspection, when the person can think about the balance between the positive and negative examples of the majority culture as well as the minority culture.

Finally, if all goes well, the person moves into Stage 5, Integrative Awareness. The introspection work has been done. The person now feels secure inside and can appreciate the majority culture as well as other cultures. There is more flexibility about moving between cultures and the person is now more accepting of diverse people.

The stage model does not always follow in sequence. Can you explain why? Do all Black people, Indigenous people, and other people of color start with Stage 1 or not?

Deaf Identity Development Framework

How well does this kind of model fit deaf people? Neil Glickman (1996) writes that deaf individuals are part of a minority group and share life experiences and oppression just as minority group members do. Chapter 8 explains what this is about. Because of these experiences, Glickman thought that the racial/cultural

identity development model could be applied to deaf people with some modifications. He created a theory of Deaf identity development that is similar to the racial/cultural identity development model. See Table 6–2 for a description of this theory/model. Note the similarities and differences with Table 6–1.

In this model, to be culturally hearing (Stage 1) is to conform to the majority culture, which is hearing. What does this mean? Looking back at the Conformity stage in Table 6–1, this stage is described as believing that one should integrate into the majority culture and conform to its values. So, to be culturally hearing means that the deaf person tries to be as much like a hearing person as possible. Hearing people often see being deaf as a medical problem to be fixed either through

Table 6–2. Glickman's Theory of Deaf Identity Development

Stages of Development	Description
Stage 1: Culturally Hearing	Being deaf is seen as a medical problem to be fixed. It is better to conform to how hearing people act with each other and to follow hearing culture. This means focusing on spoken language, not signed language, and trying to be able to understand speech through hearing aids or cochlear implants. There may be denial about being deaf.
Stage 2: Marginal	The person has trouble connecting with hearing or deaf people. There is little connection with either hearing or Deaf cultures.
Stage 3: Immersion	There is enthusiastic embrace of everything Deaf. Deaf culture is the best. Hearing culture is rejected.
Stage 4: Bicultural	There is a balanced perspective about both Deaf and hearing cultures. The person can comfortably interact in both Deaf and hearing cultures. Strengths and weaknesses in both cultures are recognized.

Source: Adapted from Glickman (1996).

medical intervention (surgery to repair a dysfunctional middle ear or to insert a cochlear implant into the cochlea, which is part of the inner ear) (see Chapter 2) or through hearing aids. To be culturally hearing also suggests that the person would have a preference for spoken language. It means that the person prefers to be part of the hearing world and interact mostly with hearing people. There is little interest in finding deaf friends or learning a signed language.

> Kim's parents never told her she was deaf. They decided she should get a cochlear implant when she was 18 months old. They worked hard to help her learn how to listen and speak. Kim grew up thinking she just had a hearing problem and that was why she had a cochlear implant. Her parents enrolled her in a mainstream school where everyone was hearing. Kim had a tutor to help her with schoolwork as she could not hear everything clearly. But the tutor knew nothing about deaf people or Deaf culture, so Kim thought she was the only person in the world with a hearing problem. She worked hard to keep her hearing friends and be part of her hearing society.

To be culturally marginal (Stage 2) means that the deaf person is sort of in limbo. The deaf person has a hard time making hearing friends. That often happens when hearing children transition from play to talking among themselves as they get older. It becomes more difficult for the deaf youngster to participate in these talking conversations. If the conversation is one-on-one, friendship can develop. But if more peers join in, the deaf youngster or teenager will become frustrated while trying to follow conversations, especially when it is noisy. Then the deaf teenager feels left out. And if there are no deaf people in the area, where does the teenager belong? That is what being in a marginal stage is all about.

> Kim is now getting older. Her hearing friends are busy among themselves. They act as if it is too much trouble to include Kim. Kim begins to withdraw. Since she is not aware that she is "deaf," she is in limbo and not part of either the hearing or deaf worlds. She goes through high school that way. She tries to participate in some activities, but because of difficulties in communicating, she becomes a loner, mostly focused on her studies.

A transformation becomes possible as the deaf person makes the transition from Stage 2 to Stage 3, which is the Immersion stage. This stage combines the Racial/Cultural Identity Model Dissonance/Encounter and Resistance/Immersion stages. In other words, there is a realization that trying to be hearing is not always worth the struggle. Deaf people may see that hearing people are not always patient with them. Hearing people do not always try to include the deaf person in events or hire them for jobs. Hearing people may think that deaf applicants cannot do well in school or on the job because they cannot easily get information or follow instructions. Those kinds of experiences can be very upsetting for the deaf person. And then, the person may meet a deaf person who has lots of Deaf friends and is part of the Deaf community. As the culturally marginal deaf person sees how connected

Deaf people are and how easy communication is through sign language, there is anger at all the time wasted struggling to be hearing. That person will start to think, "No more bothering with hearing people! Hearing people are not worth all the hassle and struggle in dealing with them." There is a new fascination with everything Deaf. Immersion into Deaf culture is an exciting new experience. There is no criticism of Deaf people or Deaf culture. Sign language is preferred over spoken language.

> It is now time for college. Kim enters a community college. This college happens to have a program for deaf students. Kim is not part of that program, but she sees deaf people signing in the hallways. Then, in one of her classes, there is a deaf person, with a sign language interpreter. This access to communication catches her attention. The deaf person is not struggling like she is. Kim stops the deaf person after class to ask about the sign language interpreter. Mike, who is culturally Deaf, explains through writing that the college provides services for deaf students. He and Kim start conversing during each class. He suggests she take an ASL class. In the ASL class, Kim learns about Deaf culture. She begins to realize how much she missed. She starts going to Deaf events and gets very excited about FINALLY being part of a community. She becomes more skilled in ASL. She tells her parents how frustrated she was previously and how happy she is now. Her life is more and more with the Deaf community and she is less involved with hearing people.

Stage 4 is labeled as the Bicultural stage. Looking at Table 6–1, this stage parallels Stage 4: Internalization/Introspection and Stage 5: Integrative Awareness in the Racial/Cultural Identity Model. In these stages, the minority identity is internalized, and the person recognizes the strengths and problems in both the minority and majority cultures. This is what happens when the deaf person enters the Bicultural stage. The deaf person now realizes that not everything Deaf is perfect. Deaf people can have problems just like hearing people have problems. Yet, the person is still proud to be culturally Deaf. There is respect for both signed and spoken languages. The deaf person is comfortable communicating and collaborating with both hearing and deaf people. Perspectives about Deaf and hearing cultures are better balanced. Well-being tends to be comparatively better (see below).

> Kim experiences problems with some Deaf individuals who criticize her ASL signs and do not accept her as a Deaf person. She gets upset and realizes that not all Deaf people are wonderful. She is still proud to be Deaf and still has some Deaf friends. She decides it is best to balance both hearing and Deaf cultural experiences. She feels okay about using her spoken English as well as ASL. She is more at peace inside herself, knowing that she is bicultural and can go back and forth between hearing and Deaf cultures. She sees the Deaf part of herself as a gain that has enriched her life.

It is important to recognize that many deaf persons do not follow the Deaf Identity Development sequence. Deaf children of culturally Deaf parents are born into the culture. Because of this, they typically start their identity development in Stage 3, Immersion. One example is that of Nyle DiMarco, an actor who has performed in the TV series *Switched at Birth* and who not only became America's Next Top Model in 2015 but also won ABC's *Dancing With the Stars* competition in 2016. His parents are Deaf and part of a multigenerational Deaf family; he grew up Deaf and went to schools for the deaf. ASL is his native language, and he uses his smartphone to text with hearing peers, as seen in excerpts from the *America's Next Top Model* show. When individuals such as Nyle get exposed to the hearing world and to spoken language, they may become Bicultural as they learn more about hearing cultural values and how to interact with hearing people. Others will start off as Marginal, especially if they cannot communicate with their hearing families, and will not know where they belong. If they go to a school where there are Deaf children, they may move into the Immersion stage and then gradually become Bicultural. There are different possibilities, depending on the person and the environment. The same is true for those who are dealing with racial identity development issues.

Can you think of other possibilities? What about the culturally Deaf person who may want to immerse into the hearing world? This rarely happens, but it is something to think about. What about hearing children of Deaf parents? They are often called CODAs, which stands for Children of Deaf Adults. What might their identity sequence be like? Could their identity development be similar to that of deaf children of Deaf parents?

The four identity categories have psychological implications. The individuals in each of these categories may be emotionally and/or socially well adjusted or have problems. Research shows a trend toward comparatively better psychological adjustment for the Bicultural and Deaf acculturated groups (e.g., Hintermair, 2008; Jambor & Elliott, 2005; Maxwell-McCaw, 2001). That is not to say that the culturally hearing group is not well adjusted. Other research shows that adolescents with or without cochlear implants are equally well adjusted, whether they are hearing acculturated or Deaf acculturated (e.g., Chapman & Dammeyer, 2016; Hardy, 2010; Leigh, Maxwell-McCaw, Bat-Chava, & Christiansen, 2009; Mance & Edwards, 2012). While deaf adolescents with cochlear implants may have more opportunities to use spoken language and thus may develop hearing or bicultural identities, some nonetheless may struggle to identify with hearing society or Deaf cultures (Leigh & Andrews, 2017; Marschark, Zettler, & Dammeyer, 2017). The key is ease of communication and having friends. If the deaf person with or without cochlear implants interacts easily with hearing peers and has friends, the person will probably be identified as a part of hearing society. If communication with Deaf peers is good and the deaf person has Deaf friends, then the identity will be Deaf. If the individual feels comfortable with both hearing and Deaf peers, the deaf person falls into the Bicultural group.

Glickman developed the Deaf Identity Development Scale to show which category the person may be categorized as after filling out the scale. He used different descriptions of Deaf and hearing cultures, as well as marginal and bicultural descriptions, for participants to choose. The score reflects the person's placement in the different categories. For example, if the person likes to go to hearing events, that item will be checked as part of the Hearing category.

Acculturation Model

This model is based on the immigration experience. In other words, this model focuses on how immigrants relate to their home culture while they are learning how to deal with the culture of their new country. Immigrants, deaf as well as hearing, know the cultural behavior of their home country. They are psychologically oriented to the culture of their home country. When they enter a new country, they have to learn new cultural behaviors and figure how to handle the psychological challenges of learning new behavior. Some will decide they only want to hold on to the home culture where they are psychologically most comfortable. The process of adjusting to the culture in a different country is called acculturation.

Table 6–3 shows four different ways that immigrants can adjust, depending on their attitudes to their home culture and the new culture. In the Assimilation Strategy, for example, Carlos wants to be as American as possible and spends a lot of time interacting with Americans. To do this, Carlos changes his name to Charles and gets away from his home culture. He feels embarrassed about his home culture. What if Carlos feels comfortable in his home culture? And what if he feels confused and overwhelmed with American culture? He may decide to stay away from American culture and just live in the area where his home culture is strong. He will then be following the Separation Strategy.

What if Carlos wants to hold on to his home culture and also be part of the new American culture by learning English, interacting with Americans as much as possible, and following American culture? This is called the Integration Strategy. And finally, if Carlos is not interested in being fully immersed in his home culture or learning how to be part of the new American culture, he can be described as marginal. This is an example of the Marginalization Strategy. It is important to remember that a lot depends on whether the new culture is welcoming of the immigrant to make the acculturation experience positive. If the American environment is not supportive of Carlos, then adjusting to American culture will be difficult. Also, we have to think of Carlos's personality. Is

Table 6–3. Four Different Acculturation Strategies

Acculturation Strategies	Description
1. Assimilation Strategy	Give up the home culture identity and work to fully interact with the new culture.
2. Separation Strategy	Hold on to the home culture identity. Avoid interacting with the new culture.
3. Integration Strategy	Hold on to the home culture identity. At the same time, work on interacting with the new culture.
4. Marginalization Strategy	Little interest in maintaining cultural identity with either the home culture or the new culture.

Source: Adapted from Berry (2002).

he timid, shy, quiet, assertive, strong, out-spoken, or what? This can also influence how Carlos will experience acculturation to the new culture. Will Americans accept Carlos or not?

Can you see how these four strategies parallel the racial identity development categories of conformity, dissonance, resistance, and integration? Deborah Maxwell-McCaw (2001) saw the parallels and started thinking about how deaf people may get into Deaf culture. She saw this not as a racial identity development process but rather as acculturation. She wrote that Glickman's deaf identity development theory focuses on internal feelings about identity, related to psychological feelings about self and others. Her theory uses the same categories as Glickman's theory: Culturally Hearing, Marginal, Culturally Deaf, and Bicultural. She felt it was necessary to add behavior types that support each specific identity.

This is because being in a culture is not just about feelings but also how well the person knows the culture and behaves in the culture. Is the person competent in the culture? Does the person use the language of the culture? Becoming culturally competent in a particular culture is part of the acculturation experience. Acculturation can be at different levels, from little or no acculturation to very heavily acculturated, depending on how the person feels. See Table 6–4 to view the different cultural/behavior types of acculturation that Maxwell-McCaw developed to show how well a person may acculturate to Deaf or hearing cultures.

The first domain is that of Cultural Identification. Maria, who happens to be deaf, is exploring Deaf culture. She knows that right now she is more comfortable with hearing people and is psychologically connected with them. She is not that comfortable with culturally Deaf people.

Table 6–4. Five Domains of Acculturation for Deaf and Hearing Cultures

Acculturation Domains	Description
1. Cultural Identification	Psychological identification with deaf or hearing people. Who are you most comfortable with: deaf or hearing people?
2. Cultural Involvement	How much is one involved in Deaf cultural activities or in hearing cultural activities?
3. Cultural Preferences	Do you prefer to be with Deaf or with hearing people?
4. Language Competence	How well does one sign and understand a signed language, for example, ASL? And how well does one speak and understand the spoken language, for example, English?
5. Cultural Knowledge	How well do you know Deaf culture, such as favorite jokes? Hearing culture, such as nursery rhymes?

Source: Adapted from Maxwell-McCaw (2001); Maxwell-McCaw and Zea (2011).

Thinking about the second domain, Cultural Involvement, how involved is Maria with hearing cultural activities compared to Deaf cultural activities? She is new to Deaf culture, so her involvement right now may be quite limited. It could increase depending on whether she can become more comfortable at Deaf cultural activities.

What about Cultural Preferences (the third domain)? Maria may prefer to be with hearing family members, partners, or school or work colleagues. Or she may be feeling very frustrated because of communication problems and start to prefer to be with deaf peers. Or is she going to prefer both hearing and culturally Deaf people, in balance? As for the fourth domain, Language Competence, it all depends on Maria's fluency in English versus her fluency in ASL. She may speak English well. As part of her exploration of Deaf culture, she is learning ASL. If her ASL is still weak, it will be difficult for her to identify with Deaf culture. And finally, the fifth domain has to do with Cultural Knowledge. How well does Maria know hearing culture ways of believing and behaving versus how well does she know Deaf culture ways of believing and behaving? For example, does she know that in hearing society, people see the ears as the only way to access language, while in Deaf culture, people say the eyes are most important in accessing language, especially through signs or the printed word?

These five dimensions are part of the Deaf Acculturation Scale, a measure that was developed to identify whether one is Hearing Acculturated (high scores on hearing items such as, "I am most comfortable with other hearing people" and low scores on deaf items), Deaf Acculturated (high scores on deaf items such as, "How well do you sign ASL?" and low

scores on hearing items), Bicultural (high scores on both hearing and deaf items), and Marginal (low scores on both hearing and deaf items) (Maxwell-McCaw, 2001; Maxwell-McCaw & Zea, 2011). This measure was developed based on a largely white sample. In a preliminary study, Nelson Schmitt and Leigh (2015) used this measure on a sample of Black deaf individuals and noted the possibility of identity concerns specific to Black deaf people that differed from the original white deaf sample and recommended ongoing research to further understand this phenomenon.

The Narrative Approach

There are researchers who feel that just figuring out identities based on surveys and measures are too limiting. They prefer the narrative approach. When people tell stories about their experiences and their feelings about themselves, researchers can get rich information about identities. They do that by examining themes from the people's life stories to describe individuals and how their interactions with others influence what identity they have.

One researcher, Stein Erik Ohna (2004), interviewed 22 deaf Norwegian adults. These interviews provided data that he analyzed. During his analysis, he looked for themes that suggested transition points or phases in the process of deaf identity development. See Table 6–5 for the phases that he identified from his interview data. Can you see the similarities between the phases in Table 6–5 and the deaf identity categories in Table 6–2? It is interesting how data from both interviews and measurements support each other.

Do keep in mind that Deaf persons with Deaf parents may start from a

Table 6–5. Deaf Identity Development Phases for Deaf Adults With Hearing Parents

Phases in Deaf Identity Development	Description
Phase 1: Taken-for-Granted Phase	Taking for granted I am like hearing people. Even if I meet deaf persons, I still feel I am like hearing people.
Phase 2: Alienation Phase	Acknowledging that hearing people don't understand me and I don't understand them.
Phase 3: Affiliation Phase	I start to recognize Deaf as an identity and want to connect with Deaf people as we understand each other. Hearing people become different.
Phase 4: Deaf-in-My-Own-Way Phase	I am more comfortable with both Deaf and hearing people. I try to help hearing people understand me as a Deaf person.

Source: Adapted from Ohna (2004).

different center. In Phase 1, the taken-for-granted phase may involve not only Ericka's feelings of similarity with hearing people but also with culturally Deaf people, starting with her Deaf parents. When communicating with hearing people becomes a problem, Ericka starts to feel alienated from them as part of the alienation phase. At the same time, she feels strongly connected with Deaf people, thus moving into the affiliation phase. Finally, similarly to deaf adults with hearing parents, Ericka starts to balance her feelings for both deaf and hearing people as part of the deaf-in-my-own-way phase.

To sum up, Ohna shows that alienation, affiliation, language and communication, and hearing and deaf environments all interact to help the individual create his or her own deaf identity. Following Ohna, Mauldin and Fannon's (2020) interviews with five deaf, racially diverse lesbians and gays revealed how affilia-tions with Deaf people and transitioning into Deaf culture happened in stages as they were exposed to other Deaf individuals on and off and reevaluating how much they accepted themselves as Deaf. As they actively inserted themselves in the Deaf community, they could actively assert their Deaf identity and demand accommodations. Mauldin and Fannon also write about obtrusiveness, meaning ways different stigmas may come in and out of focus, depending on the situation and relationships. For example, if hearing classmates do not invite their Deaf classmates to a social event and the Deaf classmates find out, they have to make a choice in how to manage future interactions with their hearing classmates depending on what Deaf identity they have internalized.

A recent study reporting on interviews with five Saudi Arabian deaf college students in the United States illustrates the complexity of acculturating to a new country (Alzahrani, 2017). Difficulty learning English, being homesick, finding halal food, and dealing with the individualistic philosophy of the United States as opposed to the collective culture in the home country complicated the acculturation experience. In contrast, recognizing that "Deaf same" helped their connection with Deaf peers at Gallaudet University plus moving from the "Deaf can't" framework of their home culture to a "Deaf can" study anything or do anything in contrast to being forced into only the deaf education track in their home country contributed to an enhanced Deaf identity. At the same time, they kept their Saudi identity and held on to their core cultural beliefs, including praying at designated times and women continuing to wear the hijab. Where do you think they fit within Ohna's phases?

Can people be boxed into categories? Every time people describe themselves, their stories or their narratives can vary. Much depends on their situation. If Dan is in the Immersion category and mistrusts hearing people because his hearing coworkers ignore him and his supervisor has not recommended him for a raise, perhaps one day he has a positive interaction with a hearing coworker who accepts him as a culturally Deaf person. He can still be in the Immersion category and avoid hearing people, but on that one day, he may be more flexible.

Deaf identities are not the only identities we must consider. As you may remember from the beginning of this chapter, everyone has multiple identities. How do these multiple identities interact with deaf identities and create feelings of oppression? This falls under the theme of intersectionality. We will explore this question in the next section.

INTERSECTIONALITY

Just like the hearing community, the deaf community is very diverse. There are differences because of race, ethnicity, religion, sexual orientation, family beliefs and values, and other factors. We start by looking at how race/ethnicity and being deaf interact with each other, using the concept of intersectionality (Crenshaw, 1989). Intersectionality is defined as how race, class, gender, and other individual characteristics intersect and create the potential for overlapping discriminatory experiences. Within the contexts of race/ethnicity and being deaf, these experiences will exacerbate feelings of oppression. Issues related to oppression are discussed in Chapter 8. Much of the literature on intersectionality has shifted its focus to how identity aspects interact with each other despite the fact that the original focus was on how racism and sexism lead to complex interactions of oppressive overlays. The sections below focus on identity aspects, while Chapter 7 describes individuals who are part of various Deaf communities within the larger Deaf community. We acknowledge that the issue of intersectionality issues for Deaf people is an area ripe for research as the literature on this topic continues to be limited (Cawthon, Johnson, Garberoglio, & Schoffstall, 2016; Mauldin & Fannon, 2020; Ruiz-Williams, Burke, Chong, & Chainarong, 2015).

Race/Ethnicity

As we wrote earlier in this chapter, when deaf children are born to hearing families, "deaf" may not be their core identity, even if they see themselves as the "different" ones in their families. Race/ethnicity as part of the family's culture is more likely to be the deaf child's first or early core identity (other than gender). The deaf child will see the parents' skin color, how the parents do various activities, and how the parents show emotions. The child will consciously and/or unconsciously absorb these. It will take time for the deaf child to see that the parents respond to "something" in the environment (sounds and spoken words) that the child cannot. As the child realizes that when the hearing aid or cochlear implant is off, hearing sound or words is not possible, that is when the child begins to understand that she or he is deaf. If the parents explain that to the child as well, the child begins to internalize the label "deaf" as part of identity development. How well this internalization happens depends on the child's exposure to family communication, support from the environment, and positive or negative reactions from people whom the child sees. The child may feel culturally Deaf if he or she sees other deaf children, particularly culturally Deaf children.

If the child has culturally Deaf parents who are also a racial/ethnic minority, it is likely that the racial/ethnic identity will develop at the same time as the Deaf identity. The parents will be able to explain to the child, once the child develops understanding of ASL, who they are and who the child is, as, for example, a Black-Afro-Latinx Deaf child or a Black Jewish Deaf child.

As time goes on, the Latinx Deaf girl will begin to learn that the two identities make her a minority within a minority. She is a minority when interacting with white Deaf people because she is Latinx. It helps to understand that the Latinx Deaf culture is not the same as the non-Latinx Deaf culture because of the different cultural backgrounds. Latinx Deaf culture is more connected to the Caribbean, Central America, and South America cultural origins, while how white Deaf culture in the United States has heretofore been described is more connected to the English/Protestant tradition. Also, she is a double minority within the white hearing society because she is Latinx and Deaf. She is also a minority within the Latinx hearing population because she is Deaf. So where is the group she can identify with? Is it easy for her to find a Latinx Deaf group? It all depends on where she lives and whether there is a large Latinx Deaf community in her area. What if she and her family migrated to the United States from another country? Latinx people from the home country are not always the same as Latinx in the United States.

Moriah sees that there are ways in which she is the same as her family. Her skin color is the same as theirs. She learns to copy her parents' behavior. They teach her to follow their ways. This is all through her eyes, as she does not have a hearing aid. She sees them running to open the door and wonders: "How did they know someone is at the door?" Her parents try to explain that they hear and she does not. They point out that the fire engine is very loud. She realizes she does not hear. Moriah's parents tell her that she is deaf. That means she cannot hear. When she goes to the school for the deaf, she begins to learn ASL and starts to see herself as Deaf.

Latinx people in the United States, at least most of them, have a little bit or more of the American ways inside them. As Reichard (2015) indicates, it is not that simple to describe who the Latinx community is; it is definitely not a homogeneous community.

Hopefully this gives you a taste of how complex it is to be of two or more minorities. Each group membership requires following different norms, behavior, and values. Native American or Indigenous, Asian, Arabic, and Black Deaf people experience similar challenges. Also, we have to remember that Native Americans or Indigenous people are part of many different tribes. Asians come from many different countries, such as Korea, Thailand, Viet Nam, Japan, Cambodia, India, and China. Blacks are part of America but claim an African heritage, and there are also Blacks from the Caribbean area and Africans from Africa who have to adjust to Deaf culture in the United States (Dunn & Anderson, (2020). The same is true of Arabs, who come from Iraq, Saudi Arabia, the UAE, Egypt, and other countries. So the identification can be more within countries of origin rather than the larger Latinx, Black, Arab, or Asian Deaf communities. Now, that is even more complex!

And much depends on the situations in which Deaf people of different racial/ ethnic backgrounds find themselves. If they are with white Deaf people, how do they behave and relate to others? If they are in situations where they are with their hearing home culture, how do they manage? And so on? That shows us how important it is for identities to be solid, yet fluid, with different ways of behaving or focusing on specific identities in different situations. Obasi (2014) provides a thoughtful analysis of, for example, how an Asian Deaf woman experiences her Deaf identity as more prominent in her hearing workplace, but in other environments, her other identities may emerge as more relevant. Obasi compares identity to a dice with many different sizes; it depends on the angle that determines which identity is being shown. But even if the other angles cannot be seen, these angles are still influencing the identity that is shown.

Some people can integrate racial/ ethnic identity and Deaf identity and not keep them separate. Ralph can say, "I am Black Deaf!" That means he has integrated the Black and Deaf cultures into who he is. He supports a Black Deaf label, which shows he is different from white Deaf people, and he takes pride in that. He also is more confident within himself. With this identity, he can connect with the hearing Black culture through his Black identity, and he can connect with both Black and white Deaf communities with his Deaf identity. Black and Deaf are equally important to him. Deaf becomes more relevant when he is in a situation where there is communication difficulty, like with hearing people at work. Black becomes more relevant when he is with white people, whether hearing or deaf, either in school or at a Deaf festival. So a lot depends on where he is at any time during the day and whom he is with.

Sexual Orientation

What does it mean to be Deaf and Lesbian, Gay, Bisexual, Transgender, Queer/Questioning, or Asexual (LGBTQA)? What does it mean to be Deaf and LGBTQA and have ethnic minority status? A lot depends on how accepting the family and friends are, as well as schoolmates and coworkers. A lot also depends on cultural perspectives about people who are LGBTQA. In the United States, the ongoing publicity on the legalization of Lesbian and Gay marriages has made the topic of sexual orientation more acceptable, especially in the media. However, there are cultures and religions that are not accepting of LGBTQA individuals. It is very difficult for individuals who live in these nonaccepting entities to feel safe about coming out and being open about their sexual orientation. If they are deaf, how much more difficult might that be, especially if they are trying to find other deaf people like themselves? It is easier in the large cities, where one can find groups of LGBTQA and deaf people. But if they are members of an ethnic minority, it probably will be much more difficult to find LGBTQA deaf individuals who belong to their ethnic minority group. Although there are chat rooms on the Internet, these are not always safe for minors or adults. Can you see how challenging that can be? Chapter 7 presents various multiple identities that Deaf individuals may have and what they have done with their lives.

However, the close-knit nature of small deaf communities may make it easier for Deaf LGBTQA individuals to feel safe and connected because of their friendships within the community. The chances of their being rejected become less. But rejection is still possible. Deaf LGBTQA can find a "home" when they find others like themselves (Gutman & Zangas, 2010).

Gender and ethnic identities tend to be clear early in life. Sometimes deaf identities develop early, sometimes later. What about Lesbian, Gay, Bisexual, and Transgender identities? These tend to develop later, at various times in one's life, and the coming-out process can happen at any stage in one's life. To be Deaf, LGBTQA, and of ethnic minority status means dealing with a lot of self-acceptance and intersectionality issues related to each minority status and hoping that others accept them. The coming-out process can be easier if there is support. If not, the coming-out process can be emotionally very difficult.

> Josiah has good speech but is on the margin at hearing parties. His Deaf friends question whether he is Deaf or hard of hearing because he socializes with hearing people a lot. Because he is Gay, he is having a hard time finding other Deaf Gay peers. He is also of Asian origin and knows no one who is Deaf, Gay, and Asian like himself. His parents are not happy with his sexual orientation. Their culture and religion are not welcoming if the person is LGBTQA. The parents also want him to be as "hearing" as possible. So he has issues with figuring out his intersectional identity and feeling comfortable internally. What might work best for him?

Disability

According to Guardino and Cannon (2016), who have taken a careful look at available demographics, approximately 40% to more than 50% of the deaf and hard-of-hearing population may have additional disabilities. Even though we call these disabilities additional disabilities, they are not just additional. Instead, these disabilities interact with the deaf part and other identities the person may have. We need to understand that conditions such as cerebral palsy, blindness, autism, amputation, and intellectual or cognitive disabilities, among others, will affect communication and social opportunities. These individuals may not always be fully accepted by the Deaf community because of their disabilities (Ruiz-Williams et al., 2015). There are also cultural perspectives on disability in general and deafness in particular depending on race/ethnicity, social class, sexual orientation, and belief systems, with some cultures accepting individuals who are deaf or who have various disabilities, some cultures hiding them, and some cultures rejecting them.

Some of these individuals may have to rely on significant others such as parents or caretakers for activities of daily living or access to information. If these significant others do not accept them, they may have difficulty developing a sense of trust in themselves and a strong identity that includes their additional dis-ability, their being deaf, and everything else about themselves. Also, more likely, Deaf persons with additional disabilities may never see another person who is like them, such as another Black Deaf person with cerebral palsy. They may then feel more like they are the only ones in the world and no one else is like them. Some will wish to get rid of the part of themselves that is unacceptable in their society, while others embrace their identity and show that they can live to the fullest with what they have. A report on studies done in Scandinavia shows how important self-determination and participation in activities are for DeafBlind students as well as their relief when they are with others like themselves (Möller & Danermark, 2007).

One important point to consider when thinking about disabilities in general is that some culturally Deaf people

---

Meredith Burke describes herself as a white, DeafDisabled, queer woman growing up with cerebral palsy (Ruiz-Williams et al., 2015). In considering which terms best fit her—*Deaf or Disabled, Deaf and Disabled, and DeafDis-abled*—ultimately, as a form of self-determination, she declared that both her identities, specifically Meredith Burke and DeafDisabled, are equal and go hand in hand together (Burke, 2013).

Lisa was puzzled with how her parents kept watching her. She was doing fine on her own as a 20-year-old Deaf person, even though she had some trouble seeing things on the side. Lisa did not know that her parents knew for a long time that she would lose her sight due to Usher syndrome (a genetic syndrome that causes one to become deaf and blind). The parents never told her because they did not want to upset her. When she finally went to the eye doctor after bumping too many times into people, the doctor told her the truth. Her trust in her parents and in herself as a culturally Deaf person was shattered. She was scared she would lose her Deaf friends, who might not want to be bothered by her changing communication needs, which involve more tactile signing, with signing on the hands. She struggled with accepting herself as not just Deaf but also DeafBlind.

view themselves as a population with its own language and culture, compared to other disability groups that may have their own disability culture but not a unique language of their own. What these groups have in common is their perception that they are part of human diversity (Couser, 2005).

CONCLUSIONS

We hope you can now see how internalizing each of the marginalized identities we discussed in this chapter will help the deaf individual to get a stronger sense of self and be more confident in facing life's challenges. There are many other types of identities, including, for example, socioeconomic grouping, work, and religion, in addition to what has been discussed in this chapter. Perhaps you can think of how these additional identities will interact within the concept of intersectionality, and how oppressive experiences related to some of these identities may affect one's life. It is important to recognize that the culturally Deaf identity will be shaped through interactions with all the other minority identities. Because of these interactions and varying social contexts, the culturally Deaf identity cannot be fixed or absolute (Paul, 2014, 2018). Furthermore, De Clerck (2018) observes that "Deaf identities are increasingly understood as part of complex, multilayered, and dynamic identities" (p. 488). Recognizing all of these identities and intersectionalities will help the Deaf person feel validated.

REFERENCES

Alzahrani, A. (2017). *Attitudes of Saudi Arabian Deaf college students: Their assimilation experiences while studying in the United States* (Doctoral dissertation). Available from ProQuest Dissertations and Theses database (Proquest No. 10616590).

Atkinson, D., Morten, G., & Sue, D. W. (1989). *Counseling American minorities: A cross-cultural perspective* (3rd ed.). Dubuque, IA: W. C. Brown.

Berry, J. W. (2002). Conceptual approaches to acculturation. In K. Chun, P. B. Organista, & G. Marín (Eds.), *Acculturation* (pp. 17–37). Washington, DC: American Psychological Association.

Breivik, J.-K. (2005). *Deaf identities in the making.* Washington, DC: Gallaudet University Press.

Burke, M. (2013). Speakout: Deaf or Disabled, Deaf and Disabled, or DeafDisabled. *The Buff and Blue.* Retrieved from http://www.thebuffandblue.net/?p=11156

Cawthon, S. W., Johnson, P. M., Garberoglio, C. L., & Schoffstall, S. J. (2016). Role models as facilitators of social capital for deaf individuals: A research synthesis. *American Annals of the Deaf, 161*(2), 115–127. https://doi.org/10.1353/aad.2016.0021

Chapman, M., & Dammeyer, J. (2016). The significance of deaf identity for psychological well-being. *Journal of Deaf Studies and Deaf Education, 22,* 187–194. https://doi.org/10.1093/deafed/enw073

Cimento, E. (2013, May/June). LOFT-y connections: Accepting my deafness and getting an internship. *Volta Voices,* pp. 44–45.

Corker, M. (1996). *Deaf transitions.* London, UK: Jessica Kingsley.

Couser, G. T. (2005). *Disability as diversity: A difference with a difference.* Retrieved from https://periodicos.ufsc.br/index.php/desterro/article/download/7325/6748

Crenshaw, K. (1989). Demarginalizing the intersection of race and sex: A Black feminist critique of antidiscrimination doctrine, feminist theory, and antiracist politics. *University of Chicago Legal Forum, 140,* 139–167.

Cross, W. E. (1995). The psychology of Nigrescence: Revising the Cross model. In J. G. Ponterotto, M. Casas, L. A. Suzuki, & C. M. Alexander (Eds.), *Handbook of multicultural counseling* (pp. 93–122). Thousand Oaks, CA: Sage.

De Clerck, G. (2018). A sustainability perspective on the potentialities of being deaf: Toward further reflexivity in Deaf Studies and deaf education. *American Annals of the Deaf, 163*(4), 480–489. https://doi.org/10.1353/aad.2018.0031

Dunn, L. & Anderson, G. (2020). Examining the intersectionality of Deaf identity, race/ethnicity, and diversity through a Black Deaf lens. In I. W. Leigh & C. A. O'Brien (Eds.), *Deaf identities: Exploring new frontiers* (pp. 279-304. New York, NY: Oxford University Press.

Fitzgerald, T. (1993). *Metaphors of identity.* Albany: State University of New York Press.

Glickman, N. (1996). The development of culturally deaf identities. In N. Glickman & M. Harvey (Eds.), *Culturally affirmative psychotherapy with deaf persons* (pp. 115–153). Mahwah, NJ: Lawrence Erlbaum.

Guardino, C., & Cannon, S. (2016). Deafness and diversity: Reflections and directions. *American Annals of the Deaf, 161*(1), 104–112. https://doi.org/10.1353/aad.2016.0016

Gutman, V., & Zangas, T. (2010). Therapy issues with lesbians, gay men, bisexuals and transgender individuals who are deaf. In I. W. Leigh (Ed.), *Psychotherapy with deaf clients from diverse groups* (2nd ed., pp. 85–108). Washington, DC: Gallaudet University Press.

Hardy, J. (2010). The development of a sense of identity in deaf adolescents in mainstream schools. *Educational and Child Psychology, 27*, 58–67.

Hintermair, M. (2008). Self-esteem and satisfaction with life of deaf and hard-of-hearing people: A resource-oriented approach to identity work. *Journal of Deaf Studies and Deaf Education, 13*, 278–300.

Jambor, E., & Elliott, M. (2005). Self-esteem and coping strategies among deaf students. *Journal of Deaf Studies and Deaf Education, 10*, 63–81.

Kluwin, T., & Stinson, M. (1993). *Deaf students in local public high schools: Background, experiences, and outcomes.* Springfield, IL: Charles C Thomas.

Lang, H. (2004). *Edmund Booth: Deaf pioneer.* Washington, DC: Gallaudet University Press.

Leigh, I. W. (2009). *A lens on deaf identities.* New York, NY: Oxford University Press.

Leigh, I. W., & Andrews, J. (2017). *Deaf people and society: Psychological, sociological, and educational perspectives* (2nd ed.). New York, NY: Routledge.

Leigh, I. W., Maxwell-McCaw, D., Bat-Chava, Y., & Christiansen, J. (2009). Correlates of psychosocial adjustment in deaf adolescents with and without cochlear implants: A preliminary investigation. *Journal of Deaf Studies and Deaf Education, 14*, 244–259.

Mance, J., & Edwards, L. (2012). Deafness related perceptions and psychological well-being in deaf adolescents with cochlear implants. *Cochlear Implants International, 13*, 93–104.

Marschark, M., Zettler, I. & Dammeyer, J. (2017). Social dominance orientation, language orientation, and deaf identity. *Journal of Deaf Studies and Deaf Education, 22*, 269–277. https://doi.org/10.1093/deafed/enx018

Mauldin, L., & Fannon, T. (2020). *They told me my name: The social processes of Deaf identity development.* https://doi.org/10.1002/symb.482

Maxwell-McCaw, D. (2001). Acculturation and psychological well-being in deaf and hard-of-hearing people (Doctoral dissertation, The George Washington University, 2001). *Dissertation Abstracts International, 61*(11-B), 6141.

Maxwell-McCaw, D., & Zea, M.C. (2011). The Deaf Acculturation Scale (DAS): Development and validation of a 58-item measure. *Journal of Deaf Studies and Deaf Education, 16*, 325–342.

Möller, K., & Danermark, B. (2007). Social recognition, participation, and the dynamic between the environment and personal factors of students with deaf-blindness. *American Annals of the Deaf, 152*, 42–55.

Nelson Schmitt, S., & Leigh, I. W. (2015). Examining a sample of Black Deaf individuals on the Deaf Acculturation Scale. *Journal of Deaf Studies and Deaf Education, 20*(3), 283–295.

Obasi, C. (2014). Negotiating the insider/outsider continua: A Black female hearing perspective on research with Deaf women and Black women. *Qualitative Research*, *14*(1), 61–78. https://doi.org/10.1177/1468794112465632

Ohna, S. E. (2004). Deaf in my own way: Identity, learning, and narratives. *Deafness and Education International*, *6*, 20–38.

Parham, T. A., & Helms, J. E. (1985). Attitudes of racial identity and self-esteem in Black students: An exploratory investigation. *Journal of Counseling Psychology*, *28*, 250–257.

Paul, P. (2014). What is it like to be deaf? *American Annals of the Deaf*, *159*(3), 249–256. https://doi.org/10.1353/aad.2014.0022

Paul, P. (2018). What's it like to be deaf? Reflections on signed language, sustainable development, and equal opportunities. *American Annals of the Deaf*, *163*(4), 471–479. https://doi.org/10.1353/aad.2018.0030

Reichard, R. (2015, March 9). *9 things Latinos are tired of explaining to everyone else*. Retrieved from http://mic.com/articles/111648/9-things-latinos-are-tired-of-explaining-to-everyone-else

Ruiz-Williams, E., Burke, M., Chong, V. Y., & Chainarong, N. (2015). "My Deaf is not your Deaf": Realizing intersectional realities at Gallaudet University. In M. Friedner & A. Kusters (Eds.), *It's a small world: International deaf spaces and encounters* (pp. 262–273). Washington, DC: Gallaudet University Press.

Sue, D. W., & Sue, D. (2008). *Counseling the culturally diverse* (5th ed.). Hoboken, NJ: John Wiley & Sons.

Tajfel, H. (1981). *Human groups and social categories*. Cambridge, UK: Cambridge University Press.

Weinberg, N., & Sterritt, M. (1986). Disability and identity: A study of identity patterns in adolescents with hearing impairments. *Rehabilitation Psychology*, *31*, 95–102.

Wijeyesinghe, C., & Jackson, B. (Eds.). (2012). *New perspectives on racial identity development* (2nd ed.). New York: NY University Press.

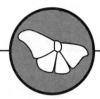

CHAPTER 7

Deaf Communities Within the Deaf Community

When people talk about Deaf people, they would often refer to Deaf people as the Deaf community. Is there really one Deaf community, or are there multiple Deaf communities? What do the Deaf communities look like? Who do you think of when you read the word "Deaf"? How often do you see Deaf people in media? What kind of Deaf people do you see? Who do you think is representing the Deaf communities? In pop culture, some of the well-known Deaf celebrities are Chella Man, CJ Jones, Marlee Matlin, Nyle DiMarco, and Shoshannah Stern, thanks to their appearances in television shows and movies and/or influence (online presence on social media).

A decade before the second edition of this book was published, a Deaf filmmaker, Wayne Betts Jr., introduced the concept of Deaf lens in his TEDxlslay presentation in 2010. Betts explained that as a film student, he created short films using concepts and techniques that he learned. The short films he created did not feel natural. Even using what he learned in his

film studies, Betts couldn't bring his Deaf world to the screen. Betts (TEDx Talks, 2010) provided more details on his experience as a Deaf filmmaker in a school taught by and for hearing filmmakers:

I followed all of the rules of film language. I tried various ways to rearrange the rules but I never got the feeling that it was natural. I wanted to watch something on the screen and say "That's my world!" right there on the screen. I had never experienced. Film language had a box around it, and I felt trapped in this box. I struggled to get out of the box by rearranging the rules. Then I realized I should just put the box aside.

At that point, Betts decided to take a new and experimental approach in filmmaking. He started with scriptwriting. Instead of writing in print or typed English, he signed scripts in ASL in front of a camera. Yes, he wrote his scripts in his language. In creating *GALLAUDET: THE*

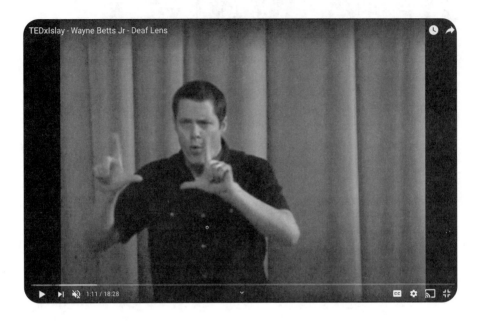

FILM (2010), he had actors, crew members, cameramen, editors, and everyone else relying on the ASL script. This is only a glimpse of what a Deaf lens really is—in filmmaking, that is.

There are multiple definitions for the word "lens." In filmography, a camera lens is an optical lens. It is essentially an eye for the camera to make pictures and/or videos. In this context, a lens means a perspective for Betts. He went to a film school. He learned from hearing filmmakers and colleagues. He had to rely on filmmaking curricula that were designed by hearing filmmakers. It didn't work quite well for him. So Betts adapted and found a filmmaking lens that could truly bring Deaf stories to the screen: a Deaf lens. Now, let's talk about you. Yes, you, the reader.

You may be a Deaf student and you may be taking a Deaf Studies course or you may be curious to learn about your own communities and cultures. You may be taking an American Sign Language (ASL) course for your personal interest or as a foreign language requirement for graduation. You may be an audiology student. Think of the textbook(s) you have to read. Who are the writers? Think beyond their names. What communities are they part of? Are they Deaf? If not, is it a hearing lens? If so, what else is part of their identities? How many lenses are there in the books you are reading about Deaf people? Who do you see in the textbook(s)? Who is missing in the textbook(s)? Through what lens(es) are you reading about our Deaf communities? Are the lenses intersectional?

Intersectionality is a term and a theoretical framework by a Black woman professor and lawyer, Kimberlé Williams Crenshaw. Crenshaw cofounded the field of critical race theory (CRT; Gary, 1995). CRT offers a lens or a perspective of the society while considering how race, law, and power altogether affect everyone (Yosso, 2005). CRT drives the social jus-

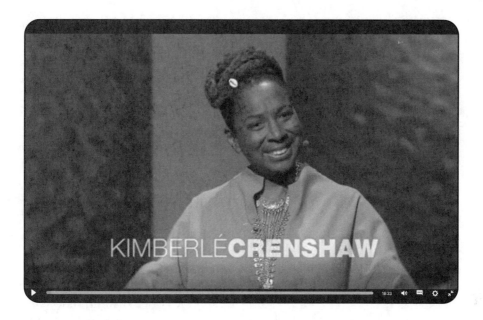

tice movement along with Crenshaw's intersectionality.

Crenshaw met Emma DeGraffenreid, a Black woman whose story led to the inception of intersectionality (TED, 2016). In 1976, Emma DeGraffenreid and other Black women filed a lawsuit against General Motors for race and gender discrimination. Their case was ultimately dismissed. The court did not believe that they could experience both race and gender discrimination at the same time (Crenshaw, 2015). For several centuries, up to the 1970s, in the United States, there was nothing noted on race and gender discrimination overlapping in the workplace or any other areas of life. Both this gap and the injustice in the lawsuit mentioned above drove Crenshaw to study the "profound invisibility in relation to the law" and find a definition for it (Crenshaw, 2015). Thus, intersectionality was born. Crenshaw (2015) described intersectionality as follows:

Intersectionality is an analytic sensibility, a way of thinking about identity and its relationship to power. Originally articulated on behalf of black women, the term brought to light the invisibility of many constituents within groups that claim them as members, but often fail to represent them. Intersectional erasures are not exclusive to black women. People of color within LGBTQ movements; girls of color in the fight against the school-to-prison pipeline; women within immigration movements; trans women within feminist movements; and people with disabilities fighting police abuse—all face vulnerabilities that reflect the intersections of racism, sexism, class oppression, transphobia, able-ism and more. Intersectionality has given many advocates a way to frame their circumstances and to fight for their visibility and inclusion.

How much of intersectionality do you see or know within the Deaf communities?

How often do you see and learn about Black Deaf women?

Candace Jones

Carolyn McCaskill

Claudia Gordon

Haben Grima

Lauren Ridloff

Laurene E. Simms

Storm Smith

Do you recognize any of these names? How often do you see and learn about any other Deaf people with intersectional identities and experiences in your textbook(s)?

As you are halfway through this book, it is important to consider what lenses are used to write this book. The four coauthors are Irene W. Leigh, Jean F. Andrews, Raychelle Harris, and Topher González Ávila. Three of the four coauthors are white and one coauthor is Brown. There are no other coauthors of Color. What does that mean for writings in this book on Black Deaf communities, Indigenous Deaf communities, Asian Deaf communities, and Deaf communities of Color? Two of the four coauthors are straight and two coauthors are Queer. What does that mean for writings in this book on the Queer Deaf communities? Three of the authors identify themselves as cisgender women and one as a cisgender man. What does this mean for the writings on gender identities and expressions in the Deaf communities? Three of the four coauthors are in their forties or older. What does that mean for the writings on different Deaf generations? One of the four coauthors is hearing. What does that mean for the writings on the Deaf communities?

The team of authors has been working hard on this book, trying to make it fair and accurate in terms of portrayal and representation of our Deaf communities. However, the coauthors cannot deny the majority of the lens used in writing this book that is white/straight/older/women. What do these lenses mean? The coauthors also must recognize that this book is heavily influenced by their implicit biases. Kirwan Institute (2014) describes implicit biases as "hidden biases operating largely under the scope of human consciousness influence the way that we see and treat others, even when we are determined to be fair and objective" (p. 9). There may be some writings in this book that do not do some of our communities justice. There may be some communities that may not be well represented in this book. There may be some communities that are not included in this book, despite the subtitle *Exploring Deaf Communities in the United States*.

It is virtually impossible to write about all Deaf communities with the lenses we have for this book while staying free of biases. There is no "the" Deaf community. There are Deaf communities. The Deaf communities are so vast and diverse that words cannot even describe these communities. For centuries, there have been "intersectional erasures" (Crenshaw, 2015). Marginalized communities are more than often excluded (whether intentionally or not) in textbooks, in media, and in our leadership positions.

With that being said, the rest of this chapter will focus on individuals from different Deaf communities and their talents and accomplishments and, most especially, the positive changes they made for us all. It's important to note that this chapter will not sufficiently explore the Deaf communities. The emphasis is on the word *sufficiently*. However, it is hoped that this new chapter will spark interest for you, the readers, to expand your exploration of our Deaf communities.

Yashaira "Yash" Romilus. Yash is DeafBlind Latinx. She works at DeafBlind Interpreting National Training & Resource Center as a protactile trainer and a mentor for interpreters nationwide (DeafBlind Interpreting, n.d.-a, n.d.-b). Yash also cofounded Protactile Theater, a theater where DeafBlind patrons have full access and can enjoy theatrical performances (AJE-DC, 2019). See Chapter 11 for a full description of this type of theater.

Victoria Monroe. Victoria is Black Deaf Queer. Victoria founded Transformative Deaf Education, a nonprofit organization, after a 16-year-old Black Deaf male student was expelled from school (Transformative Deaf Education, 2020). At that point, she aimed to "become an agent of change to transform Deaf Education and deaf programs for equity and inclusive atmosphere in a school setting."

Victor Magide. Victor was Deaf gay Cuban and an out Leatherman. Victor was known for his photography (Rentería, 2017). He graduated from Rochester Institute of Technology with a Fine Arts degree. He owned a photography studio in Miami, Florida, and he specialized in fashion, editorials, and male erotica. He worked as a celebrity photography for Sony Music Latin.

Talila "TL" Lewis. TL is a Black Disabled Queer Genderfluid hearing community lawyer who cofounded HEARD (Helping Educate to Advance the Rights of Deaf Communities) together with incarcerated people and deaf/disabled community members. HEARD is a national volunteer-dependent nonprofit organization, serving Deaf and Disabled people affected by mass incarceration and injustice in the U.S. criminal legal system. HEARD created the only national database of deaf/disabled incarcerated people and of police violence against deaf/disabled people. At the time of the writing of this book, TL serves as the volunteer Director for HEARD. See Chapter 10 for additional information about criminal justice issues for Deaf defendants, as well as imprisoned and returned people.

Storm Smith. Storm is a Black Deaf woman filmmaker. She is the first deaf woman to work at BBO, a leading advertising agency (Hassler, 2018). She has filmed, produced, and directed films and videos. She worked with Apple in creating coding concepts in ASL (Smith, n.d.). Smith advocates that "much more needs to be done in order to bring people with disabilities into the fold, and create content that is easily accessible to anyone and everyone" (Heusner, 2019).

Sarah A. Young Bear-Brown. Sarah is a Deaf Meskawki woman activist. She was awarded the Hamilton Relay 2016 Deaf Community Leader Award for her advocacy for service gaps for the Deaf communities, especially the Deaf Indigenous communities ("Sarah Young Bear-Brown," 2016). She was a part of the #NoDAPL protest at Standing Rock, North Dakota, to support the Water Protectors (Mehta, 2016). The protest was in response to President Trump's approval on building the 1,200-mile-long Dakota Access Pipeline on Indigenous land, more specifically, the Standing Rock Sioux Tribe's reservation (Sisk, 2017).

Roberto Cabrera. Roberto is second generation DeafBlind, Dominican, and Queer. He earned a master's degree in Counseling with an emphasis in Mental Health and Marriage and Family Therapy. Roberto is a member of the core team for the DeafBlind Interpreting National Training and Resource Center and one of the leading mentors for the DeafBlind Interpreting Training Institute. Throughout his career as an advocate, he's been involved with various community and educational projects at local, state, and national levels. He collaborated with organizations in obtaining state grants to improve accessibility via CoNavigators trainings for California's DeafBlind community. He aims for full accessibility in the DeafBlind community.

Najma Johnson. Najma is a Black-DeafBlindDisabled TransMasc Panqueer folk. Najma is well known for their people-centered community advocacy. At the time of the writing of this book, Najma works as the Executive Director for DAWN (formerly known as Deaf Abused Women's Network) in Washington, DC. DAWN is a trauma-informed, healing-centered, culturally responsive, and transformative justice-based, community-based agency focused on providing multifaced services to the survivors and the community, understanding and addressing power-based violence by providing direct services and education to reduce violence in the Deaf communities (DeafDawn, 2020).

Mervin Primeaux-O-Bryant. Mervin is a Black, Deaf, gay man. He is an actor, artist, and activist. He founded the Mervin P. O'Bryant Foundation, whose mission is to advocate for and improve the quality of life of LGBTQ Deaf people through the performing and creative arts (Primeaux-O'Bryant, n.d.). Besides his theatrical performances, Mervin travels worldwide to provide education on HIV/AIDS and to support Deaf People of Color impacted by HIV/AIDS.

Melissa Kelley Colibrí. Melissa is Deaf queer mixed Latinx femme whose pronouns are they/them. Melissa is a full-time activist advocating for accessibility within the LGBTQ community in San Diego (San Diego Pride, n.d.). At the time of the writing of this book, Melissa is the accessibility manager for San Diego Pride, San Diego Trans Pride, and SheFest. Melissa also serves on the Transgender Law Center's national Disability Project Advisory Board.

Laurene E. Simms. Laurene is an African American Deaf woman (Gallaudet University, n.d.). She is a Professor at Gallaudet University's Department of Education. Laurene is also one of the founders of the National ASL/English Bilingual Consortium for Early Childhood Education (NASL-ECE), a nonprofit organization that provides training for families of young Deaf children birth to 8 years. She cofounded Deaf Women of Color and served as the Program Coordinator for the first two Deaf People of Color Conferences (Deaf People, n.d.).

Lauren Ridloff. Lauren is a Deaf Black Mexican woman. Lauren is an actor and a teacher. Lauren is known for her numerous roles: her performance as Sarah Norman in the 2018 Tony-nominated Broadway play, *Children of a Lesser God*, and her role as Connie in the AMC television series, *The Walking Dead*. She worked at the New York Deaf Theater, where she codirected *Sign Me Not* and directed the first Deaf version of *The Vagina Monologues*

(Iryna, 2019). Lauren is confirmed to portray Makkari in the 2021 Marvel film, *The Eternals*, marking her the very first Deaf superhero for Marvel (Peck, 2019).

Joseph "LJ" Williams. LJ is Black Deaf. LJ is a teacher, a mentor, a Deaf interpreter (DI), and an advocate. LJ has worked at several schools and at a local Deaf ministry. His mission is to "support students in reaching their highest potential and helping them discover that they can do anything they set their minds to" (FASLTA, n.d.).

Joseph Hill. Joseph is a Black Deaf man. Dr. Joseph Hill is Associate Professor in the National Technical Institute for the Deaf's Department of American Sign Language and Interpreting Education at Rochester Institute of Technology. He was the first Black Deaf person to earn his doctorate degree in linguistics at Gallaudet University in Washington, DC in 2011. His research interests include sociohistorical and sociolinguistic aspects of African American variety of American Sign Language and attitudes and ideologies about signing varieties in the American Deaf community. His contributions include *The Hidden Treasure of Black ASL: Its History and Structure* (2011), which he coauthored with Carolyn McCaskill, Ceil Lucas, and Robert Bayley, and *Language Attitudes in the American Deaf Community* (2012).

John H. L. Wilson Jr. John was a Black DeafDisabled man. John's wrongful conviction story was the impetus for the creation of HEARD (Helping Educate to Advance the Rights of Deaf Communities). In the early 1990s, DC Metropolitan Police Department officers interrogated John and interviewed other Black Deaf people without interpreters. Due to inevitable and avoidable miscommunications, as well as other common errors found in wrongful conviction cases, John was sentenced to life in prison for a crime he always maintained he did not commit (Lewis, 2018). He spent 24 years, 5 months, and 14 days in the Federal Bureau of Prisons, where he experienced abuse, neglect, and extreme isolation for the entirety of his time behind bars. HEARD advocates fought for his freedom for 12 years. He was finally able to return home on March 6, 2019. Like many formerly incarcerated people, he passed away soon thereafter, on September 6, 2019.

Janette Durán-Aguirre. Janette is Deaf Mexicana. Janette is a fierce advocate always fighting for Deaf education. At the time of the writing of this book, Janette serves on the Board of Directors of Council de Manos and is the current president-elect for California Educators of the Deaf. Janette also works as a school counselor for Marlton School in Los Angeles, California. In 2019, Janette and many other teachers, students, and supporters protested and participated in the largest United Teachers of Los Angeles Strike against the Los Angeles Unified School District (Mernit, 2019). One of the reasons for the protest was against the possibility of privatization of education that would ultimately shut down many schools, including Marlton. #EnLaLucha4DeafEd.

Jade Bryan. Jade is a Black Deaf woman. Jade is a filmmaker who produced and directed award-winning documentaries, including *Listen to the Hands of Our People, On and Off Stage: The Bruce Hlibok Stories, 9/11 Fear in Silence: The Forgotten Underdogs*, and *Reaching Zenith: A Black Deaf Filmmaker's Journey*" (IMDB, n.d.). At the time of the writing of this book, Jade is working on a documentary, *Black and Deaf in America*, that covers issues faced by Black Deaf people who are impacted by racism, police brutality, black erasure, and oppression.

Haben Girma. Haben is a Black Deaf-Blind woman. Haben is one of the first known DeafBlind people to graduate from Harvard Law School (Girma, n.d.). Haben works as an advocate for equal opportunities for people with disabilities. President Barack Obama named her a White House Champion of Change. She has written a best-selling book, *Haben: The Deafblind Woman Who Conquered Harvard Law*, that was featured in the *New York Times*, *Oprah Magazine*, *People*, *The Wall Street Journal*, and the *Today Show*.

Drago Rentería. Drago is a Deaf disabled Chicano transgender man and long-time LGBTQ/social justice activist, leader, and educator. Drago has devoted much of his life toward making the world a better place for marginalized LGBTQ communities. Drago is also notably one of the first out Deaf transgender people in the United States and frequently educates on transgender issues to audiences nationwide; he is listed in the "Inaugural Trans 100," a list of 100 notable transgender people. At the time of the writing of this book, Drago serves as Executive Director of Deaf Queer Resource Center, a national organization for Deaf LGBTQ communities he founded and has run since 1995. In addition to his LGBTQ activism work, Drago is also a photojournalist and documentary photographer and uses his photography to bring more awareness to issues such as racism, housing injustice, police brutality, and gentrification.

Claudia Gordon. Claudia Gordon is a Black Deaf woman. Claudia Gordon is one of the first known Black Deaf women to be a lawyer. Claudia Gordon worked with President Barack Obama as one of his key advisors for disability issues in the United States (Yeheyes, 2018). Claudia also worked with the

Department of Homeland Security as a Senior Policy Advisor in the mid-2000s. She supported the government in enforcing executive orders for people with disabilities in emergency preparedness situations, including Hurricane Katrina in New Orleans.

CJ Jones. CJ is a Black Deaf man. CJ is an actor. He's most known for his part as Joseph in the 2017 summer hit, *Baby Driver*. Because of this film, he became one of the first known Black Deaf actors to work in an international blockbuster film (Jones, n.d.). At the time of the writing of this book, CJ is set to play in the movie sequels for the *Avatar* series directed by James Cameron. He has worked in numerous movies and television shows. He has also performed in theaters and even produced the International Sign Language Theater Festival, which hosted theater artists from all over the United States, Russia, and Mexico.

Chella Man. Chella Man is Jewish Chinese Deaf Genderqueer Queer. He is an artist, a model, and an advocate. Chella Man plays Jericho, a crime fighter in *Titans*, a DC Universe television show (Burack, 2019). He also started a popular YouTube channel to document his transition, his identity, and his love life. His main focus is to educate others on issues regarding being queer and disabled within a safe space (Them, n.d.).

Carolyn McCaskill. Carolyn is a Black Deaf woman. Carolyn is the second Black Deaf woman to graduate from Gallaudet University with a doctorate degree (National Black Deaf Advocates, n.d.). Carolyn is well known for her coauthoring of the book, *The Hidden Treasure of Black ASL: Its History and Structure*. Carolyn traveled through the country to share her expertise and to educate about the Black Deaf community and their language, Black ASL, and their culture.

Candace Jones. Candace is a Black Deaf woman. Candace is a news anchor for Sign1News, an educator, an ASL poet, and a motivational speaker. Working with Sign1News, Candace delivers local, regional, and national news and information in ASL online (Deaf Women United, 2018). Candace worked with Accessible Material Projects (AMP) in bringing accessibility through English-to-ASL translation. She also provides consultant support for the Research and Development Center on Literacy and Deafness (CLAD) at Georgia State University (National Black Deaf Advocates, 2016).

Carla García-Fernández. Carla is a proud native of New Mexico. [Currently, García-Fernández is an assistant professor in the Deaf Studies department at California State University Northridge.] Carla's research interests center around intersectionality, social justice—particularly in education, critical race studies, Deaf- Chicanx & Latinx critical studies, and Ethnic Studies. In Carla's free time, she values spending time with her family, unearthing the roots of her family tree, and she truly enjoys the outdoors as a way to stay spiritually connected to Mother Earth (UTexas, n.d.).

Armando Castro-Osnaya. Armando is a Deaf Mexican. Armando is a professor at several colleges and universities, where he teaches Lengua de Señas Mexicaña (LSM) and ASL. Armando and one of the coauthors, Topher, codeveloped Gallaudet University's very first hybrid LSM course. Armando travels throughout the United States and Mexico to teach LSM and to educate about Mexico's Deaf communities and cultures, as well as LSM and five Indigenous sign languages used in Mexico.

> Discuss with your classmates what you learned and how you felt after reading the spotlights. Who did you read that surprised you and why? What kind of people and communities would you like to learn more about that were not included or discussed enough here in this chapter or this book? If more people and communities were represented well in our textbooks and in media, how different would our view of the Deaf communities be?

The spotlights you just read aren't enough. These are far away from enough for a chapter on the Deaf communities. The descriptions of the individuals above emphasize the point made at the beginning of this chapter, namely, that there are multiple Deaf communities with their own languages, cultures, and identities.

How often do you read about all these different Deaf communities? How often do you read about the many different Deaf languages and cultures, apart from the Eurocentric ASL and the "mainstream" white Deaf culture? How often do you read about the victories and the struggles within the Deaf communities with intersectional identities and experiences? Did you know about any of the 14 Black Deaf people in the United States with a PhD (O'Donnell, 2017)? What was it like for them to deal with racism and audism in school and out in the real world? In the age of Trump, what is/was it like for Deaf people with intersectional identities and experiences?

Francis Anwana. Francis is a Black DeafDisabled man, who came to the United States on a student visa for education. He enrolled at the Michigan School for the Deaf in the city of Flint. He spent 34 years in the United States until he was detained by U.S. Immigrant and Customs Enforcement (ICE). If he were to be deported to his home country in Nigeria, he would not have survived due to his medical conditions and need for access to communication (Warikoo, 2018).

Speaking of Flint, what was it like for Black Deaf people during the infamous Flint Water Crisis? Since 2014, people in Flint, Michigan have been suffering health issues due to severe water contamination (Denchak, 2018). At the time of the writing of this book, people of Flint are still waiting for a governmental response to this citywide health crisis.

Raul Alcocer. Raul is a Deaf Latino man who has been living in the United States since he was a baby. He is now the father of a baby Deaf girl. He was only 24 years old when ICE detained him and took him away from his family (DPAN, 2018). He did not have access to communication with the ICE officers and was detained for at least 4 months with still no access to communication. He was eventually released with public support. There are many Black and Brown Deaf migrants who were not as fortunate. Where are their stories?

In the wake of the pandemic in early 2020, one of President Trump's responses was to refer to COVID-19 or the coronavirus as the "Chinese virus" (Rogers, Jakes, & Swanson, 2020). This label has targeted specifically a group of people, and because of that, it has led to an increase of xenophobia and racism in the United States, especially toward Asian Americans (Somvichian-Clausen, 2020). How did this impact the experiences of Asian Deaf people in this time of a worldwide pandemic? Where are their stories?

With closures of schools and non-essential businesses and social distancing during this pandemic, how did this impact DeafBlind people who rely on touch to communicate? In Vargas's (2020) interview, James Groff, Ali Goldberg, and Haben Girma described their experience as DeafBlind people during this time. James is a graduate student at Gallaudet University, and he and other DeafBlind students were informed by their school in an e-mail that services from Support Service Providers (SSPs) and Certified Deaf Interpreters (CDIs) would be terminated effective April 3, 2020. Groff explained that he was working on his master's thesis, and losing access to these services made this "even more difficult." Ali Goldberg, a freshman, talked about the growing isolation and the sense of depression it brings. Haben explained that while she had always struggled with isolation all her life, the isolation brought back the old fears, and she couldn't resort to Netflix, a form of escapism for many people. She pointed out that transcripts to Netflix shows and movies are "not easy to get." Where are more stories like James's, Ali's, and Haben's?

The age of Trump had a devastating impact on the LGBTQIA+ communities. The Trump administration announced that the Affordable Care Act would not cover 1.5 million transgender Americans and that they would not be guaranteed health care protections (Ring, 2019). The Trump administration denied U.S. embassies from flying the pride flag on flagpoles during the LGBTQ Pride Month in June (Lederman, 2019). The Trump administration cut federal funding for the University of California's HIV and AIDS research program (Goldstein, 2019). Where are the stories of Lesbian, Gay, Transgender, Bisexual, and Queer Deaf people during this time?

Again, the Deaf communities deserve much more than what has been described in this book. The Deaf communities deserve to be written about and represented by their own communities and in their own lenses, rather than through someone else's lens. In February 2020, Crenshaw was asked to explain what intersectionality means today. In her answer, Crenshaw saw intersectionality as a lens:

These days, I start with what it's not, because there has been distortion. It's not identity politics on steroids. It is not a mechanism to turn white men into the new pariahs. It's basically a lens, a prism, for seeing the way in which various forms of inequality often operate together and exacerbate each other. We tend to talk about race inequality as separate from inequality based on gender, class, sexuality or immigrant status. What's often missing is how some people are subject to all of these, and the experience is not just the sum of its parts. (Steinmetz, 2020)

While it is true that there are implicit biases in this book, this book should not serve as the one-stop center for information on the Deaf communities. The book does not hold all lenses for all Deaf communities. Although Wayne Betts Jr.'s Deaf lens of filmmaking is groundbreaking and revolutionary, it is a white Deaf man's lens. Through the lenses of Deaf filmmakers of Color, what would filmmaking look like? Through the lens of Black Deaf authors, Indigenous Deaf authors, and Deaf authors of Color, what would our textbooks and curricula look like? How different would everything be? It goes without saying that the book does not sufficiently portray or represent our Deaf communities and their intersectional identities and experiences. The book needs more lenses. What you can do instead is make this book one of the first steps in your journey in embarking and learning about our Deaf communities. Rezenet Moges Riedel (National Deaf Center, 2020) emphasized that there are not enough documented stories that explain the diverse range of deaf experiences. Intersectionality will shed light on, and bring understanding to, various experiences. The fact that we generalize everything is a problem. In generalizing, we focus on the majority, and neglect the variety of bodies and human experiences, which is why it is important that teachers are aware of the diversity of their students, whether hearing or deaf.

There are so many people and communities to meet, so many languages and cultures to know, and so much to learn beyond this book. As readers, you are always and forever encouraged to continue your journey and to explore our Deaf communities.

In closing, the coauthor of this chapter, Topher González Ávila, dedicates his recognition and appreciation to and for Kimberlé Williams Crenshaw, a Black woman, for her impactful and necessary research works on the framework of intersectionality. Intersectionality brought greater understanding of U.S. systematic injustice and oppression against Black women and Black communities. While intersectionality has benefited all other communities of Color, the coauthors recognize that intersectionality was designed by a Black woman and to understand and validate Emma DeGraffenreid and all Black women's experiences of multiple systematic oppression.

Moges-Riedel et al.'s (2020) open letter in ASL about intersectionality—signed

and transcribed by Rezenet Moges-Riedel, Socorro Garcia, Octavian Robinson,
Shazia Siddiqi, Anna Lim Franck, Kailyn
Aaron-Lozano, Salatiel Pineda, and Ashlea
Hayes—addressed the use of intersectionality. In the letter, authors explained how
the term intersectionality has become a
buzzword inside and outside the Deaf
communities. People are quick to use
intersectionality to describe their experiences without careful consideration.

While it is absolutely valid that Deaf
people can experience multiple oppressions at once, intersectionality doesn't
always apply to everyone. For example,
a white Deaf woman can experience sexism and audism, but intersectionality
would not apply to this scenario. This is
because the said person's race is a systematic privilege itself. People who are white
could experience two or more systematic
oppressions at once. However, because of
the societal implications, their race plays
a significant role in the power dynamics.
That being said, the coauthors want to
recognize the origin and the drive behind
intersectionality.

More important, the emphasis goes
to the fact that intersectionality was
designed by a Black woman and for Black
women. It is also of utmost importance
that the deepest recognition, respect, and
appreciation go to and for Kimberlé Williams Crenshaw and all Black women.

REFERENCES

AJE-DC. (2019, April 26). *ProTactile theater in DC.* Retrieved from http://www.aje-dc.org/2019/04/26/protactile-theater-in-dc/

Burack, E. (2019, July 18). *18 things to know about Chella Man.* Retrieved from https://www.heyalma.com/18-things-to-know-about-chella-man/

Crenshaw, K. (2015, September 24). *Why inter-sectionality can't wait.* Retrieved from https://www.washingtonpost.com/news/in-theory/wp/2015/09/24/why-intersectionality-cant-wait/

DeafBlind Interpreting. (n.d.-a). *Core team.* Retrieved from https://www.dbinterpreting.org/core-team.html

DeafBlind Interpreting. (n.d.-b). *Deafblind mentors.* Retrieved from https://www.dbinterpreting.org/deafblind-mentors.html

DeafDawn. (n.d.) *About—Dawn.* Retrieved from https://deafdawn.org/about/

Deaf People. (n.d.). *Deaf person of the month—Lauren E. Simms.* Retrieved from https://www.deafpeople.com/dp_of_month/SimmsLaureneE2019.html

Deaf Women United. (2018, March 26). In Face-book [Photo file]. Retrieved from https://www.facebook.com/DeafWomenUnited/posts/26-of-31-candace-jones-atlanta-ga-deaf-women-herstory-month-dwhm-dwhm2018-deafwo/1881688508532242/

Denchak, M. (2018, November 8). *Flint water crisis: Everything you need to know.* Retrieved from https://www.nrdc.org/stories/flint-water-crisis-everything-you-need-know

DPAN. (2018, January 12). *Deaf man detained by ICE.* Retrieved from https://www.facebook.com/watch/?v=766155186910214

FASLTA. (n.d.). *Conference 2020 | Faslta.* Retrieved from https://www.faslta.org/copy-of-conference-2020-2

Gallaudet University. (n.d.). *Lauren Simms—My.gallaudet.* Retrieved from https://my.gallaudet.edu/laurene-simms

Girma, H. (n.d.). *Haben Girma—Disability rights, author, speaker.* Retrieved from https://habengirma.com/

Goldstein, A. (2019, June 5). *New restriction on fetal tissue research 'was the president's decision'.* Retrieved from https://www.washingtonpost.com/health/trump-administration-imposes-new-restrictions-on-fetal-tissue-research/2019/06/05/b13433c0-8709-11e9-a491-25df61c78dc4_story.html

Hassler, C. (2018, March 6). *Storm Smith didn't see Deaf women of color making films, so she made her own—now, she's changed the ad industry forever. Retrieved from https://chelsea adelainehassler.com/2018/03/06/storm-smith-didnt-see-deaf-women-of-color-making-films-so-she-made-her-own-now-shes-changed-the-ad-industry-forever/

Heusner, M. (2019, November 7). *Deaf bbdo creative: 'Your work may win awards, but is it accessible to everyone?'* Retrieved from https://www.campaignlive.com/article/deaf-bbdo-creative-your-work-may-win-awards-accessible-everyone/1664989

IMDB. (n.d.). *Jade Bryan. Biography.* Retrieved from https://www.imdb.com/name/nm0116894/bio?ref_=nm_ov_bio_sm

Iryna, S. (2019, March 3). *The Walking Dead: Get to know Lauren Ridloff.* Retrieved from https://undeadwalking.com/2019/03/07/walking-dead-get-know-lauren-ridloff/

Jones, C. (n.d.). *CJ Jones | About.* Retrieved from https://www.cjjones.com/about

Kirwan Institute. (2014). *State of the science: Implicit bias review 2014.* Retrieved from http://kirwaninstitute.osu.edu/wp-content/uploads/2014/03/2014-implicit-bias.pdf

Lederman, J. (2019, June 7). *Trump admin tells U.S. embassies they can't fly pride flag on flagpoles.* Retrieved from https://www.nbcnews.com/politics/national-security/trump-admin-tells-u-s-embassies-they-cant-fly-n1015236

Lewis, T. (2018, November 14). *Support John Wilson's return home!* Retrieved from https://www.gofundme.com/f/johnwilsondeafreentry

Mehta, S. (2016, December 31). *#Nodapl: Sarah Young Bear-Brown.* Retrieved from https://sarikadmehta.com/2016/12/31/nodapl-sarah-young-bear-brown/

Mernit, J. (2019, January 21). *Deaf school's chants are heard loud and clear in teachers strike.* Retrieved from https://capitalandmain.com/deaf-schools-chants-are-heard-loud-and-clear-in-teachers-strike-0121

Moges-Riedel, R., Garcia, S., Robinson, O., Siddiqi, S., Lim Franck, A., Aaron-Lozano, K., Pineda, S., & Hayes, A. [muckymuddy].

(2020, March 11). *Open letter in ASL about intersectionality* [Video]. YouTube. Retrieved from https://youtu.be/JcTYXpofAI0

National Black Deaf Advocates. (n.d.). *Dr. Carolyn McCaskill.* Retrieved from https://www.nbda.org/spotlight/dr.-carolyn-mccaskill

National Black Deaf Advocates. (2016, February 16). In Facebook [Photo file]. Retrieved form https://www.facebook.com/NBDAdvocates/photos/16-of-29-blackdeafstars-candace-jones-georgia-educator-blackdeafhistorymonth-day/1149004848467228/

National Deaf Center. (2020, January 29). In Facebook [Photo file]. Retrieved from https://www.facebook.com/nationaldeafcenter/photos/a.226823901078575/840226896404936/?type=3&theater

O'Donnell, B. R. J. (2017, August 16). *We have 14 Black Deaf Americans with Ph.D.s—14: A conversation with a deaf-studies professor and a student she's been supporting throughout his academic career.* Retrieved from https://www.theatlantic.com/business/archive/2017/08/gallaudet-franklin-jones-carolyn-mccaskill/536949/

Peck, P. (2019, July 23). *Meet Lauren Ridloff, the marvel cinematic universe's first deaf superhero.* Retrieved from https://www.buzzfeed.com/patricepeck/lauren-ridloff-marvel-eternals-deaf-actress-walking-dead

Primeaux-O'Bryant, M. (n.d.). In Facebook [About page]. Retrieved from https://www.facebook.com/kijijijijj/about/

Rentería, D. (2017, January 10). In Facebook [Photo file]. Retrieved from https://www.facebook.com/photo.php?fbid=10154709596505428&set=a.10154709596305428&type=3&theater&comment_id=10157904971080428&force_theater=1&notif_t=photo_comment&notif_id=1583765249729480

Ring, T. (2019, May 24). *New Trump health care rule will harm 1.5 million trans people.* Retrieved from https://www.advocate.com/transgender/2019/5/24/new-trump-health-care-rule-will-harm-15-million-trans-people

Rogers, K., Jakes, L., & Swanson, A. (2020, March 18). *Trump defends using 'Chinese* virus' label, ignoring growing criticism. Retrieved from https://www.nytimes.com/2020/03/18/us/politics/china-virus.html

San Diego Pride. (n.d.). *Melissa Kelley Colibrí*. Retrieved from https://sdpride.org/melissa-kelley-colibri/

Sisk, A. (2017). *Timeline: The long road to #nodapl*. Retrieved from http://insideenergy.org/2017/01/23/timeline-the-long-road-to-nodapl/

Smith, S. (n.d.). *Works of magic*. Retrieved from https://www.officialstormsmith.com/works-of-magic

Somvichian-Clausen, A. (2020, March 25). *Trump's use of the term 'Chinese virus' for coronavirus hurts Asian Americans, says expert.* Retrieved from https://thehill.com/changing-america/respect/diversity-inclusion/489464-trumps-use-of-the-term-chinese-virus-for

Steinmetz, K. (2020, February 20). *She coined the term 'intersectionality' over 30 years ago. Here's what it means to her today.* Retrieved from https://time.com/5786710/kimberle-crenshaw-intersectionality/

TED. (2016, October). *Kimberlé Crenshaw—The urgency of intersectionality* [Video file]. Retrieved from https://www.ted.com/talks/kimberle_crenshaw_the_urgency_of_intersectionality?language=en

TEDx Talks. (2010, June 22). *TEDxIslay—Wayne Betts Jr—Deaf Lens* [Video file]. Retrieved from https://youtu.be/ocbyS9-3jjM

Them. (n.d.). *Chella Man*. Retrieved from https://www.them.us/contributor/chella-man

Transformative Deaf Education. (2020, February 19). In Facebook [Video file]. Retrieved from https://www.facebook.com/watch/?v=524770728145192

UTexas. (n.d.). *Carla García-Fernández*. Retrieved from https://education.utexas.edu/departments/curriculum-instruction/graduate-programs/cultural-studies-education/alumni/carla-garc%C3%ADa-fern%C3%A1ndez

Vargas, T. (2020, April 8). *They are deaf and blind, and social distancing has now taken their ability to touch.* Retrieved from https://www.washingtonpost.com/local/they-are-deaf-and-blind-and-social-distancing-has-now-taken-their-ability-to-touch/2020/04/08/de5a9d42-79ae-11ea-9bee-c5bf9d2e3288_story.html

Warikoo, N. (2018, September 8). *Deaf and disabled immigrant faces deportation after 34 years in the United States.* Retrieved from https://www.usatoday.com/story/news/nation-now/2018/09/08/deaf-immigrant-deportation-francis-anwana/1243524002/

Yeheyes, T. (2018, February 10). *First deaf African American lawyer Claudia Gordon, anti-discrimination advocate.* Retrieved from https://www.respectability.org/2018/02/first-deaf-african-american-lawyer-claudia-gordon-anti-discrimination-advocate/

Yosso, T. J. (2005). Whose culture has capital? A critical race theory discussion of community cultural wealth. *Race Ethnicity and Education, 8*(1), 69–91.

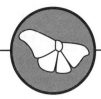

CHAPTER 8

Navigating Lives

INTRODUCTION

Shanna Sorrells (2006) remembers that when she was in the eighth grade and waiting in the cafeteria line, a hearing friend told her she had overheard a boy talking about how dumb Shanna was because she was deaf. Shanna's eventual response was to write the winning essay for the Rockville (Maryland) Human Rights Commission student essay contest that starts with:

Don't laugh at me

Don't call me names

Don't get your pleasure from my pain

In god's eyes we're all the same!

(Sorrells, 2006, p. B21)

Although we are all the same in that we are human beings, none of us are exactly the same. Most people do not realize that to be different is part of the human condition of diversity. We are all different in our own ways. But still, many people are not comfortable if they see someone they think is too different.

What about deaf people? Individuals may say that they are comfortable with deaf people. A research study showed that hearing people who had never met deaf people may score as bicultural on a questionnaire, meaning they think they can be comfortable with deaf people as well as hearing people (Leigh, Marcus, Dobosh, & Allen, 1998). But is this true in reality? As opposed to visible disabilities, people tend not to notice if a person is deaf until the person starts to communicate. If the communication does not go smoothly, will hearing people feel a sense of discomfort? Does that feeling reinforce opinions that deaf people are limited in their ability to function? This is something for you to think about.

> Would you go to a Deaf doctor? A Deaf lawyer? A Deaf car mechanic?

Society tends to have a hard time believing that deaf people can live full lives like hearing people can or do things that hearing people can do. Historically, deaf people have been marginalized,

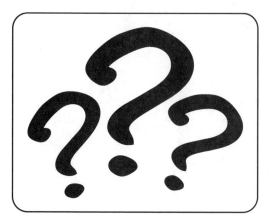

Figure 8–1. Image credit to Alexander Wilkins. Used with permission.

silenced, ignored, or sidelined by society (Cleall, 2015). We have discussed this problem throughout the book. As a result, deaf people have had to show their resilience, their confidence in themselves, and their ability to stand up for themselves in the face of discrimination and oppression, as Shanna did. Why does this keep happening again and again?

FORMS OF DISCRIMINATION

When the word *normal* pops up, people usually will think of others like themselves. They do not think of people who are "different" from themselves. If they meet a signing deaf person for the first time, they probably will see that person as "different" or as a person with a disability. This is a typical response because people tend not to understand how Deaf people can see themselves as being just like hearing people except that they use a different language. Interestingly, there was one place in the United States where hearing people did not view deaf people as abnormal. This was on Martha's Vine-

yard, where there was a high incidence of hereditary deafness starting in the 18th century through the early part of the 20th century. As Nora Groce (1985) explains it, everyone on Martha's Vineyard spoke sign language. Hearing people comfortably interacted with deaf people and sometimes even signed among themselves.

However, this was not so elsewhere. For example, in the 1800s, prominent Deaf people organized famous banquets in Paris, France, to discuss critical issues of the day. Yet, at the same time, deaf people were often described as "incomplete" (Mottez, 1993), clearly suggesting stigma. And during that period, deaf teachers in different countries usually were paid less than hearing teachers who taught in schools for the deaf and were often assigned to teach less academically inclined students (Sayers, 2017), a perfect example of oppression in which an unjust exercise of power serves to keep a specific group of people down. Lennard Davis (2000) wrote that during the 1950s, his culturally Deaf parents had to prove to others that they could do what hearing people could do. Even to this day, Deaf people have been asked if they can drive a car because they can't hear! In the United States, deaf people have been driving for decades, although in some countries, they are still not allowed to drive. Highly qualified deaf people who dreamed of becoming medical doctors were denied entry into medical schools (see Donald Ballantyne's example below). Others such as Philip Zazove (1993), a very successful family medicine physician, fought to get into medical schools and finally succeeded in getting into one. All these anecdotes are examples of discrimination and oppression, which happens when there are barriers that limit opportunities in education, career development, and entertainment just because the person is deaf.

A deaf young woman who was able to speak clearly was interviewed for a senior position in a major library system, for which she was well qualified. Her interview went very well. It looked like she would be offered the job. The top executives invited her for drinks at a noisy bar. She was unable to follow the conversations and did not get the job (Bouton, 2013). Is this discrimination?

Why do deaf people have such problems? This is because communication and language barriers between deaf and hearing people create a stereotypical picture of deaf people as not capable because they do not speak, or if they speak, many may not be fluent in spoken language, or if they are in noisy environments, may look incompetent because they cannot follow conversations. Stereotyping happens when a person makes a judgment that is supported by that person's group and becomes a belief system that generalizes to everyone in the stigmatized group, whether true or not. In the U.S. government, we now have the National Institute on Deafness and Other Communication Disorders. This title clearly suggests that deafness is a communication disorder. But if deaf people are fluent in a sign language, do they have a communication disorder? Does communication have to be spoken? Clearly, this stereotyping of deaf people as having a communication disorder has been harmful for Deaf people who are fluent users of ASL and therefore are not communication disordered.

Such stereotyping leads to discrimination. Discrimination happens when there is some negative action against members of a group or, in this case, deaf people. Discrimination can be obvious or indirect. Direct discrimination happens when being deaf itself is listed as a disqualification. Indirect discrimination is more subtle, such as being ushered out of a doctor's office more quickly than a hearing patient might have been. If a deaf person mentions being deaf on a job application, might this red flag lower the chances of that person being invited for a job interview? Is this direct or indirect discrimination?

On half of her 20 or so applications for a psychology internship in a very competitive process, Christen Szymanski mentioned that she was deaf. Despite being highly qualified, she was not invited for any interviews. On the other half of her applications, she did *not* mention she was deaf. For every one of these applications, she was invited for interviews and obtained a year-long internship (Szymanski, 2010).

Would you consider this discrimination obvious or indirect?

There is a civil rights law called the Americans With Disabilities Act of 1990 (ADA) (see Chapter 10 for additional details). It prohibits discrimination based on disability. Because the courts judged efforts to minimize the disability (for example, using cochlear implants; see Chapter 2) as resulting in the person no longer falling under the ADA (for example, because the person can now "hear" with a cochlear implant), the law was changed in 2008 to emphasize that even with technology or medication to minimize the disability, the person still had a disability (even with cochlear implants, the person is still deaf). This law is now called the Americans With Disabilities Amended Act of 2008.

Employers may hesitate to hire deaf people, including culturally Deaf people, because of concerns about language and communication access (e.g., Task Force on Health Care Careers for the Deaf and Hard-of-Hearing Community, 2012). They may not be aware that they have internalized subtle biases, such as "hearing superiority." Because of this, they may discriminate, thinking they will minimize problems by not hiring that person. They likely do not realize that there are deaf people who have the potential to meet or even exceed their expectations, whatever the situation is. Deaf people know how to make communication happen and can teach employers this if they are given the chance. Too often, deaf people have to fight for this chance.

This hearing superiority attitude has been defined as a part of audism. Audism represents a system of advantage based on hearing or speaking ability (Bauman, 2004; Eckert & Rowley, 2013). One prime example of audism is that spoken language is superior to sign language and represents a higher level of language use. This can be a real problem for culturally Deaf individuals even though linguists have documented that ASL is a real language just as spoken English is a real language (e.g., Petitto, 2014). When communication breaks down, the blame is placed on the deaf person's inadequacy in spoken language and not the hearing person's inadequacy in sign language. When hear-

ing people see or hear the word *deaf*, they often assume the person will be unable to function as hearing peers do. These are examples of audism.

> In 1988, the Gallaudet University Board of Trustees chose a hearing candidate over two deaf candidates to be president of Gallaudet University. Is this an example of audism? Note that this resulted in the Deaf President Now protest that ended with I. King Jordan, a deaf man, becoming the president (see Chapter 1).

Although the word *audism* was coined in 1975, its concept is not new as it represents hearing privilege or hearing superiority that has happened for centuries to people who are deaf, especially to people who are culturally Deaf.

> Eckert and Rowley (2013) describe different aspects of audism.
>
> Overt audism: Hearing superiority is assumed. There is no effort to disguise discrimination.
>
> Covert audism: Audism is more difficult to identify.
>
> Aversive audism: Despite belief in equality, the practice is to socially exclude the Deaf population or target and minimize their values.
>
> Can you suggest examples of each type of audism?

Only recently has the relationship between audism and racism been explored. Lisa Stapleton (2016) reports on a long history of dual discrimination/oppression due to being both Deaf and Black. For example, professors may not want to have ASL interpreters in their classrooms because it is distracting for them. Their excluding Deaf students from classroom discourse is a form of oppression and audism. And when Deaf culture is taught based only on examples of white Deaf populations, this renders Black Deaf culture invisible when in fact there are thriving Black Deaf communities (see Chapter 7 for examples of Deaf individuals who are part of different Black Deaf communities).

RESILIENCE

Deaf people have shown resilience when dealing with society's stereotyping, oppression, discrimination, and audism. The fact that signing deaf communities all over the world have existed for centuries proves that these communities are very resilient.

What does resilience mean? Brooks (2006) defines resilience as facing risk and seeing the possibility of achieving positive outcomes. It reflects the ability to bounce back despite difficult situations or setbacks. If the deaf person feels capable of doing things despite the doubts of hearing persons and works to prove that capability, that is a form of resilience. This strength to face being stigmatized and achieve goals has to come from within the person.

What are examples of resilience? Elisa Cimento (see her story in Chapter 6) decided that the negative attitudes of other people were the problem, not her. Shanna Sorrells, whose poem introduces

this chapter, felt pain because her peers bullied her for being "different." She fought back with a positive attitude and wrote an essay expressing her feelings and her inner strength.

Here's another example. Alec, a culturally Deaf man, wishes to attend a professional conference and do a presentation. He requests sign language interpreter services. The conference organizers say no; it is Alec's responsibility to provide interpreters if he needs them.

Question: What is really happening here? Who is the problem?

Obviously, the conference organizers feel that because Alec does not use spoken English, he has to fix his problem. Alec decides to attend the conference, bring his own ASL to English interpreter, and do his presentation on stage. He tells his interpreter to turn off the microphone and not translate his ASL into spoken English. He starts his presentation using ASL. The audience sits in stunned silence for a few minutes, and then some audience members call out for an interpreter. The interpreter tells Alec. He responds, "Oh, you all need an interpreter? If you knew ASL, there would be no problem." That is an example of resilience, inner strength, and creativity in problem solving while dealing with people who make things difficult for the deaf person.

One of the authors of this book, Irene W. Leigh, had to stand up for herself when at the age of 13 she was denied entry to an honors program in her mainstream high school and then again was denied entry to the university of her choice, even while students below her in class rank and extracurricular activities were accepted. She was told upfront, "You are deaf. This is going to be too hard for you." She successfully fought against this overt discriminatory attitude. Where did this resilience come from?

To understand how deaf people succeed in standing up to society's expectations that they are "not good enough," we have to look at how they see themselves positively, how they get support from their families and schools (Leigh was supported by her hearing parents and elementary school principal), and how they use positive self-talk to fight the frustrations created by a society that does not always understand them. The book, *Resilience in Deaf Children* (Zand & Pierce, 2011), demonstrates how relationships based on families and school settings can influence and strengthen resilience in deaf children.

The Role of Relationships in Strengthening Resilience

Genetics, the environment, and one's cultural background contribute to resilience. Genetics and the environment play a role in the development of intelligence and personality. In the environment, did the deaf person have access to language? For the culturally Deaf person, that means access to sign language as well as written language. For other deaf people, that means access to both spoken and written languages. Does the deaf person have a good internal language system because of that access? Does he or she sign or speak fluently? Does the culture of the person provide good support systems? It's really all about relationships.

Again, it all starts in the family. Relationships with the caregiver(s) are the foundation for access to language. Caregivers, including parents and extended family members, establish relationships with deaf babies and young children through physical contact such as hugs, holding the child, and so on, while talking, signing, and/or gesturing with the child. If families and peers are supportive and find ways to communicate easily with the deaf child, this helps the deaf child feel good inside, even if things are tough outside the family. Having a sense of

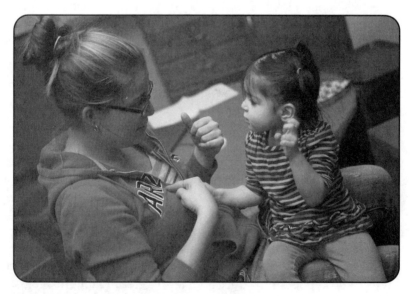

Figure 8–2. Used with permission.

humor; being able to adapt to different situations, make decisions, articulate feelings, solve problems, and be open to talking about communication and Deaf culture; and feeling comfortable with their deaf identities all count in making the deaf child resilient.

The Deaf children of culturally Deaf parents grow up with consistent access to sign language and communication. They see how their Deaf parents deal with hearing people outside of the home. As long as the parents are sensitive to child development issues, communicate well with their Deaf children, and adequately support their Deaf children in feeling proud of themselves, this strengthens the development of resilience.

In most families (approximately 96%; Mitchell & Karchmer, 2004), the parents of a deaf child are hearing. Because of this, the path to a culturally Deaf identity for the child usually takes longer, if at all. Much depends on how quickly the parents adjust when they are told the baby is deaf. Do the parents or the family try to get information about how to feed language to their baby? Do they try to learn about Deaf culture? Do they find out about sign language classes, like Darby's mother did in Chapter 1? Are they able to meet culturally Deaf adults through Deaf mentor programs that help them communicate with their baby? Do they find out about early intervention programs that focus on bilingualism (both signed and spoken languages)? Are they happy with and attached to their signing Deaf child? Do they encourage their child to play with other Deaf children? All of these will help to strengthen resilience in the child when the child starts to experience challenges in different life situations.

If the Deaf child has friends who also sign, that helps to reinforce connections and strengthen the culturally Deaf identity. Often, culturally Deaf friendships happen if the child goes to a school where the language of teaching is sign language, together with written language. Figure 8–3 shows a group of three children showing pride in ASL through

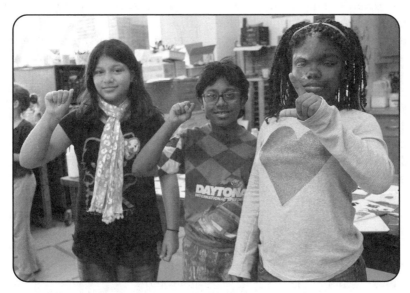

Figure 8–3. Students fingerspelling ASL. Used with permission.

fingerspelling the letters. Teacher and peer influences provide opportunities for supporting Deaf relationships. If teachers, particularly hearing teachers, are very supportive of Deaf culture and help the child learn about Deaf culture and the Deaf community, this can be a very powerful influence.

The majority of deaf children are now educated in the mainstream, not in schools for the deaf (e.g., Marschark, 2018). Many of these children may never see another deaf child. Despite stories of friendships with hearing peers at school, it is still a fact that many deaf children find themselves isolated (Leigh, 2009; Oliva, 2004). Classmates will interact with them less often than they would with hearing peers. These deaf children may be embarrassed about being deaf, as Elisa Cimento was (see above). To minimize social problems, some deaf children will try to hide their being deaf, but that creates lots of stress in being something they are not. Bullying is also a problem that may emerge, as children are often cruel without really understanding the impact of what they are doing. Being deaf can be even more difficult during the teenage years when adolescents want to be like everyone else, thereby leaving deaf friends out of the loop.

There are camps such as Camp Mark Seven in Old Forge, New York, where ASL predominates. At this camp, these deaf children who are alone in the mainstream can see that they are not the only deaf children in the world and can share their experiences with other Deaf peers. This helps build their confidence in how they handle different situations when they return to school. Deaf parents will also send their hearing children to Camp Mark Seven in order to share experiences and know they are not alone.

When deaf children who are isolated in their schools become adolescents and young adults, they may become curious about other deaf people (e.g., Leigh, 2009). With good Internet access, they can learn more about the Deaf community and Deaf events. If they know ASL, it is much easier to connect with Deaf sports events, social gatherings, and other places where Deaf people congregate. They will want to learn more about Deaf culture and the Deaf community as they see how easily accessible communication with other Deaf people can be compared with more difficult situations with hearing people. This creates opportunities for more positive self-esteem as Deaf people who take pride in their sign skills and learn different ways of being a Deaf person. This also strengthens their resilience as proud members of American Deaf culture.

THE WORLD OF WORK

> Can you think of jobs that deaf people cannot do? Are you sure there is no way they can do the job? What about the role of technology?

Resilience definitely comes in handy as deaf people enter the working world. It helps to know that there are numerous success stories of deaf women and men who have entered fields that were long thought to be impossible for them, such as law. We have already discussed the experience of deaf people who applied to medical school in the past. Two inspiring success stories out of many teach us the importance of resilience when things get tough.

Dr. Donald Ballantyne was a top premedical student at Princeton University in the 1940s. Every medical school he applied to rejected him because he was deaf. He finally got a PhD in animal biology. What is amazing is that he eventually became an expert in microvascular and plastic surgery and was an instructor for medical doctors (Lang & Meath-Lang, 1995).

Dr. Nathie Marbury (WPSDAA, 2013) came from a poor Black family in Mississippi. She had 15 brothers and sisters. Western Pennsylvania School for the Deaf saved her life. She was the first in her family to attend college. Her doctoral research focused on Black Deaf American identity contributors and challenges (Marbury, 2007). She broke barriers as the first Black Deaf person to teach in some schools and became a well-known ASL professor and storyteller. This is important because of the history of segregation that many schools for the deaf had before desegregation was ordered subsequent to the 1954 Supreme Court decision in *Brown v. Board of Education of Topeka*.

Yes, thanks to those resilient early pioneers, job opportunities for Deaf people have increased. We now have Deaf nurses, doctors, lab technicians, school administrators, teachers, cooks, architects, engineers, psychologists, lawyers, stockbrokers, baseball players, actors, janitors, computer technicians, and so on. We can see Deaf workers interacting in schools, agencies, and organizations for deaf people. Starbucks opened its first Signing Starbucks in Washington, DC, following the one established in Malaysia. This is a fully accessible workplace, with an all-Deaf staff who cater to both hearing and Deaf customers (Siegel, 2018). As for Deaf entrepreneurs, Austin, Texas, has claimed roughly 30 Deaf-owned businesses (Brandeis, 2015). Garberoglio, Palmer, Cawthon, and Sales (2019) report that a higher percentage of deaf people (11.6%) are self-employed compared to hearing people (9.8%) or are business owners (4.1% compared with 3.8%). As noted in Chapter 9, technology advances have made communication access far easier for deaf people who want to succeed at jobs or run their own businesses.

Three deaf entrepreneurs have started a Lost River Vacations company that will build vacation cabins in the West Virginia woods. Their first house was built by a Deaf carpenter; its walls are decorated with artwork done by Deaf artists, and a Deaf-owned company is designing hiking trails on the property (Smith, 2019).

More typically, there are Deaf workers who are the only Deaf workers in hearing workplaces. Even though we have numerous success stories in both deaf and hearing workplaces, there are still many Deaf people who struggle in the workplace.

Trish Nolan, a medical records technician, applied for promotion to become a supervisor. She had seniority, having been there longer than anyone else. She was turned down each time she applied, even though she had good job evaluations. She believes it was because she is deaf (Task Force on Health Care Careers for the Deaf and Hard-of-Hearing Community, 2012). Might this be an attitudinal barrier?

Underemployment and lack of employment are issues for many Deaf as well as hard-of-hearing workers, including those of minority status. It is sobering to note that 47% of deaf people are either not employed or not part of the labor force and that deaf people are looking for work to a greater extent than hearing people (Garberoglio et al., 2019). Fewer African American and Native American/Indigenous deaf individuals are working compared with white deaf individuals. Those who do not go on to higher education, vocational schools, or vocational training programs have more difficulty finding jobs than their hearing peers. A review of the 2011 American Community Survey that examines national data indicates that deaf individuals confront barriers to and within the labor market, leading to lower employment rates and reduced earnings (Benito, Glassman, & Hiedemann, 2016). Their statistics indicate that roughly 40% is due to educational level, limited experience, race/ethnicity, and marital status, while the remaining 60% is attributed to communication issues, occupational segregation, labor market discrimination, and stigma. Contributing factors include difficulties accessing the English language, too few graduating with high school diplomas that represent solid academic achievement, and attitudinal barriers on the part of employers as well as educational settings that provide career training opportunities (Punch, Hyde, & Creed, 2004).

Attitudinal barriers are created by authorities who doubt the abilities of deaf people and have limited expectations for them. Attitudinal barriers are a significant problem that is very difficult to deal with because these can be expressed in subtle ways. The stories of Trish Nolan and Christen Szymanski (see above) are examples of subtle barriers that later become obvious.

Employers do not always see how Deaf people can do a good job at work because of communication issues (Task Force on Health Care Careers for the Deaf and Hard-of-Hearing Community, 2012). They often are not aware of ADA regulations requiring that employers provide reasonable accommodations for workplaces that have 15 or more employees. Employers worry that reasonable accommodations will be too expensive. For example, ASL interpreting costs tend to be never-ending as that is an ongoing need. At the same time, employers do not realize that Deaf people have lifelong experiences in figuring out how to communicate and how to use technology to improve communication. They can provide suggestions to manage communication in cost-effective ways and use interpreters only when necessary, such as for group meetings. However, Deaf workers will often miss out on informal worker conversations, which can be important for networking.

The presence of additional disabilities will impact work opportunities for Deaf people. Statistics show that approximately

79% of deaf people were in the labor force compared with 39% of deaf people with additional disabilities (Garberoglio et al., 2019). DeafBlind individuals have difficulties in finding jobs after graduating from high school. Those DeafBlind individuals who want to work struggle to get accommodations for their disabilities (Arndt & Parker, 2016). Cmar, McDonnall, and Markoski (2018) found that DeafBlind people with paid high school work experiences and/or vocational education services, no additional disabilities, and positive parent expectations did better in getting jobs after high school.

Training program directors in either vocational or professional tracks tend to be skeptical that Deaf people can succeed in their programs. They often believe that Deaf people should be trained to work with computers or do lab work, for example, rather than with people. That can be a significant attitudinal barrier that Deaf people have to overcome. Deaf people often have to go the extra mile to prove their competency in working with people and teach supervisors to be more open-minded about their potential.

In conclusion, Deaf students do benefit from exposure to different career possibilities before making a final decision. They need support during the transition from high school to career training and preparation for the world of work. Schools and vocational rehabilitation agencies play an important role in this transition phase.

HEALTH ISSUES

Deaf people, resilient or not, have to deal with life issues such as health and mental health issues, just as hearing people do. Research on the health of deaf individuals confirms that there are differences when compared with the general population of typically hearing people. For example, Barnett and Franks (2002) found that deaf adults report poorer health and are less likely to see doctors and receive health care services. They are less likely to have accurate information about health-related conditions, such as breast cancer (Cumberland et al., 2018). This can be due to difficulty in communicating directly with medical people or difficulty in getting sign language interpreting services.

Not only that, in another study, Barnett and Franks (1999) also reported increased mortality (deaths) in deaf adults. They found this by linking National Health Interview Survey data that included information from deaf people with the National Death Index. More recently, Barnett and researchers (2011) used an ASL-accessible survey to get health-related information from Deaf participants. On the positive side, they found that there were fewer deaf smokers. On the negative side, they found higher risks for high cholesterol, prediabetes, and heart disease.

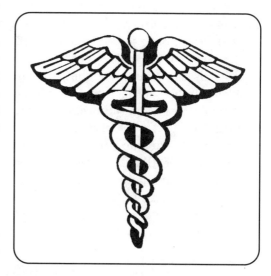

Figure 8–4. Public domain.

Significant health problems included obesity, partner violence, and suicide. A Swedish study of DeafBlind individuals found physical and mental health issues, particularly headaches and shoulder, neck, and back pain (Wahlqvist, Möller, Möller, & Danermark, 2016).

Although there are a number of reasons for the health problems experienced by many Deaf and DeafBlind persons, including family history, medical problems at birth, education, socioeconomic status, income, sexual orientation, ethnicity, and race, one significant reason has to do with limited English literacy[1] and lack of access to English-based health-related information that is printed or delivered through television, radio, or the Internet via captions or text information about health practices (to maintain good health) and healthy relationships (to lower stress in the home) (e.g., Harmer, 1999; Kelleher, 2017). Many may misunderstand instructions for medicine after they see doctors, either because they do not understand the advanced words doctors use or because sign language interpreters were not provided or were not qualified for the job, meaning they did not know the terms or interpret these correctly. Without knowing ASL or without good ASL interpreters, doctors may misdiagnose medical symptoms. This can lead to ongoing health problems. In-hospital lack of accommodations will increase communication issues, making Deaf patients feel discriminated against (Sirch, Salvador, & Palese, 2017). As Deaf and DeafBlind people get older, they tend to need more medical care and are even more disadvantaged due to communication challenges. If they were able to get information (such as through ASL

videos about health issues or technology to convert text to Braille) or explain themselves through ASL with the use of ASL interpreters as needed, it could improve their health literacy. One study based on four in-depth interviews found that health care providers who were sensitive to the needs of Deaf patients and who were willing to use ASL interpreters provided better experiences for their patients (Blackaby, 2018). Blackaby also noted that his participants felt they must educate health care providers on the importance of interpreters. Another study in the United States that included Deaf women with lower levels of education demonstrated that a breast cancer educational program developed for them was successful in increasing awareness (Cumberland et al., 2018). A survey/interview project of 26 tribal vocational rehabilitation service providers serving Deaf, DeafBlind, and hard-of-hearing tribal members investigated the nature of their services (Paris, 2020). Results confirmed that the biggest problem they faced was the lack of resources, most importantly interpreter services and access to communication, especially for consumers with limited literacy. Additionally, in terms of health care services, 10% of those interviewed reported that they consult with their own medical providers who were knowledgeable about traditional healing practices in order to provide appropriate services, while another 10% mentioned traditional gatherings involving medicinal herbs and healing. Activities such as these gatherings enhance physical health.

It seems that politicians are waking up to the ASL needs of their deaf constituents related to health issues. According to

---

[1]Caveat: We want to emphasize that there are bilingual Deaf people who were given opportunities to access both ASL and English and master both while growing up. This should not be overlooked when looking at statistics for literacy rates in Deaf people.

a video message sent out by the National Association of the Deaf (2020), during the coronavirus (COVID-19) pandemic, governors of 47 different states had ASL interpreters present during their press conferences to update the public regarding efforts to contain the pandemic.

MENTAL HEALTH ISSUES

Mental health is generally understood as a state of well-being in which individuals realize their potential, cope with typical life stresses, work productively, and can contribute to their communities (World Health Organization, 2014). According to this definition, yes, many Deaf people are mentally healthy (Leigh & Pollard, 2011). They manage very well, are resilient, have jobs, raise families, join organizations, connect on the Internet, and so on, as this book demonstrates. However, Deaf adults have been reported to associate the term *mental health* not with health but with psychological problems, insanity, or mental health services (Steinberg, Loew, & Sullivan, 1999). Mental health symptoms can be viewed as stigmatizing when Deaf people are trying to be accepted as part of the general society (Leigh & Pollard, 2011). Still, more Deaf people need mental health services compared to the general population (Fellinger, Holzinger, & Pollard, 2012). This happens when they have emotional or behavioral issues that require psychiatric or psychological attention. Trained professionals need to acknowledge the variety of D/deaf experiences and be aware of the interface of Deaf culture and mental health. This enables them to appropriately diagnose and treat these individuals (Brenman, Higginga, & Wright, 2017). For this reason, the National Association of the Deaf website (http://www.nad.org)

has several position papers on culturally affirmative approaches for health care and mental health access.

Whether these deaf individuals have problems or not depends on a variety of factors (Du Feu & Chovaz, 2014). Their problems could be because they are more vulnerable to stress in their daily lives. Or they may have had difficulties growing up and learning how to manage a complex environment. Or they may have been born with genetic or birth issues that make it difficult for them to learn to understand what is going on and behave appropriately in their environment. This can cause problems for them at home or outside the home.

> One example of birth issues: CMV is a popular abbreviation for cytomegalovirus. When the mother gives birth, she may pass this virus to the baby. Some of these babies will have neurologic or developmental problems that can result in psychological difficulties (see Leigh & Andrews, 2017, for a brief review).

One research study asked Deaf participants what they thought caused mental health problems (Steinberg, Loew, & Sullivan, 2010). Most of them felt that problems were caused by communication breakdowns with family while growing up. Some blamed poor family communication for their own problems with addiction or psychological issues. If parents have difficulty communicating with their deaf child because of the language barrier, this can cause the deaf child to feel isolated at home. Such experiences reinforce the perception that lack of communication causes mental health problems. Deaf people often have lifelong problems in communicating with hearing family members as well as hearing people outside the family.

> Mara's parents never learned ASL, even though Mara attended a school for the Deaf where she lived in the dorms and went home on weekends. Mara was very angry with her parents because they never explained to her what had happened to a younger sister who "disappeared" while Mara was at school. She was shocked when she finally found out that the sister had committed suicide. She started taking drugs to escape from this painful knowledge. Getting family support and therapy might have helped her.

Sadly, it is often hard for Deaf people to get mental health help when they need it (Gerke, 2016; Glickman, 2013; Glickman & Hall, 2019). How do they find out where to go? Few mental health service programs throughout the United States serve primarily Deaf clients. If they live in rural areas, it is almost impossible to get services. Video technology (see Chapter 9) can help them connect with service providers (Crowe, 2017; Gournaris, 2009). One example of a video technology service provider is that of National Deaf Therapy (https://nationaldeaftherapy.com/). If Deaf clients are part of the Deaf community in large cities, they can find out where there are good Deaf mental health service agencies. A lot of information is shared when culturally Deaf people get together, including where to go for help and feedback about the quality of agencies.

Lots of talk happens when Deaf people get together. Some individuals may want to keep their mental health issues private, fearing their information will get out. What is talked about in California may be talked about in Florida almost immediately because of the famous Deaf cultural trait of information sharing. This is especially true now that the Internet and social media make it easy for Deaf people to communicate with each other. For that reason, some Deaf people will not look for help because they are afraid their information will be shared.

How many mental health clinicians know ASL? How many understand that Deaf people may know mental health vocabulary in ASL but not in English? How many mental health clinicians know about Deaf culture and can work with Deaf people? Deaf people of color? Deaf immigrants? Deaf Transgender people? Not many (Gerke, 2016; Joharchi, 2017; Leigh & Pollard, 2011). This was clear in the research study in which Steinberg et al. (2010) (described above) asked for feedback about mental health services. That is also why many Deaf people may be nervous about getting mental health services. Will they be understood? Will they be correctly diagnosed so that they can get appropriate treatment and medications? They also do not trust clinicians who think they sign well when they really do a minimal level of signing.

Because of the shortage of ASL-fluent clinicians, it is often necessary to use ASL interpreters in mental health settings (Leigh & Pollard, 2011). These interpreters may have little training in how to work in mental health clinics and may not have the interpreting expertise to understand the wide range of signing skills used by Deaf clients (Wattman, 2019). This may require adding a Deaf Interpreter (DI) to team with the interpreter. The DIs are Deaf and can translate what the ASL interpreter signs into linguistic terms that match the Deaf person's language because of their ability to codeswitch between varieties of sign language (Leigh & Andrews, 2017). When interpreters are effective, mental health sessions can be helpful and Deaf clients appreciate that. They would prefer using ASL interpreters rather than struggle to directly communicate with non-ASL-fluent mental health clinicians. However, they often are concerned about confidentiality. They may risk seeing those interpreters and DIs in Deaf social situations or at work if employers provide ASL interpreting services and feel uncomfortable because of the sensitive information shared in mental health sessions. Interpreters are legally required not to disclose confidential information, but it is possible that some interpreters may breach confidentiality, thereby negatively affecting client feelings of safety.

> Leslie wanted an ASL-fluent therapist for her psychological problems. She couldn't find any, so she met with a therapist and an ASL interpreter. She revealed very private sexual relationship problems during her sessions. One day, there was an important meeting at work, and that interpreter showed up to interpret. Leslie was very embarrassed and wished she could escape from that meeting.

Another issue of concern is that unfortunately, many mental health clinicians do not know how to use interpreters appropriately (Leigh & Pollard, 2011; Steinberg et al., 2010). They may speak too fast, use language that may be difficult for interpreters to translate in ways that cli-

ents understand, or talk to the interpreter and not to the client. Because clients must look at the interpreter, the connection with the mental health clinician who is really leading the session will be weaker. It is very important for the clinician and the interpreter to work together as a team to make sure that the client has some eye contact with the clinician and gets good services. In this way, the Deaf client will feel validated as a person and not struggle with communication issues.

DOMESTIC VIOLENCE

Domestic violence includes rape, sexual assault, robbery, and assault committed by intimate partners, family members, or other relatives. Statistics show that this type of violence happens too often. The average annual number of domestic violence is over a million, with intimate partner violence accounting for approximately 15% of all violent victimizations (Truman & Morgan, 2014). This represents a greater percentage than that for family members or other relatives. Only about half of all domestic violence is reported to the police.

Deaf people are not immune from this type of violence. In the study on health-related information obtained through an ASL-accessible survey reported in the Health Issues section above, Barnett and researchers (2011) found that partner violence was a significant health concern. Additional research reports indicate that partner violence, emotional abuse, and forced sex (rape) are higher in the deaf population (e.g., Anderson, Leigh, & Samar, 2011; Pollard, Sutter, & Cerulli, 2014). Deaf and hard-of-hearing females and males on a college campus were 1.5 times more likely to be victims of sexual harassment, sexual assault, psychological abuse, and physical abuse than their hearing peers (Anderson & Leigh, 2011; McQuiller Williams, & Porter, 2010). And in 2018, there were 1,547 calls to the National Deaf Hotline Center from Deaf survivors of domestic violence and sexual assault (M. Erasmus, personal communication, May 20, 2019). Those individuals who are DeafBlind feel especially vulnerable to abuse (Simcock, 2017).

What are examples of aggression when the abuser is deaf or knows ASL? If the abuser signs very close to the victim's face when angry or stomps on the floor, this is intimidation. Emotional abuse involves insults such as making fun of the victim's ASL skills, saying the victim is a terrible mother, or threatening to take the children away. Forced isolation occurs when the abuser constantly checks the victim's smartphone, e-mail, and/or videophone or prevents the victim from socializing or meeting family members. If the police become involved, they will listen to the hearing abuser's version rather than the deaf victim's version. This is also an example of hearing privilege or audism. All this information and more about deaf victims can be obtained from both the DeafHope's website (http://www.deaf-hope.org) and the ADWAS (Abused Deaf Women's Advocacy Services) website (http://www.adwas.org).

Victims experience barriers that make it difficult to seek help. Language, communication, health literacy, and confidentiality are significant barriers. The deaf victim may fear retaliation from the perpetrator or Deaf community members, fear that the police or other service providers may not be helpful due to lack of communication accessibility, or be afraid to report an intimate partner despite serious injury (Barber, Wills, & Smith, 2010;

Mastrocinque et al., 2017). They often will have limited knowledge of available and accessible resources, keeping in mind that these resources are scarce and located mostly in large urban areas. The Internet has created more opportunities for Deaf victims to get help, that is, if the victims are allowed to access the Internet. The Internet provides information sources that individuals can share with victims.

CRIMINAL JUSTICE ISSUES

For most Deaf people, life issues do not include criminal activities. However, there are Deaf people who do enter the criminal justice system. Deaf and hard-of-hearing detainees should have the same rights as their hearing peers in terms of access at hearings and participation in prison programs, services, and activities. In reality, they face serious barriers at every step in the system. Many professionals in the legal system create barriers because they do not understand Deaf culture or what Deaf people are like, do not understand how to make sure Deaf people know what is going on, and do not care (Vernon & Miller, 2005). This section serves as a brief introduction, with Chapter 10 providing more details.

Police who handcuff Deaf people are unwittingly limiting the ability of Deaf persons to communicate using their hands (Novic, 2018). At the time of arrest, an ASL interpreter is rarely present, even though this is a legal requirement supported by the ADA (see explanation above) and some states. Many police officers are unaware of this requirement. Even though Deaf people have a right to avoid self-incrimination based on the Miranda warning and other legal-related documents, they will have a hard time understanding these without qualified and competent ASL interpreters who understand complicated legal vocabulary and can make sure that Deaf people know what is going on (Hoopes, 2003). Few ASL interpreters are qualified to interpret in legal settings. There are also Deaf Interpreters (DIs, see above explanation) who can translate what the ASL interpreter signs into a linguistic format that the Deaf person in the legal system can understand (Leigh & Andrews, 2017). It has been found that one-fourth of Deaf people do not have an interpreter during legal procedures (Miller & Vernon, 2002).

When Deaf people sign legal documents or forms without really knowing or understanding the contents, this often traps them into situations that can cause a lot of issues. For example, they may easily agree to a plea bargain without understanding what it is and what their charges are (Leigh & Andrews, 2017). If it includes jail time, they may be in for a shock. Even if they know their rights and can assert themselves, it is very hard to do this while one is in prison and is subject to prison rules regarding how to communicate with guards and supervisors. Even if correctional centers have policies in place for treating deaf inmates, personnel may not provide Deaf people with equal access to communication for many reasons, including not understanding communication needs, costs, and not respecting prisoners (e.g., Zapotosky, 2015).

Prisoners have to follow commands that are often spoken, or orders conveyed through auditory signals such as loudspeakers. That makes it hard for Deaf prisoners to respond appropriately, so they may be punished for not immediately doing what they are supposed to do. If they complain about treatment in prison, they also run the risk of being punished. If they are subject to solitary confinement,

on top of already being socially isolated within the hearing prison system, they are doubly isolated. They are essentially in a prison within a prison, and suicide becomes a real possibility (Morgan, 2017). Because of these experiences, often documented by HEARD, an advocacy organization for Deaf prisoners, the American Civil Liberties Union and the NAD filed a lawsuit against the Georgia Department of Corrections, the State Board of Pardons and Paroles, and several individual defendants, alleging discrimination and abuse of its deaf and hard-of-hearing inmates (Novic, 2018).

Jerry Coen, a former inmate, remembers how cruel his guards were. For example, one of them got mad at him, grabbed his hearing aid, and crushed it. Even though Coen filed a grievance over this incident, the Georgia Department of Corrections rejected the complaint because, in their words, the destruction of his property does not affect him. He was repeatedly denied access to inmate programs because interpreters were not provided and was disciplined for bad behavior because of rules he could not hear or follow. When a hearing on his case was held, he was handcuffed with his hands behind his back, thus preventing him from using ASL to communicate. Because of lack of access, he had anger problems and experienced 1 week of solitary confinement without any explanation of what caused this placement (Novic, 2018).

An increasing number of states, including Texas, California, and New York, among others, have established centralized units for Deaf prisoners (Talita Lewis, personal communication, May 28, 2019).

AGING ISSUES

We know that the population of people who have become eligible for Social Security or pensions is one of the fastest growing populations in the United States. Currently, this group represents about 15% of the U.S. population and is projected to increase to 24% by 2060 (Mather, 2016). This group is also increasingly racially and ethnically diverse. The probability that individuals will face health, financial, and social issues increases with age. What are the implications for culturally Deaf people who fall into the aging category?

Although gerontology (the study of aging and the problems of older people) is a growing field, not enough attention or research has been directed at the aging Deaf population (Feldman, 2010). This is a serious concern because Deaf people are also living longer and confronting issues associated with growing older (Lesch, Burcher, Wharton, Chapple, & Chapple, 2018). If they are undereducated and underemployed, they face financial struggles in accessing services, which then becomes a serious barrier to positive healthy aging.

The good news is that financial advisors who are themselves Deaf are now providing accessible financial information. The Social Security Administration provides sign language interpreters for Deaf people who are investigating their Social Security benefits. However, on the downside, as health issues increase with age, older Deaf people are struggling with barriers to health care access, including communication with medical service pro-

viders (Lesch et al., 2018; Witte & Kuzel, 2000). In their focus groups of elderly Deaf participants, Witte and Kuzel noted that the participants seemed resigned to their difficulties. Feldman (2005) reports that these types of individuals just stop going for treatment, whether for primary health care or mental health care. As Feldman (2010) notes, the overwhelming majority of social service agencies and organizations do not necessarily have expertise in working with older Deaf people. Most gerontologists who work with older patients rarely have the skills to diagnose or accurately evaluate older Deaf clients (Feldman, 2010). This becomes critical in situations when Deaf people have strokes that impact their signing ability and service providers cannot competently assess them. It is important to search for service providers such as Jaime Wilson, a Deaf Board Certified neuropsychologist in Tacoma, WA. However, Feldman also reports that current culturally Deaf baby boomers are much more aware of their rights compared to Deaf people of earlier generations, thanks to recent disability rights laws, including the ADA. They are less likely to accept professionals who do not provide adequate access and will pursue legal action to achieve functionally equivalent access, meaning access equivalent to the services provided to hearing peers. They likely will join organizations such as Deaf Seniors of America (DSA), an organization whose goals are to improve the quality of life of deaf seniors, disseminate resource information, and enhance awareness among the general public regarding the needs of Deaf senior citizens. Its biennial conferences include seminars focused on providing information that will empower Deaf senior citizens to advocate for themselves and promote healthy aging.

As older Deaf individuals face possible moves into assisted care facilities and nursing homes, they fear increased isolation if peers and staff are not able to communicate with them. One poignant example is that of the coronavirus pandemic. Due to restrictions that do not allow visitors in order to prevent contagion, this has caused isolation for hearing nursing home residents, and even more isolation for deaf nursing home residents with staff unable to communicate with them due to mask requirements that prevent speechreading and limited to no knowledge of ASL. Should Deaf seniors be unable to drive or use public transportation, they are less able to connect with social support groups, and we know that social support is important for quality of life as people age. However, the advent of videophones (see Chapter 9) has helped many homebound Deaf people connect with their friends and relatives, thereby improving their morale. In the state of Ohio, Columbus Colony is one of all too few facilities that provide skilled nursing and care for older Deaf individuals. Efforts are under way in other areas of the United States to establish similar facilities to address the needs of this growing population.

CONCLUSIONS

Deaf people deal with life events, just as hearing people do. They face more obstacles due to barriers in communicating with their hearing families and getting information about critical areas such as health, medical, and mental health settings, as well as educational and employment opportunities. Nonetheless, with the support of families who understand, support from employers who are willing to take advantage of their skills, and support from the Deaf community who share stories and explain about opportunities, the chances for Deaf people to be resilient and enjoy good quality of life throughout the life span are greatly improved.

REFERENCES

Anderson, M., & Leigh, I. W. (2011). Intimate partner violence against deaf female college students. *Violence Against Women, 17,* 822–834.

Anderson, M., Leigh, I. W., & Samar, V. (2011). Intimate partner violence against deaf women: A review. *Aggression and Violent Behavior: A Review Journal, 16,* 200–206.

Arndt, K., & Parker, A. (2016). Perceptions of social networks by adults who are deafblind. *American Annals of the Deaf, 161*(3), 369–383. https://doi.org/10.1353/aad.2016.0027

Barber, S., Wills, D., & Smith, M. (2010). Deaf survivors of sexual assault. In I. W. Leigh (Ed.), *Psychotherapy with Deaf clients from diverse groups* (pp. 320–340). Washington, DC: Gallaudet University Press.

Barnett, S., & Franks, P. (1999). Deafness and mortality: Analyses of linked data from the National Health Interview Survey and National Death Index. *Public Health Reports, 114,* 330–336.

Barnett, S., & Franks, P. (2002). Health care utilization and adults who are deaf: Relationships with age at onset of deafness. *Health Services Research, 37,* 105–120.

Barnett, S., Klein, J. D., Pollard, R. Q, Samar, V., Schlehofer, D., Starr, M., . . . Pearson, T. (2011). Community participatory research with deaf sign language users to identify health inequities. *American Journal of Public Health, 101,* 2235–2238.

Bauman, H.-D. (2004). Audism: Exploring the metaphysics of oppression. *Journal of Deaf Studies and Deaf Education, 9,* 239–246.

Benito, S. G., Glassman, T. S., & Hiedemann, B. G. (2016). Disability and labor market earnings: Hearing earnings gaps in the United

States. *Journal of Disability Policy Studies, 27*(3), 178–188. https://doi.org/10.1177/1044207316658752

Blackaby, J. (2018). *Can you hear me now? Being deaf and healthcare experiences.* (Master's thesis). Available from ProQuest Number 10747623.

Bouton, K. (2013). Quandary of hidden disabilities: Conceal or reveal. *New York Times.* Retrieved September 24, 2013, from http://www.nytimes.com/2013/09/22/business/quandary-of-hidden-disabilities-conceal-or-reveal.htm

Brandeis, A (2015). *Austin a top city for deaf-owned businesses.* Retrieved from https://www.kxan.com/news/local/austin/austin-a-top-city-for-deaf-owned-businesses/1049427048

Brenman, N. F., Hiddinga, A., & Wright, B. (2017). Intersecting cultures in deaf mental health: An ethnographic study of NHS professionals diagnosing autism in D/deaf children. *Culture, Medicine, and Psychiatry, 41*(3), 431–452. https://doi.org/10.1007/s11013-017-9526-y

Brooks, J. (2006). Strengthening resilience in children and youths: Maximizing opportunities through schools. *Children and Schools, 28,* 69–76.

Cleall, E. (2015). Silencing deafness: Displacing disability in the nineteenth century. *Portal: Journal of Multidisciplinary International Studies, 12*(1), 115–130.

Cmar, J. L., McDonnall, M. C., & Markoski, K. M. (2018). In-school predictors of post-school employment for youth who are deaf-blind. *Career Development and Transition for Exceptional Individuals, 41*(4), 223–233. https://doi.org/10.1177/2165143417736057

Crowe, T. (2017). Telemental health services as a targeted intervention for individuals who are deaf and hard of hearing, *JADARA, 51*(1). Retrieved from https://repository.wcsu.edu/jadara/vol51/iss1/2/

Cumberland, W. G., Berman, B. A., Zazove, P., Sadler, G. R., Jo, A., Booth, H., . . . Bastani, R. (2018). A breast cancer education program for D/deaf women. *American Annals of the Deaf, 163*(2), 90–115. https://doi.org/10.1353/aad.2018.0014

Davis, L. (2000). *My sense of silence.* Urbana: University of Illinois Press.

Du Feu, M., & Chovaz, C. (2014). *Mental health and deafness.* New York, NY: Oxford University Press.

Eckert, R. & Rowley, A. (2013). Audism: A theory and practice of audiocentric privilege. *Humanity and Society, 37*(2), 101–130. https://doi.org/10.1177/016059761381731

Feldman, D. (2005). Behaviors of mental health practitioners working with culturally deaf older adults. *Journal of the American Deafness and Rehabilitation Association, 39,* 31–54.

Feldman, D. (2010). Psychotherapy and Deaf elderly clients. In I. W. Leigh (Ed.), *Psychotherapy with Deaf clients from diverse groups* (pp. 281–299). Washington, DC: Gallaudet University Press.

Fellinger, J., Holzinger, D., & Pollard, R. (2012). Mental health of deaf people. *The Lancet, 379*(9820), 1037–1044. Retrieved from https://www.thelancet.com/pdfs/journals/lancet/PIIS0140-6736(11)61143-4.pdf

Garberoglio, C., Palmer, J., Cawthon, S., & Sales, A. (2019). *Deaf people and employment in the United States: 2019.* Washington, DC: U.S. Department of Education, Office of Special Education Programs, National Deaf Education Center on Postsecondary Outcomes. Retrieved from https://www.nationaldeafcenter.org/sites/default/files/DeafEmploymentReport-2019.pdf

Gerke, A. C. (2016). *A phenomenological examination of disability, microaggressions, and the experiences of deaf adults in mental health services* (Doctoral dissertation). Available from ProQuest #10108925.

Glickman, N. (Ed.). (2013). *Deaf mental health care.* New York, NY: Routledge.

Glickman, N., & Hall, W. (Eds.). (2019). *Language deprivation and deaf mental health.* New York, NY: Routledge.

Gournaris, M. J. (2009). Preparation for the delivery of telemental health services with individuals who are deaf. *Journal of the American Deafness and Rehabilitation Association, 43,* 34–51.

Groce, N. (1985). *Everyone here spoke sign language.* Cambridge, MA: Harvard University Press.

Harmer, L. (1999). Health care delivery and deaf people. *Journal of Deaf Studies and Deaf Education, 4,* 73–110.

Hoopes, R. (2003). Trampling Miranda: Interrogating Deaf suspects. In C. Lucas (Ed.), *Language and the law in Deaf communities* (pp. 21–59). Washington, DC: Gallaudet University Press.

Joharchi, H. (2017). *Negotiating access to mental health services: Deaf people with immigrant roots* (Doctoral dissertation). Available from ProQuest #10674033.

Kelleher, C. (2017). *When the hearing world will not listen: Deaf community care in hearing-dominated healthcare* (Master's thesis). Available from ProQuest #10264695.

Lang, H., & Meath-Lang, B. (1995). *Deaf persons in the arts and sciences.* Westport, CT: Greenwood Press.

Leigh, I.W. (2009), *A lens on deaf identities.* New York, NY: Oxford University Press.

Leigh, I. W., & Andrews, J. (2017). *Deaf people and society: Psychological, sociological, and educational perspectives.* New York, NY: Routledge.

Leigh, I. W., Marcus, A., Dobosh, P., & Allen, T. (1998). Deaf/hearing cultural identity paradigms: Modification of the Deaf Identity Development Scale. *Journal of Deaf Studies and Deaf Education, 3,* 329–338.

Leigh, I. W., & Pollard, R. Q. (2011). Mental health and deaf adults. In M. Marschark & P. Spencer (Eds.), *Oxford handbook of Deaf studies, language, and education* (Vol. 1, 2nd ed., pp. 214–226). New York, NY: Oxford University Press.

Lesch, H., Burcher, K., Wharton, T., Chapple, R., & Chapple, K. (2018). Barriers to healthcare services and supports for signing deaf older adults. *Rehabilitation Psychology.* https://doi.org/10.1037/rep0000252

Marbury, N. (2007). *Influences of challenges and successes on identity for Black Deaf Americans* (Doctoral dissertation). Retrieved from https://search.proquest.com/openview/ 98ac916862750b4b04397e5c07b1d5e2/1? pq-origsite=gscholar&cbl=18750&diss=y

Marschark, M. (2018). *Raising and educating a deaf child.* New York, NY: Oxford University Press.

Mastrocinque, J. M., Thew, D., Cerulli, C., Raimondi, C., Pollard, R. Q., & Chin, N. P. (2017). Deaf victims' experiences with intimate partner violence: The need for integration and innovation. *Journal of Interpersonal Violence, 32*(24), 3753–3777. https:// doi.org/10.1177/0886260515602896

Mather, M. (2016). *Fact sheet: Aging in the United States.* Retrieved from https://www .prb.org/aging-unitedstates-fact-sheet/

McQuiller Williams, L., & Porter, J. (2010, February). *An examination of the incidence of sexual, physical, and psychological abuse and sexual harassment on a college campus among underrepresented populations.* Paper presented at the Western Society of Criminology Conference, Honolulu, HI.

Miller, K., & Vernon, M. (2002). Qualifications of sign language interpreters in the criminal justice system. *Journal of Interpretation, 12,* 111–124.

Mitchell, R., & Karchmer, M. (2004). Chasing the mythical ten percent: Parental hearing status of deaf and hard of hearing students in the United States. *Sign Language Studies, 4,* 138–163.

Morgan, J. (2017). *Caged in: Solitary confinement's devastating harm on prisoners with physical disabilities.* New York, NY: American Civil Liberties Union. Retrieved from https:// www.aclu.org/sites/default/files/field_ document/010916-aclu-solitarydisability report-single.pdf

Mottez, B. (1993). The deaf-mute banquets and the birth of the deaf movement. In J. Van Cleve (Ed.), *Deaf history unveiled* (pp. 27–39). Washington, DC: Gallaudet University Press.

National Association of the Deaf. (2020). *Access during coronavirus public briefings.* Retrieved from https://www.nad.org/2020/03/19/ access-during-coronavirus-public-brief ings/

Novic, S. (2018, June 21). *Deaf prisoners are trapped in frightening isolation*. Retrieved from https://www.cnn.com/2018/06/21/opinions/aclu-georgia-deaf-abuse-lawsuit-novic/index.html

Oliva, G. (2004). *Alone in the mainstream*. Washington, DC: Gallaudet University Press.

Paris, D. (2020). Perspectives of tribal vocational rehabilitation providers serving D/DB/HOH. *ADARA Update, 1*, 3–5. Retrieved from https://www.adara.org/uploads/7/3/3/7/73376615/adara_update_january_2020.pdf

Petitto, L. (2014). Three revolutions: Language, culture, and biology. In H.-D. Bauman & J. Murray (Eds.), *Deaf gain* (pp. 65–76). Minneapolis: University of Minnesota Press.

Pollard, R. Q., Sutter, E., & Cerulli, C. (2014). Intimate partner violence reported by two samples of Deaf adults via a computerized American Sign Language survey. *Journal of Interpersonal Violence, 29*(5), 948–965. Retrieved from https://journals.sagepub.com/doi/abs/10.1177/0886260513505703

Punch, R., Hyde, M., & Creed, P. (2004). Issues in the school-to-work transition of hard of hearing adolescents. *American Annals of the Deaf, 149*, 28–38.

Sayers, E. (2017). *The life and times of T. H. Gallaudet*. Lebanon, NH: ForeEdge Press.

Siegel, R. (2018, October 23). Starbucks opens first U.S. sign language store—with murals, tech pads, and fingerspelling. *The Washington Post*. Retrieved from https://www.washingtonpost.com/business/2018/10/23/starbucks-opens-first-us-sign-language-store-with-murals-tech-pads-fingerspelling/?utm_term=.6fa17e281940

Simcock, P. (2017). One of society's most vulnerable groups? A systematically conducted literature review exploring the vulnerability of deafblind people. *Health & Social Care in the Community, 25*(3), 813–839. https://doi.org/10.1111/hsc.12317

Sirch, L., Salvador, L., & Palese, A. (2017). Communication difficulties experienced by deaf male patients during their in-hospital stay: Findings from a qualitative descriptive study. *Scandinavian Journal of Caring Sciences, 31*(2), 368–377. https://doi.org/10.1111/scs.12356

Smith, E. E. (2019, May 8). Celebrating the silence. *The Washington Post*, pp. B1, B2.

Sorrells, S. (2006, October 4). Rockville student rails against stereotypes. *The Gazette*, p. B-21.

Stapleton, L. (2016). Audism and racism: The hidden curriculum impacting Black d/Deaf college students in the classroom. *Negro Educational Review, 67*(1–4), 149–169.

Steinberg, A., Loew, R., & Sullivan, V. J. (1999). The diversity of consumer knowledge, attitudes, beliefs, and experiences. In I. W. Leigh (Ed.), *Psychotherapy with deaf clients from diverse groups* (pp. 23–43). Washington, DC: Gallaudet University Press.

Steinberg, A., Loew, R., & Sullivan, V. J. (2010). The diversity of consumer knowledge, attitudes, beliefs, and experiences. In I. W. Leigh (Ed.), *Psychotherapy with deaf clients from diverse groups* (2nd ed., pp. 18–38). Washington, DC: Gallaudet University Press.

Szymanski, C. (2010). An open letter to training directors regarding accommodations for deaf interns. *APPIC E-Newsletter*, pp. 1–5. Retrieved from http://www.rit.edu/ntid/hccd/system/files/An%20Open%20letter%20to%20Training%20Directors.pdf

Task Force on Health Care Careers for the Deaf and Hard-of-Hearing Community. (2012). *Building pathways to health care careers for the deaf and hard-of-hearing community: Final report, March 2012*. Rochester, NY: Gallaudet University, Rochester Institute of Technology/National Technical Institute for the Deaf, University of Rochester Medical Center, & Rochester General Health System.

Truman, J., & Morgan, R. (2014). *Nonfatal domestic violence, 2003–2012. Special Report.* Washington, DC: U.S. Department of Justice, Office of Justice Programs, Bureau of Justice Statistics.

Vernon, M., & Miller, K. (2005). Obstacles faced by Deaf people in the criminal justice system. *American Annals of the Deaf, 150*, 283–291.

Wahlqvist, M., Möller, C., Möller, K., & Danermark, B. (2016). Implications of Deafblindness: The physical and mental health and social trust of persons with Usher syndrome Type 3. *Journal of Visual Impairment & Blindness, 110*(4), 245–256. https://doi.org/10.1177/0145482X1611000404

Wattman, J. (2019). Interpreting for deaf people with dysfluent language in forensic settings. In N. Glickman & W. Hall (Eds.), *Language deprivation and deaf mental health* (pp. 210–234). New York, NY: Routledge.

Witte, T., & Kuzel, A. (2000). Elderly deaf patients' health care experiences. *Journal of the American Board of Family Practices, 13,* 17–22.

World Health Organization. (2014). *Mental health: A state of well-being.* Retrieved from https://www.who.int/features/factfiles/mental_health/en/

WPSDAA. (2013, April 16). *In memory of Nathie Marbury, class of 1962.* Retrieved from http://www.wpsdalumni.org/2013/04/in-memory-of-nathie-marbury-class-of-1962/

Zand, D., & Pierce, K. (Eds.). (2011). *Resilience in deaf children.* New York, NY: Springer.

Zapotosky, M. (2015, September 13). Judge rules redress be paid to deaf ex-inmate. *The Washington Post,* p. C5.

Zazove, P. (1993). *When the phone rings, my bed shakes: Memoirs of a deaf doctor.* Washington, DC: Gallaudet University Press.

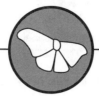

CHAPTER 9

Technology and Accessibility

When a baby cries, how do Deaf caregivers know? When someone knocks on the door? When an emergency vehicle has its siren on? When their name is being called at the local coffee shop to inform them their coffee is ready?

Those questions are rooted in the fundamental nature of "access," or "accessibility." Accessibility refers to enabling access for a wider range of people, be it a product, a device, the environment, or services (Ginnerup, 2009). You may have used those accessibility features, such as the curb cuts (Figure 9–1), which persons in wheelchairs use to roll down from the curb to the street, or to roll up to the sidewalk from the street.

You might have also appreciated the number display on the wall informing you of the number being called after you take a number from the dispenser. You might have run your fingertips across a

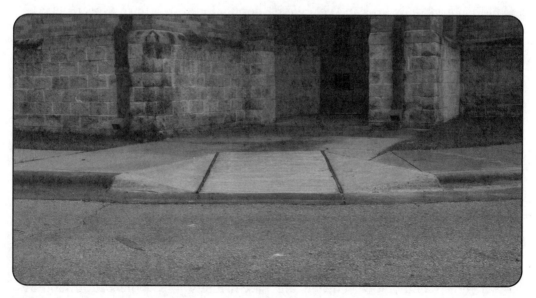

Figure 9–1. An example of a curb cut. Photo credit: John Moore Jr. Used with permission.

tactile braille floor number sign while in the elevator. You might have liked the color contrast between the halls and the carpeting, especially the borders of the carpeting at your school. All of those are products or designs that aim to be utilized by people with diverse ranges of abilities (Gold, 2011).

HISTORY: FOUNDATIONS FOR ACCESS

When did the accessibility movement in the United States start? In the early 1800s, people with disabilities were often forced to enter institutions and asylums or were used as entertainment in traveling circuses, which were also called "freak shows." Freak shows were popular in Europe and America, and focused on disabled people with physical oddities doing normal things despite their disabilities (NFCA, 2020). The thinking at that time was about the purification of the American people—people wanted to see "normal" people in their daily lives. People with disabilities were segregated and hidden from daily lives and yet ogled at with fascinating disgust and revulsion in freak shows and traveling circuses (NFCA, 2020). Some people with disabilities were sterilized to make sure they could not produce more babies with disabilities. This is called "eugenics," specifically the belief that the human population could be improved through having the more superior humans breed and the inferior, problematic humans be removed or sterilized. Inferior humans often included people with disabilities and people of certain ancestry, national origin, and race (Winzer, 2009). In contrast, characteristics of superior humans were often white people, with no disability, blue-eyed, and tall, all of which were considered desirable

qualities. Chapter 2 provides an introduction to this topic as well.

In the late 1800s through the early 1900s, the eugenics movement spread rapidly. This type of thinking led to former German Chancellor Adolf Hitler's delusion of the "pure race" in the 1930s and during World War II by removing "inferior" humans from the human race, not by sterilization but instead by euthanasia (Fleischer & Zames, 2011; Pelka, 2012). Between 1907 and 1958, 30 U.S. states had eugenic sterilization laws in place. Around that time, the American Breeders Association explored the idea of sterilizing people with disabilities, particularly intellectual disabilities, in the United States. After witnessing the horrors of Nazi Germany in the late 1930s and 1940s, the eugenics movement in the United States was quickly condemned by the public, but not before 70,000 Americans were sterilized without their consent and often without their knowledge (Cohen, 2016).

Public schools funded by taxpayers proliferated in the 1940s and 1950s, and students that did not fit the general population were put in "special classes" within the school. Those special classes often included deaf, blind, cognitively challenged, and students with other disabilities who were grouped together in one class (Winzer, 2009).

The 1960s included a major shift in thinking for the American public, including civil rights and desegregation, leading to the Architectural Barriers Act of 1968, signed into law by President Lyndon B. Johnson. This law requires that facilities built by the government must be accessible (Fleischer & Zames, 2001). This movement continued well into the 1970s with many states passing laws requiring accessibility for people with disabilities. In 1973, President Richard Nixon signed the Rehabilitation Act. This act prohibited federal agencies and agencies receiving federal funding from discriminating against people with disabilities in their hiring practices. This act also provided civil rights to children and people with disabilities, including reasonable accommodations. In 1975, the United States led the world in the passage of Public Law 94-142, Education for All Handicapped Children Act, requiring schools to provide an "appropriate education to children with disabilities," signed into law by President Gerald Ford (Winzer, 2009, p. 127).

Much more landmark legislation regarding access and equality for people with disabilities followed, but the most pivotal one for the American disability rights movement was the Americans With Disabilities Act (ADA) of 1990, signed into law by President George H. W. Bush (Pelka, 2012). As seen in Figure 9–2, people rallied to support the ADA legislation on March 12, 1990. The ADA was signed 4 months later, on July 26.

ADA is a wide-ranging civil rights law that prohibits discrimination based on disability, including requiring employers to provide reasonable accommodations to employees with disabilities, and accessibility requirements for public accommodations (McNeese, 2014). Also see Chapter 10 for additional details on overall legislation,

DEAF COMMUNITY AND ACCESS

Even with the ADA in effect, the National Association of the Deaf (NAD) and other disability rights organizations continue to remain proactive and pave ways for equal access for the Deaf community.

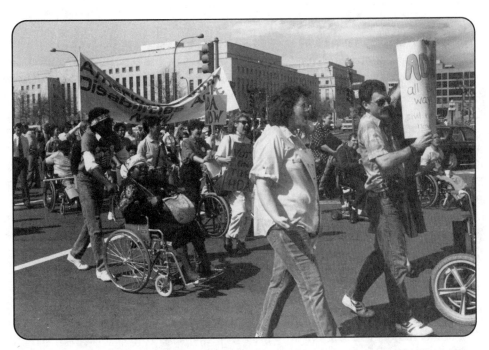

Figure 9–2. People rallying for the passage of the Americans With Disabilities Act on March 12, 1990, at the Capitol. Courtesy of Gallaudet University Archives.

For instance, in February 2013, Deaf and hard-of-hearing truck drivers were finally allowed to obtain commercial drivers' licenses (CDLs) through the U.S. Department of Transportation. In July 2014, Pacific Northwest University of Health was ordered to allow a Deaf medical student to be admitted to their program. In February 2015, the NAD sued Harvard University and Massachusetts Institute of Technology (MIT) for not captioning their public online videos. In May 2015, a Girl Scouts local chapter was ordered to provide an ASL interpreter for Girl Scout troop meetings (NAD News, 2015). The lawsuits were won in 2019 and 2020. In January 2017, the Department of Justice issued regulations requiring movie theaters to provide equipment necessary to provide closed captioning. Such events show progress in making our society a more equitable one for everyone.

> In 2014, the NAD participated in an investigation to determine if apartment complexes treated hearing and deaf renters differently. They found 86% of the apartments gave less information to deaf individuals compared to hearing individuals, 56% informed deaf individuals that additional background and financial checks would be needed, and 40% hung up on deaf callers at least once. The NAD, along with other organizations, filed complaints against 715 apartment complexes in seven different states (NAD News, 2014).

There are still many more battles to be fought. For instance, in 2015, Nicki, who is Deaf, and Kris Runge, a married couple trying to become pregnant, encountered problems with interpreting services. When they attended a doctor-sponsored group therapy session with other couples, they discovered that the interpreter was not certified and couldn't adequately interpret the meeting. When Nicki went in for a uterine exam, the interpreter sat next to the gynecologist—which was highly inappropriate considering the situation. Not only that, Nicki was on a complex course of fertility medication with strict dosing rules—it was important that the information interpreted was accurate. Instead of suing the doctor or the doctor's office as traditionally done in the past, they decided to sue the interpreting agency for providing unqualified interpreters. Their attorney, Amy Robertson, working with the Civil Rights Education and Enforcement Center, says, "Go after the supply, not the demand" (Cheek, 2015, p. 1). This case was settled out of court early January 2016, with the interpreting agency promising that they "would hire and assign only RID-certified sign language interpreters" (Goodland, 2016, p. 1).

During the coronavirus pandemic of 2020, the NAD CEO, Howard A. Rosenblum, Esq., declared that "the U.S. Government has failed to make information accessible in ASL," explaining that many of the announcements coming from the White House and other government agencies often will not include captions and/or a Deaf interpreter (NAD Coronavirus, 2020, p. 1). On March 18, 2020, after many weeks of media communications about coronavirus at the local, regional, state, and national levels, *Sign1News* posted that a board-certified and ASL-fluent family physician, Dr. Deborah Gilboa, asked what one of her Deaf patients was doing to prepare for the coronavirus. The Deaf patient responded, "What is that?" (Sign1News, 2020, p. 1).

For the novel coronavirus crisis, particularly COVID-19, the NAD prepared two guidelines, one for Deaf and Deaf-Blind people and one for hospitals. In their statement, the NAD painted a very grim picture of little or zero access for the Deaf person when hospitalized, saying, "Many hospitals will not allow for in-person interpreters, family members or visitors to come in the hospital" (NAD Communicating, 2020, p. 1). NAD cautioned that with COVID-19, medical personnel wear masks, full protective suits, and gloves, making it impossible to read lips, understand gestures, or try to write with a pen back and forth. Most of them try to talk to you behind a window, a door, or a curtain, not simply to protect themselves from the virus but to preserve the limited, dwindling supply of personal protective equipment (PPE, which includes masks, gloves, and suits) and to prevent cross-contamination from visiting and caring for multiple patients in the same period of time. NAD recommended that Deaf people bring an emergency bag with items to help them communicate with medical personnel, including paper, pens, plugs and chargers for their smartphone, emergency contact information, and a copy of their advance medical directive (NAD Communicating, 2020, p. 1). Sadly, rationing intensive care beds and ventilators happens when there are more sick people than there are beds and machines to help them (Camosy, 2020). But what happens if there's only one bed, or one ventilator, and two patients with novel coronavirus: a Deaf person and a hearing person? In the guidelines for hospitals, the NAD emphasized, in bold, that "hospitals must not consider patients' disabilities in making triage decisions" (NAD Communicating, 2020, p. 1). This is a critical ethical issue.

In the mid-1990s, some people argued that there was a need to go beyond "accessibility" and create designs that benefited all people, rather than inventing something and *then* adding adaptions to accommodate people with disabilities. There were several names for this, including "Design for All," "Barrier-Free" concept, and "Universal Design" (Ginnerup, 2009; Vanderheiden, 1996). Televisions are one example. When movies with sound appeared in the late 1920s, people did not think of including (or knew how to include) readable captions of the voices and sounds. The same thing happened with TV when it became broadly available in the early 1950s (NAD Movie Captioning, 2006).

> Captions and subtitles are not the same thing. Subtitles assume the viewer can hear but cannot understand the language. For instance, a French-speaking film in the United States would be subtitled in English. However, the sounds of someone knocking, running, or even speaking English in that same movie would not be subtitled. Captions include all audio, including spoken English as well as music and sound effects.

Captions

In the 1970s, people who wanted captions for their TV had to purchase an additional box (as seen in Figure 9–3) the size of a briefcase for $200.

The first show with closed captions occurred in 1972 with reruns of *The French Chef* with Julia Childs (Boboltz, 2015). *ABC News* offered a captioned version

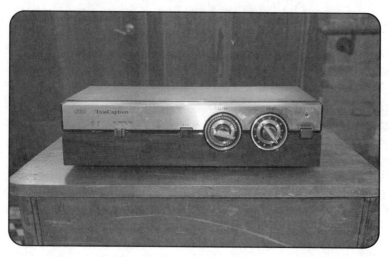

Figure 9–3. A captioning device from the 1980s, about the size of a briefcase. Photo courtesy of Texas School for the Deaf Heritage Center and John Moore Jr.

of its newscast in 1973 and was the only captioned news show for approximately the next 10 years (NCI, 2015). At that time, TVs and a caption box were approximately the same cost. So people who wanted to watch TV shows with captions would need to pay double—for the TV and the caption box. And not all shows had captioning. In fact, very few programs were captioned. To caption a show was expensive and time-consuming, so many TV shows chose not to incur additional expenses to caption their shows.

The National Captioning Institute (NCI), a nonprofit corporation, was created in 1979 and went to work in developing a mechanism for offline captioning with accurate timing that could be used by TV shows to caption their shows before airing them. On March 16, 1980, there were a limited number of regularly scheduled shows that used captions for all of their shows—*ABC Sunday Night Movie* (ABC), *Disney's Wonderful World* (NBC), *Masterpiece Theater* (PBS), *3-2-1 Contact* (PBS), and the first captioned commercial

from IBM. This was an overnight sensation for the Deaf community! In 1982, NCI invented a way to caption real-time, live broadcasts and announcements where captioners type up to 250 words per minute using a special machine. In 1984, the Democratic and Republican national conventions were captioned for the first time, using real-time captioning. Super Bowl 1985's commentary was the first real-time captioned sports event. *Family Ties* was the first corporate-funded TV series, funded by the Kellogg Company. The year 1986 saw the first daytime soap opera series captioned *Search for Tomorrow*. The first daytime talk show that was captioned was *The Oprah Winfrey Show*. In 1987, *Jeopardy* and *Wheel of Fortune* were the first game shows that had captions. The year 1991 saw the first congressional floor proceedings by the U.S. House of Representatives captioned (NCI, 2015). More and more programs caught on and started adding captions to their shows but not after countless requests for access through activism and advocacy by the

Deaf community. The earliest closed captioning icon would come with the text, *Closed captioned for the hearing impaired*, on various TV channels.

With the passage of the Television Decoder Circuitry Act of 1990, pushed through by NCI and other organizations, this law mandated that all televisions 13 inches or bigger would need to include a caption-decoding microchip (NCI, 2015). No additional purchase of a caption box was needed anymore! Deaf people could go anywhere, be it motels, bars, or fitness gyms, and ask that the captions be turned on. This is an example of universal design —not only Deaf and hard-of-hearing people benefited from this, but now children and people who were learning English could too and patrons in noisy environments such as trains, bars, and gyms could still follow the dialogue on the TV or viewers could still watch movies in an ultra-quiet environment such as in a library, with a nearby sleeping baby or a cranky roommate. Those are examples of ordinary people benefiting from technology originally designed for Deaf people. That is what universal design is all about.

> Did you notice the outdated and inappropriate term earlier, *Closed captioned for the hearing impaired*? And now we know captions are for everyone, not just Deaf people.

More changes happened and more laws were passed, including the Telecommunications Act of 1996, which required that digital television receivers also include caption technology. The year 2001 saw the very first real-time Spanish captioning with mixed case and accent marks during CNN en Español news. In 2002, NCI developed the Described Video service, translating visual media into an accessible format for blind or low-vision consumers. The Twenty-First Century Communications and Video Accessibility Act of 2010 required broadcasters to include captioning for cable television programs that are shown again on the web. This law also required HD TV boxes to include a closed caption button. In 2012, more legislation including closed captioning for programs delivered through the Internet was passed (NCI, 2015). In 2020, there was a class-action lawsuit against Pornhub for not captioning the dialogue in their videos (Steinbuch, 2020).

> Closed captions and open captions mean two different things. Closed captions mean you need to turn it on using the remote or click a button on the screen. Closed captions do not show up automatically—it has to be turned on (or off) manually. Open captions are permanently included in the video itself, cannot be turned off or removed, and will always be visible. Figures 9–4A and B show the current icons for closed captioning (cc) and open captioning (oc). And Figures 9–4C and D show what both closed captioning and open captioning look like on the screen, although there are more variations today than ever before.

Even today, there are still problems with captions and accessibility, particularly for public venues and videos on the Internet. In 2009, the NAD successfully achieved a settlement with Ohio State University's athletic department after this department failed to provide captioning

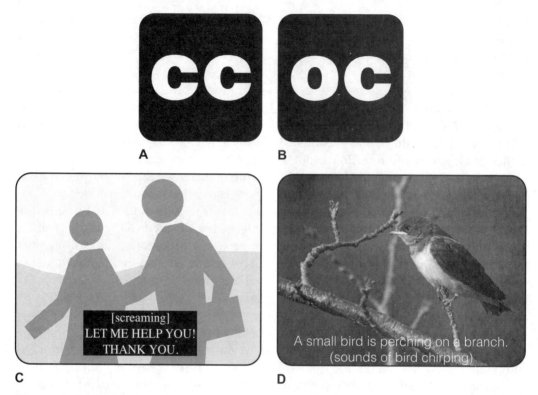

Figure 9–4. A. Current icon for closed captioning. **B.** Current icon for open captioning. **C.** Closed captioning on a screen. **D.** Open captioning on a screen. Photos courtesy of Wikimedia Commons.

at its stadium. Letters were sent to the remaining universities that were part of the Big Ten Conference informing them that they would need to adopt similar practices to ensure equal access to all fans in their stadiums. More lawsuits were to come, against the Arizona Cardinals, the University of Maryland, and the Washington Redskins (Charmatz, Hedges-Wright, & Ward, 2011; NAD OSU, 2010; Schoepfer-Bochicchio, 2013). This has created a market for businesses providing solutions for stadiums unsure how to provide accessibility to their patrons (Vitac, 2017).

Other public venues with accessibility issues may include movie theaters, concerts, planetariums, demonstrations, and theatrical performances. Movie the-

aters have had a long history in experimenting with different ways for Deaf people to fully access movies with spoken dialogue, starting in 1927 when talking pictures replaced silent films, which had been accessible for the Deaf community. This change meant that the moviegoing experience was now inaccessible for the Deaf community. There were and are several captioning organizations established, with some renamed over the decades, including Captioned Films for the Deaf, Captioned Films and Videos, Captioned Media Program, The Caption Center, Tripod Captioned Films, Movie Access Coalition, Media Access Group, and Coalition for Movie Captioning. Various captioning approaches were devised, including open captioned film prints (where captions are printed on the movie itself), screen-based caption projection systems (where captions are added by a second projector superimposed on the movie itself), seat-based caption systems, and wearable captioning systems, such as glasses that display captions in the lens and amplifications of the sound built in the temples of the glasses (NAD Movie Technologies, 2006; New Tech, 2013). To search for movies providing captioned access, http://www.captionfish.com is widely used.

Open-captioned film prints (where open captions are permanently embedded in the film itself) are favored by most members of the Deaf community because the format is most similar to captions on television (King, 2009). The cost to embed captions on the film itself and make duplicates to ship nationwide was excessive. Screen-based caption projection systems were a cost-effective alternative. However, some film footage would be heavily white, for example, such as a desert scene, rendering the projected captions (which are white) nearly impossible to see. Sadly, most movie theaters were afraid that open captions would be too intrusive for hearing viewers—in fact, Hollywood has been resistant to including open captions, arguing that seeing captions on the screen would drive away hearing viewers (Boboltz, 2015; Robitaille, 2001). Ironically, as Boboltz (2015) points out, there does not seem to be an official survey of hearing people and their opinions of open captioning on the screen, especially when captions are more and more commonplace in noisy places like restaurants, bars, and gyms or where sound needs to be muted such as libraries, red-eye flights, or with a sleeping infant.

At the 2020 Oscars, Bong Joo Hoo, the director of *Parasite*, which won four Oscars (Best Picture, Best Original Screenplay, Best Director, and Best Foreign Language Film) said, "Once you overcome the 1-inch-tall barrier of subtitles, you will be introduced to so many more amazing films" (Hong, 2020, p. 1). Ticket sellers for *Parasite* warned everyone waiting in line to purchase tickets to see the movie that the film was in Korean to prevent having to give refunds to those who didn't know and walked out demanding a refund (Hong, 2020).

The current option most movie theaters use is a seat-based caption system called Rear Window Caption (RWC) and CaptiView. Wearable glasses come in a close second. Deaf people go to the customer service desk to pick up the device. Seat-based caption systems have a thick bottom that fits in the cup holder of your seat and a black flexible rod with a reflective panel (RWC) or a LED display on top (CaptiView), roughly the size of a large envelope. Sitting down, the person using an RWC would adjust the rod and panel to be able to see the captions, as seen in Figure 9–5.

There are quite a few problems with those devices, such as batteries running out in middle of the movie, someone standing up behind you and blocking the captions being reflected on your screen, waiting for the movie to start only to discover the captions have not been activated by the theater (Note: movie previews rarely, if ever, are captioned), the flexible rod not staying in place and slowly dipping downward during the movie, exhaustion on the viewer's part in constantly refocusing eyes between the screen and the display in front of you, glasses weighing on/slipping down the bridge of your nose, inability of viewers to move in their seat without losing view of the captions, and, finally, if you go to the theater with a large group of people,

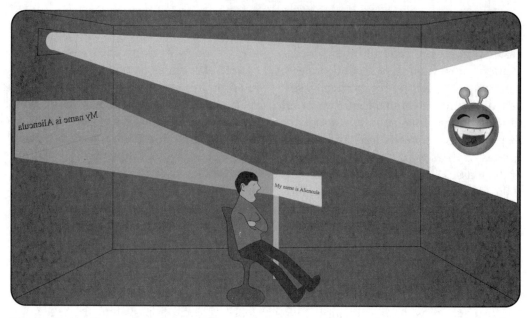

Figure 9–5. The rear window caption system. Photo courtesy of Wikimedia Commons.

often the theater does not carry enough of the devices for everyone (King, 2009; Pierpoint, 2018).

> When you go to a movie theater, ask to see and touch one of these devices. Ask how many they have in stock ready to loan out (not counting the ones that are being recharged).

Unfortunately, the current interpretation of the 1990 Americans With Disabilities Act (ADA) says that movies are not required to present open captions. Advocates claim that alternatives must be explored (NAD Movie Captioning, 2006). Access for deaf and hard-of-hearing viewers in m2wovies with 3-D effect and IMAX theaters is also sometimes inconsistent and problematic.

Other struggles regarding captioning videos on the Internet involve Netflix.

NAD sued Netflix in 2011 because not all of their streaming movies were captioned (Netflix Sued, 2011), and worse, they weren't captioned accurately—some sentences would be shortened or simplified. Swearing was often censored within captions, even though the audio track was not censored (Christian, 2014). One recent example from Netflix's *Bloodline* series, Season 1, Episode 13, had actor Kyle Chandler speak the line, "I don't know. Why don't you get to the fucking point?" The captions on the screen were, "I don't know. Why don't you get to the point?" (Bloodline, 2015).

Netflix requested that the judge dismiss the lawsuit on the basis that the Americans With Disabilities Act applies only to physical places and since Netflix is online, the ADA should not be applied to website-only businesses (Netflix Precedent, 2012). A few months later, Netflix and NAD agreed on a timetable in which Netflix would ensure all streaming content would be captioned by 2014 (Netflix Agreement, 2012). Thanks to Netflix agreeing to caption 100% of their content by 2014, NAD was able to enter into agreements with Amazon, Apple, Gogo, Hulu, and Vudu to caption their content (Television and Closed Captioning, 2020).

On Tumblr, there is a blog titled "Awkward Netflix Captions" with screenshots of actual Netflix movies with incorrect subtitles such as "sheik," while the actual spoken word is "chic." The Huffington Post comedy section has quite a collection of closed captioning fails, including an article suggesting that the captioning by the FOX network at the Republican Primary Debate on August 6, 2015, included a cat walking on their keyboard (McDonald, 2015). Another captioning fail example included a cooking show discussing refried penises, instead of beans (Wabash, 2019).

What about user-generated uploaded videos on an online platform such as YouTube? In 2006, Google purchased YouTube, and a Deaf Google captions software engineer, Ken Harrenstein, worked with a team of engineers to add the closed caption symbol to the bottom of YouTube videos, allowing people to turn captions on and off as indicated in Figure 9–6.

That was an amazing breakthrough at that time because there were no other free, public online video platforms that included the closed caption button. A few years later, Harrenstien announced that YouTube was able to add many new features, including machine-generated automatic captions and search functionality—both rooted in universal design concepts. Machine-generated automatic captions use Google's automatic speech recognition (ASR) technology within YouTube to automatically generate captions, or auto-caps for short. Although the captions may not be perfect, they are editable by the owner of the video. Also, if you happen to have a transcript of the spoken information in the video, you can upload the transcript and YouTube will use their ASR to help with auto-timing the captions throughout the video. Not only that, captions enable people speaking different languages to access video content in 51 different languages, further dismantling the Babel tower concept. Also, by making all videos captioned, this increases the power of the search function when searching for videos that discuss specific content (Harrenstien, 2009). People uploading to YouTube are more likely to add captions if the process makes it convenient, with

---

Although people may find closed captioning fails funny, think about how frustrated you would be if you couldn't understand people speaking while watching television and movies. Accurate captioning is very important in providing equal access to all. If you have Deaf friends, think carefully when you repost or share video content on social media without captions. Or add a transcript of the audio content yourself, then share. In fact, don't stop there—add image and video descriptions as well. If you'd like to learn how, search "how do I add video and image descriptions on [name of social media app]," and you'll find plenty of resources showing how you how to. Those are also called "alt text" (alternative text). Those efforts will provide access for your DeafBlind, DeafDisabled, and Deaf friends on social media.

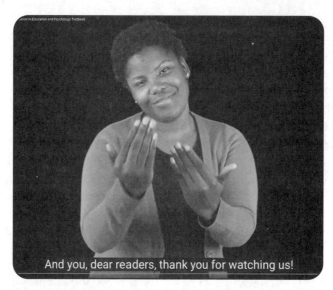

Figure 9–6. A screenshot of a YouTube video with closed captions. Photo courtesy of ASLChoice and Felicia Williams.

ASR, auto-caps, and auto-timing. Harrenstien explained at VidCon2017 conference, "Using captions is just the right thing to do" (Schumacher-Rasmussen, 2017, p. 1). YouTube continues to pave the way when it comes to accessibility and universal design.

Other than captions, what are the types of accessibility technology available? How do deaf people make phone calls? How do deaf people wake up for work? What about smoke alarm systems? Emergency alerts? There are different types of accessibility technology that are visual, auditory, and/or tactile based.

Visual-based accessibility technology tends to utilize visual alerts such as a flashing light, text-based communicative devices, or changing color hues. Auditory accessible technology is mostly rooted in amplification or closed-circuit frequencies to make it easier for hard-of-hearing people to access sound.

Most tactile-based accessibility technology for Deaf people is of the vibrating type, and DeafBlind people utilize more of this type of technology, including embossed symbols and braille, truncated domes (also called cement bubbles), and rumble strips that can be considered assistive devices (Cook & Polgar, 2014). Eight DeafBlind adults, ages 47 years and older, with various degrees of vision and hearing levels were surveyed for their preferred accessibility devices. They preferred devices including but not limited to a braille reader, talking book players, and videophones. A full list of preferred accessibility devices is shown in Table 9–1 (Ingraham, 2015).

Telephones

What about the telephone? Alexander Graham Bell's patent for his telephone

Table 9–1. Preferred Accessibility Devices for DeafBlind Adults

Braille typewriter

Talking book player

Videophone/video chat programs, apps, and software

Texting and video messaging

Large-screen video monitors and televisions (for use with VRI)

TTY with large visual display

Amplified and large button telephones

Large print calculator

Braille, talking, large display or vibrating watches, clocks, and timers

Desktop and handheld Video Magnifiers (formerly known as CCTV)

Tablet (e.g., iPad) with zoom features

Braille, tactile, and voice label systems

Screen reading software

Vibrating signaling system for doorbell, smoke detector, and telephone calls

Screen enlargement software

Raised flooring, added handrails, and grab bars

Captioned telephone with large display

Refreshable braille display

Electronic tablets using zoom feature

Barcode readers

Digital voice recorders

Bump dots/braille labels (for marking appliances)

Modified flooring, grab bars, additional handrails, lever doorknobs

Task and balanced lighting

Source: Adapted with permission: Ingraham (2015).

was granted on March 7, 1876, and 3 days later, on March 10, 1876, Bell made his first phone call to his assistant, Mr. Watson[1] (Shulman, 2008. By 1902, there were over 81,000 pay phones spread across the country, mostly in train stations and drug stores (Payphone, 2000). The telephone was improved over time, and by 1904, there were over three million phones in the United States. The first coast-to-coast

---

[1]It has been speculated that Bell bribed the patent officer to reveal Elisha Gray's initial patent (called a "caveat") and patented the telephone before Gray could (Shulman, 2008).

call was in 1915, when more and more telephone switchboards and networks were set up. The first mobile phone call occurred in 1973 (Raum, 2008).

How do deaf people make calls? For a very long time, deaf and hard-of-hearing people had to depend on hearing people, mostly family members, friends, or neighbors, to make phone calls for them. Those calls would often be for their doctor or their children's schools or to call in sick for them. When a deaf person wanted to visit another deaf person, they would often stop by unannounced and hope someone would be home. If not, they would leave a note. During that time, the invention of the telephone was the most formidable, social, and cultural obstacle for the Deaf community (DeVinney, 2015).

> Can you imagine having someone else make personal calls for you? How about having your mother call your boyfriend or girlfriend, or even their mother, to schedule a date? This actually happened many times. How would you feel?

Deaf people also depended on hard-of-hearing members of their community to try to make calls. Inventions to amplify the sound (make the sound louder) in the early 1930s required the hard-of-hearing person to put the receiver in a device so the sound coming from the device would be amplified for the entire room, giving both telephone participants no privacy. Often all environmental sounds on the other end would also be amplified, not just their voice, rendering the conversation impossible to understand. The first in-telephone receiver amplifier that

amplified the other end's voice for the listener was patented in 1964. People could increase (or decrease) the amplification using a small wheel in the middle of the telephone handset (Sanders, 1964). This was installed on most payphones in the early 1970s, as shown in Figure 9–7.

There were also portable amplifiers that hard-of-hearing people could carry around and add to the payphone or to phones in the area (DiPietro, Williams, & Kaplan, 2007).

Because of the widespread reliance on using the telephone among people who can hear, the Deaf community was set backward for decades without direct access to use of the telephone. The first breakthrough came when Robert Weitbrecht, a deaf scientist, developed the teletypewriter (TTY) in the 1960s (DeVinney, 2015). The teletypewriter looks like a typewriter with special cups designed to fit both ends of the telephone. Callers type their message on the TTY, and the message is delivered through the telephone line to the other end's TTY. That person reads the message as the other party types, and then they type back and so on.

At the beginning, it took some time for the TTY to finally gain acceptance among the telecommunications industry and the Deaf community (Lang, 2000). The telecommunications industry did not recognize that this new development would mean new customers and additional revenue. The very first machines were extremely large, similar to the size of a dishwasher, however, with an additional a foot or two on top. They were also very heavy and difficult to find and/or purchase, as supplies were limited. Older Deaf people fondly remember how loud those machines were—pressing one key would make the entire machine shake.

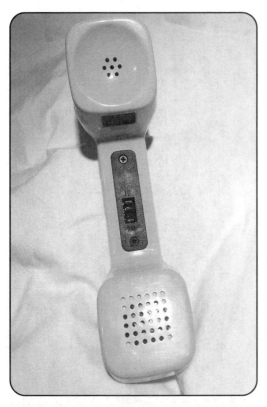 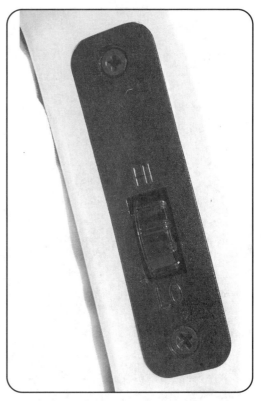

Figure 9–7. An Amplified Telephone, with the scroll increasing the volume on middle of the phone handle. Photo credit: Nick Ogrizovich. Used with permission.

A picture of one of the oldest TTYs is shown in Figure 9–8.

> Can you imagine having one of these, a large standing TTY, the size of a medium refrigerator, in your home to make calls?

In 1968, there were only 25 machines in the entire United States. A nonprofit organization, Telecommunications for the Deaf, Inc., was established in 1968 to handle the distribution of TTYs and maintain a national directory of TTY numbers for Deaf people, companies, and schools.

Their national directory went from 145 listings in 1968 to 810 listings by 1970 (TDI Milestones, 2015). Other organizations, resource groups, and people, such as the Telephone Pioneers of America, pushed forward the TTY movement by providing training on the use and maintenance of TTYs. Deaf Americans, particularly Alfred Sonnenstrahl, and on the state level Paul Taylor (New York) were also instrumental in lobbying for state support and legislation supporting the Deaf community and telecommunications from the 1970s through the 1990s. Karen Peltz Strauss, formerly Deputy Bureau Chief of the Consumer and Governmental Affairs Bureau at the Federal Communications

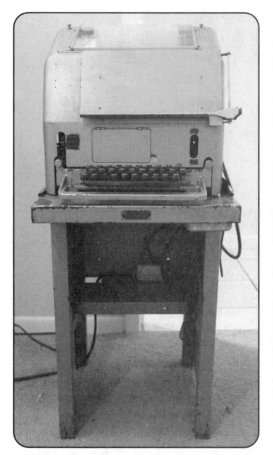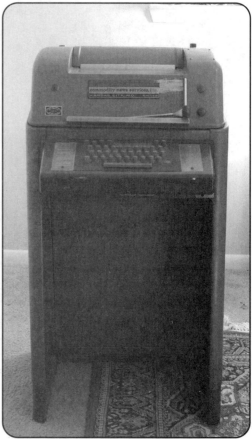

Figure 9–8. Old TTY machines in the late 1960s. Photos courtesy of Misty Morris.

Commission, worked very closely with the pioneers in this effort. She has written extensively about these legislative efforts (Peltz-Strauss, 2006).

By 1974, 7,000 TTYs were in use worldwide, and nearly all were used in deaf homes. Deaf people were thrilled to be finally able to communicate with each other directly (Lang, 2000). There was still a huge barrier—Deaf people weren't able to call hearing people, and hearing people weren't able to call Deaf people, unless they had a TTY too (Graham, 1988). Despite efforts in providing training for offices, companies, agencies, and schools to purchase a TTY and maintain a sepa-

rate number for deaf people, difficulties persisted. Sometimes, the person receiving the training would move on to other opportunities and the agency would not know what to do with the TTY. Some TTYs were hidden in a cabinet collecting dust, and when a TTY call was made, people there would run around wondering where the TTY was.

A solution was proposed: The Telecommunications Relay Service (TRS) was created first as a volunteer program. Hearing people at a specific center would volunteer to receive TTY calls and, using the telephone, deliver the spoken message to the other end, and then type back the information spoken to the Deaf caller. This would mean hearing organizations and agencies would not need to purchase a TTY, provide TTY training, and maintain the TTY line. The first statewide relay service was established in 1974 in Connecticut. More soon followed.

Then in the 1980s, newer, smaller, and more ergonomic TTYs were also produced and marketed, as seen in Figure 9–9.

Around this time, more and more adaptations were added to the telephone for hard-of-hearing people, including amplifier handsets for public phones. Some phones were also modified for compatibility with hearing aids (DiPietro et al., 2007). Deaf people were finally able to call their hearing family members and friends, make their own doctor's appointments, and even order pizza! In 1990, the ADA passed, and a nationwide relay service became available 24/7 in every state and territory (TRS, 2015).

Carrying TTYs around or looking for TTYs to make calls (or receive calls) became cumbersome. People started using the instant messaging (IM) feature. Some TRS providers capitalized on this opportunity, using a similar format to instant messaging to create what is called an Internet Protocol Relay Service—usually abbreviated as IP Relay Service. Deaf callers would type in the number on a TRS-based website providing IP Relay Services, and the relay operator would translate from text to spoken words and spoken words to text. This meant anyone with Internet access would be able to make calls through the web (FCC IP Relay, 2015). Deaf people finally were able to make calls from anywhere with an Internet connection. There were many advantages with this option, including making multiple calls or participating in conference calls. Not only that, Deaf people could type at the same time the operator was typing, which could not be done on the TTY.

Yet, TTY and IP Relay consumers were not able to connect with 911 emergency centers directly, nor were they able to connect to 911 using the relay service

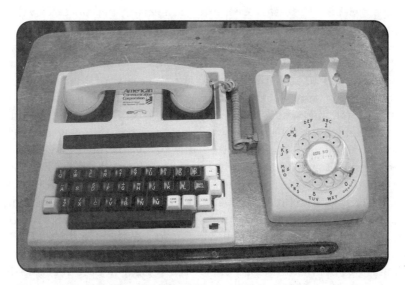

Figure 9–9. Modern TTY machine used in the 1980s, with a rotary phone. Photo courtesy of Texas School for the Deaf Heritage Center.

due to different reasons, such as a 911 operator hanging up on them thinking it was a child playing with a touchtone phone. Deaf people would run to the nearest hearing person and have them call 911 for them or call a Deaf friend with a hearing person in their house to make the call for them. Sadly, because of this, Deaf people experiencing emergencies often did not receive needed services in a timely manner, resulting in death for some (Scott, 1987). In 2008, the Federal Communications Commission (FCC) released requirements for all relay services to connect consumers with 911 for emergencies (FCC 911, 2008). In 2014, the FCC ordered that text-to-911 must become more widely available in all cities and states and that all service providers must support text-to-911. This benefits not only Deaf people but also hearing people in dangerous situations such as when a crime is happening and using voice calls could be dangerous for hearing people. AT&T, Sprint, T-Mobile, and Verizon are already voluntarily providing text-to-911 service. Although the majority of 911 call centers cannot accept text-to-911 messages yet in 2020, it is anticipated all 911 call centers will accept text-to-911 messages in the near future (FCC Text 911, 2020).

Variations in the use of TTYs also were created to accommodate diverse Deaf community members, such as voice carryover (VCO), where a Deaf person with understandable speech would do the speaking while spoken words on the other end would be typed back. The reverse was also available for people who could hear but who could not speak, called hearing carryover (HCO). Shared non-English language relay services were also available for Spanish-to-Spanish calls, among other variations. Those TRS services are

available in specific areas of the United States, with limited hours (FCC, 2020).

Although the advent of the TTY and TRS was a blessing for many Deaf Americans, there was still a language barrier for many who consider sign language to be their primary and preferred language of communication. Using a TTY meant they would need to type in English. In 1995, Ed Bosson and the Public Utility Commission of Texas tested the use of videophones with what was called Video Relay Services (VRS)—a video-based relay service where the callers would connect with an interpreter who would relay the signed message to spoken English and interpret the spoken message back to sign language. In 2000, the FCC recognized video-based relay services, and TRS companies could provide VRS (Convo, 2015). The Deaf person calls the VRS using a video-based software; an interpreter appears on the video and dials the hearing caller, who responds by phone to the interpreter. The interpreter signs the message back to the Deaf person, who then signs back and so on. The reverse also works—when the hearing person calls VRS to contact the Deaf person and dialogue ensues, as shown in Figure 9–10.

VRS was immediately embraced by the majority of the sighted, Deaf, and DeafDisabled community members who considered ASL to be their primary language of communication. Unfortunately, the needs of the DeafBlind community were neglected. Many DeafBlind people stayed with TTYs, instant messaging, or IP Relay Service (either using enlarged text or braille). While VRS expanded and improved their services, TTY products and maintenance were slowly closing up. Many Deaf people recycled their TTYs. Companies made more money off VRS

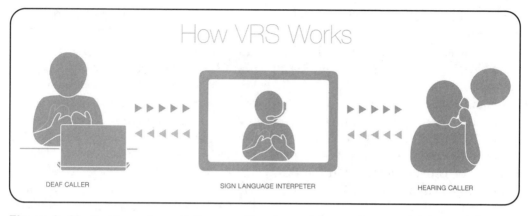

Figure 9–10. A video relay call diagram. Courtesy of Convo Communications, LLC.

and closed their IP Relay Services because the revenue was too low (Cullen, 2014; SIPRelay, 2013).

The closing down of IP Relay Services and the popularity of VRS, unfortunately, did harm against DeafBlind consumers. DeafBlind consumers find IP Relay Services to be more accessible than VRS because there are large-screen adaptations as well as braille variations for text. DeafBlind consumers need an interpreter in the room with them when using VRS, in order for the interpreter to interpret the content signed by the other party to the DeafBlind consumer. FCC regulations prohibit an additional interpreter in the room (DBTT, 2012). Currently, only one city provides interpreters to work with DeafBlind VRS calls (DBSC, 2015). As of 2014, only one VRS service has attempted to propose VRS services customized for the DeafBlind community. In 2015, a VRS company called CAAG VRS announced that the very first DeafBlind Video Relay Services (DBVRS) alpha testing was successful and that they would begin beta testing (Laird, 2014, 2015). Unfortunately, in 2016, CAAG VRS submitted a letter to FCC informing them that they will cease

VRS services for Deaf and DeafBlind customers due to financial difficulties (FCC CAAG, 2016). In 2019, CAAG VRS was bought out by Sorenson VRS, and in Sorenson's press release, DeafBlind VRS interpreting services were not mentioned (SVRS, 2019). At the first DeafBlind International conference on April 14–18, 2018, it was reported DeafBlind people with low vision can magnify or narrow the interpreter's video screen with any VRS provider. DeafBlind consumers can also request change of interpreters to one that complies with their needs (e.g., lighting, color contrast between shirt and hands, and background). MYMMX DB, a software developed by a Swedish company, attempts to address this issue on Windows (Apple versions are not available). The DeafBlind person can sign to the video interpreter and the video interpreter will speak to the other party and then type back the information to the DeafBlind consumer, who reads via braille (Davert, 2018).

Trilingual Video Relay Services (TVRS) is emerging as a full-service option for consumers who speak Spanish and other languages. A large number of deaf children from Spanish-speaking households reside in the United States. TVRS was first piloted in Austin, Texas, in 1995 (Quinto-Pozos, Casanova de Canales, & Treviño, 2010). The state of Texas was the first to successfully petition the FCC for TVRS compensation in 2000, which was then reversed in 2005, then approved again in 2006 with a condition that the ASL-to-Spanish VRS must be provided 24/7 to be eligible for compensation from the FCC (FCC ASL-Spanish, 2005; QuintoPozos et al., 2010).

In the latter half of the 2000s, rampant misuse of VRS services by the service providers themselves resulted in over seven VRS service provider closures and 26 arrests and convictions. The Federal Bureau of Investigation (FBI) arrested individuals in New York, New Jersey, Florida, Texas, Pennsylvania, Arizona, Nevada, Oregon, and Maryland who would knowingly place fraudulent calls in order to increase the amount of reimbursement from the government. This cost the government millions of dollars. FCC Chief of Staff Edward Lazarus said, "The tragedy is the unfortunate truth that a significant number of unscrupulous individuals, at great cost to the nation, have preyed on a very important program for delivering essential telecommunications services to persons with hearing disabilities" (DOJ, 2014).

Sweden was the first nation in the world to provide VRS services in 1997, and the United States was second in early 2000. VRS services are now provided worldwide, including countries such as Brazil, Chile, Denmark, Finland, France, Germany, Italy, Norway, Russia, Slovak Republic, Spain, and the United Kingdom (VRS, 2015). Read about the possibility of a career working with the VRS industry as a sign language interpreter in Chapter 12.

Alerting Devices or Systems

How do deaf people know when someone is at the door? When their baby is crying? When to wake up for work? When the fire or security alarm is going off? When someone is calling them? When there is a city-wide emergency alert? They need alerting devices or systems. What works for them?

In the old days, there were many ingenious (albeit fascinating) inventions Deaf people used to communicate with or be alerted. A tactile version of the doorbell can be seen in this 1956 photo of dorm rooms at Gallaudet University. The visitor would pull a knob in the hallway, which made the weight suddenly drop and thump on the floor. The Deaf student would be alerted that someone was at the door, as shown in Figure 9–11.

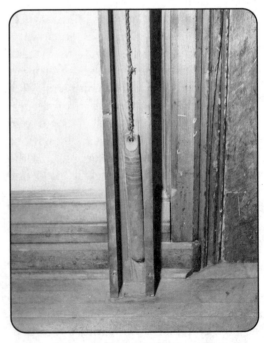

Figure 9–11. Tactile doorbell at Gallaudet University College Hall dorm room, 1956. Courtesy of Gallaudet University Archives.

Thankfully, Deaf people of today have more practical ways of being alerted when someone knocks on the door. There are many types of wireless home alerting systems that can cost between $50 and $200 when ordered online. Most alerting systems work with the existing doorbell by attaching a transmitter to the wiring. When the button is pressed, the transmitter sends a signal to a receiver (or several receivers) in the home, which turns on the light repeatedly or sets off the vibrating device (Figure 9–12).

Another creative way to alert Deaf people is to have the information transmitted to a vibrating watch (such as an Apple Watch) that the Deaf person wears.

Some Deaf people train their pets or use service dogs to alert them if someone is at the door. Some Deaf people choose to

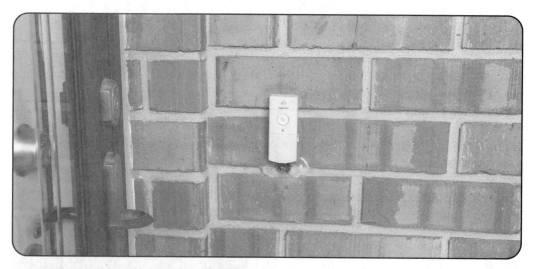

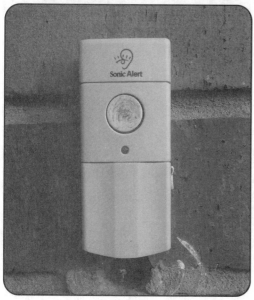

Figure 9–12. A flashing doorbell near a front door. Photo credit: John Moore Jr. Used with permission.

forego the doorbell alerting systems and rely on being texted whenever company arrives. Typical ways Deaf people get each other's attention without a doorbell include banging hard on the door with the fist or the heel, waving and shining a light through windows, or moving a piece of paper underneath a door.

VRS devices also have signaling systems. In the 1990s and 2000s, specific VRS companies would produce and install their own devices in Deaf people's homes and offices. Those devices would include a small red flashing light to inform people in the area that someone was calling. Users can check a missed calls list to see who called and/or review video messages. In the 2010s, more and more VRS companies developed software apps for desktops, laptops, and smartphones. Those software apps also often include e-mail and text alerts if someone is calling. Desktops and laptops tend to include a brief "notification" on the screen that someone is calling. Smartphones can be set up to vibrate when receiving a call. However, those aren't enough—and many Deaf people express frustration that they feel they have to keep their phones in their pockets even at home just so they are aware if someone is calling (Kolodny, 2014). That is where additional purchase for equipment such as wireless light signalers connected to home lamps can be useful.

Wake-Up Devices

How do Deaf community members wake up for work? Using a lamp by your bedside or a vibrating box beneath your mattress (also called a bed shaker) and plugging them into a clock. You set the alarm time, and the clock time, and go to bed. Simple. There are also miniature travel-

ing alarm clocks, vibrating watches, and vibrating timers. Prices range between $50 and $100 for one. Figure 9–13 provides an example.

As another example of universal design, more and more smartphones and smartwatches already include vibrating alarms and alerts, useful for Deaf, Deaf-Disabled, and DeafBlind people as well as for hearing people preferring the tactile avenue over the auditory avenue.

Baby Alerting Devices

But what about infants? How are Deaf parents or caregivers able to leave their babies in a crib or a playpen and take a shower? Cook breakfast? Change clothes? Sleep through the night? Hearing care-

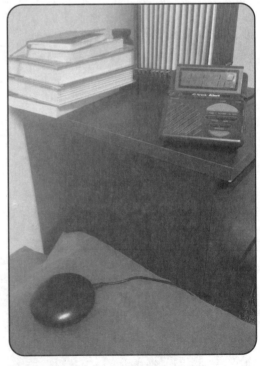

Figure 9–13. A vibrating alarm. Photo credit: Don Miller. Used with permission.

givers could purchase a baby monitor as early as 1937—at that time, the baby monitor was a radio unit where the transmitter unit (with a microphone) was placed near the child, and the sounds in this area would be transmitted by radio waves to a receiver unit (near the caregiver(s)) with a speaker, so the caregivers would be alerted by the baby's cries. This product, called the Radio Nurse, was high in demand because of the 1932 Charles Lindbergh baby kidnapping—caregivers wanted to be able to listen and protect their children in the house. At that time, the baby monitor cost $19.95, which is about $325 today—so not many people had the baby monitors in their houses until the 1980s, around the same time wireless phones came on the scene (Lammle, 2013).

How did Deaf caregivers care for their infants up until the early 1970s? Deaf caregivers would sleep with their babies (often resting their hands on the baby's chest to make sure they were breathing), bring their babies everywhere with them using a carrier or playpen, and use creative ways to make them comfortable and secure (often during their naptime) while the caregivers did their errands. During the 1970s, light-based baby monitors were reasonably priced and available for purchase through companies selling accessibility products for Deaf people—those companies would sell products including doorbell flashers, sleep alarms, smoke alarms, and baby monitors. Deaf caregivers would put the transmitter unit in the child's room and the receivers in the parents' room attached to the lamp, and whenever the baby cried, the lamp would flicker according to the cries and sounds in the infant's room. Often the lamp would flicker and the Deaf caregivers would rush into the room only to find the infant sound asleep. They had to move the microphone really close to the infant in order to make sure the light went off based on the infant's cries (and not something else!).

In the 1990s, there were new baby monitors on the market that included video—called baby cams. Parents could carry around a small device and check on their sleeping child without even going into the child's room! Figure 9–14A shows the baby monitor and baby cam side by side. Figure 9–14B shows Deaf mom Misty playing with her infant (not visible) on her baby cam.

This product was a blessing for the Deaf community. For DeafBlind people, there are baby monitors with a vibrating pager (much like what you see at restaurants when waiting for your seat) that you can attach to your pants, although this option is not as widespread or as available as the video-based baby monitor.

Residential Security and Alarm Systems

What about home security alarms? Most security alarm systems are sound-based and require voiced phone calls to and from the residence to disable the alarm or to send emergency service personnel to the residence. How does that work with Deaf people? Most of the larger security system providers have adaptations for their devices, including lighting (color coded or flashing lights) or vibrotactile (vibrator alert). Some of the advanced wireless security systems can send a text message alert to the homeowner's phone. Some will accept a text response from the homeowner instead of a voice-based phone call.

For home fire and smoke alerts, there are strobe-based and vibrating (bed shaker) systems. Some of the fire and smoke alerts

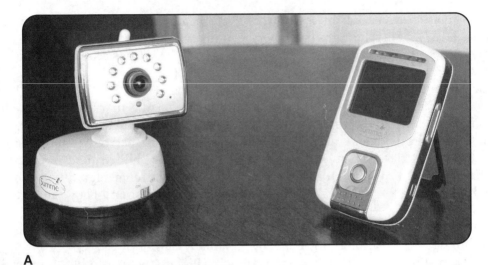

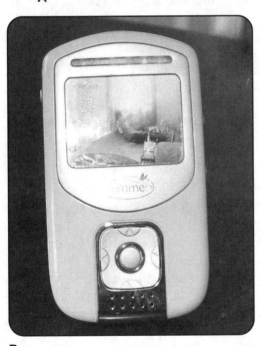

Figure 9–14. A. Baby monitor and baby cam side by side. **B.** Deaf mom Misty Morris with her baby in the baby monitor. Used with permission.

include carbon monoxide detectors. Prices range from $100 for one to $500 for a kit consisting of multiple alarms. Some cities and states have free fire and smoke alert signaler distribution programs through local fire departments for Deaf and hard-of-hearing residents, often made avail-able through federal grants or state funds. There are also weather alert radios that work with the National Weather Service broadcasts that are attached to a strobe light and/or a bed shaker.

Outdoor and indoor security cam-eras are often used as a way to alert us to someone ringing the door, a delivery person walking up to the door, a friend driving up the driveway, and more. A popular product among Deaf people is the Ring Video Doorbell product (Banks, 2019).

Emergency Announcements

As for city, state, or nationwide emergencies, such as a tornado, earthquake, hurricane, forest fire, spill of dangerous chemicals, or a shooter/terrorist—how are those communicated to the public quickly? Often they are done using television announcements, radio announcements, warning sirens, and police loudspeakers.

The FCC requires that television broadcasters, including cable operators and satellite television services that provide local emergency news, include captions or visual display of information along with their programming. For instance, if a television station displays a simple short crawl announcement along the bottom of the TV screen stating a list of schools that are closed due to snow, and the information voiced is more detailed (e.g., road closings, shelters, advice to prevent accidents), the information voiced must be immediately captioned using a live real-time captioner or an onsite stenocaptioner. Those captions cannot block any other visual information such as the crawl announcement on the bottom of the screen (NAD Emergency, 2020).

In 2020, the Federal Emergency Management Agency (FEMA) released a statement explaining their commitment to providing preparedness, response, and recovery information in formats accessible to the deaf community, including the use of a Certified Deaf Interpreter (CDI), local sign language interpreters, and workshops for emergency personnel on how to request interpreting services (FEMA Deaf, 2020).

Some state mayors and governors include interpreters on the stage with them as they announce emergency information to their residents via television. Although the emergency announcements are required by the FCC to be captioned, Deaf interpreters provide very important access for people who use ASL as their primary language, but not only that, when captions aren't functioning correctly (e.g., typos) or delayed, people who know ASL can also fall back on the Deaf interpreter to understand the message. Figure 9–15 shows Mayor Bill de Blasio with Deaf interpreter Jonathan Lamberton by his side.

New York City Mayor Michael Bloomberg and then, later, Mayor Bill de Blasio, Maryland Governor Martin O'Malley, and Massachusetts Governor Deval Patrick all have used Deaf interpreters, although many Deaf people have expressed frustration that not all mayors and governors include a qualified Deaf interpreter on stage with them yet (ASL Interpreter When?, 2015; NAD Hurricane Sandy, 2012). In 2017, when Hurricane Irma was nearing Florida, officials announced a mandatory evacuation, with the interpreter signing "pizza" and "bear monster." The NAD chief executive, Howard A. Rosenblum said, "It was atrocious," referring to the inept interpreter (Caron, 2017).

> Search on YouTube for "Hurricane Irma Emergency Fake Interpreter" and watch the captions of what the interpreter actually said. Is this appropriate during an emergency? Or is this appropriate anywhere?

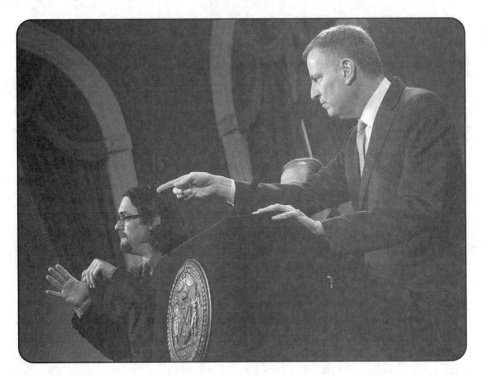

Figure 9–15. Certified Deaf Interpreter (CDI), Jonathan Lamberton, interpreting for Mayor Bill de Blasio of New York. Photos courtesy of Ed Reed and Demetrius Freeman, Mayoral Photography Office.

Weather warning systems have historically been done through radio, provided by the National Oceanographic and Atmospheric Administration (NOAA), a federal agency. There are modified radio receivers, also called "special-needs NOAA Weather Radio," that provide text-based (and large print/braille version) information from NOAA National Weather Service radio broadcasts that cost between $70 and $200.

Other types of emergency alerts include adding strobe lights on top of civil defense sirens, which tend to be installed in tornado corridors in the United States (NAD Emergency, 2020). More and more universities, organizations, and cities include paging alert signup service where you can sign up your cell phone to be notified in case of emergency via text or e-mail.

Assistive Systems and Devices

Is there technology that can assist with accessibility for live situations where Deaf and hard-of-hearing people interact with people who may not know sign language? Is there technology that provides Deaf and hard-of-hearing people with access to spoken language in a group setting? Yes—there are assistive listening systems and devices for situations like these. Hard-of-hearing people and people with cochlear implants often struggle with hearing people speaking in groups and large rooms due to background noise and room reverberation. There are many variations of assistive systems and devices to help eliminate background noise and amplify the speech of people who are talking, such as Audio Loop Systems, AM Systems, FM Systems, and Infrared Systems. All have two important components—(1) a transmitter that carries the spoken information from the speaker to the receiver and (2) a receiver that receives that information and amplifies the sound levels for the recipient, either through their residual hearing or through their hearing aid/cochlear implant (DiPietro et al., 2007). Those systems and devices aren't only for Deaf or hard-of-hearing people. Hearing people use those devices too, in different ways. For instance, when the language spoken at a conference or a meeting is in ASL, and there are hearing participants who know ASL and do not want to hear the interpreter voice the meeting in spoken English—it can be disorienting for some to listen to an ASL speaker and hear the interpreter's delayed spoken English (translation lag time) simultaneously. Hearing people who want access to the spoken version pick up a device (possibly an earphone) and sit in the back. The interpreter speaks quietly into a transmitter, and the hearing people wearing the earphones are able to follow the ASL being used in the room.

Can you imagine trying to listen to two languages at the same time?

There are additional types of technology that can be used to assist in live interaction between people who do not know sign language and Deaf people who prefer to use sign language primarily. One type of technology is called video remote interpreting (VRI). Sometimes interpreters are not immediately available in your area, so using a VRI can be a temporary solution until the interpreter arrives (NAD VRI, 2020). For example, if a Deaf person arrives at the hospital with a broken arm and cannot write back and forth because of the broken arm, the hospital can roll in a machine that looks like a TV, connected to the Internet. The machine is turned on, and an interpreter appears on the TV—often provided by the local interpreting call center. The Deaf person signs with their nondominant (and with their nonbroken arm!) to the interpreter in the video, and the interpreter voices the translation to the other party, possibly nurses and doctors in the room, and continues to interpret the session between the patient and the health care workers. A diagram showing the process can be seen in Figure 9–16.

Some people, not fully understanding the concept of VRI, attempt to use VRS services while both parties (the deaf person and the hearing nonsigner) are in the same location. If the VRS interpreter notices both are in the same room, the interpreter will then terminate the call due to FCC regulations, as federal taxes are collected for facilitating phone calls between deaf and hearing people, not to interpret between deaf and hearing people in the same room. VRI is best used with a limited amount of adults and simple conversations. For more complex interactions and large groups, an onsite interpreter would be a more appropriate choice. Also, VRI is not accessible for Deaf people with low vision or DeafBlind people. VRI is also not appropriate for young children, foreign-born individuals, and those who have minimal language skills in both or either ASL or English. Not only that, many organizations includ-

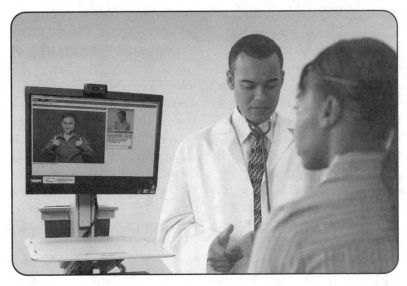

Figure 9–16. Video Relay Interpreting between the Deaf patient, interpreter on screen, and the hearing, nonsigning medical professional. Photo courtesy of Purple Communications, Inc.

ing hospitals and police stations are not familiar with the VRI setup and often struggle with getting the equipment running. High-speed Internet connectivity is often an issue. The screen may not be large enough or mobile enough to fit the visual field of the deaf person, who may also be bedridden. Some argue that signing reduced from three-dimensional form to two-dimensional form does not work (NAD-DSA VRI, 2016; Napier & Leneham, 2011).

INNOVATIVE TECHNOLOGY

Another technology some Deaf and hard-of-hearing people use involves apps that are or resemble instant messaging. There are many free apps or software programs that include two-way typed communication on phones, laptops, and computers such as iMessage, Google Chat, and AIM.

Those are usually used by Deaf and hard-of-hearing people who feel comfortable communicating in English text.

One stand-alone equipment, called UbiDuo 2, sold by sComm for over $2,000, made headlines in the Deaf community when the company proclaimed that its device should replace live, signing interpreters. The device consists of two keyboards and screen, which are connected via a wire (or wirelessly for a higher fee) and used by both the hearing and Deaf person typing to each other, back and forth. UbiDuo 2 customers include Walmart, Wells Fargo, the White House, Coca-Cola, Goodwill, the U.S. Postal Service, NASA, the U.S. Army, and the Pentagon. The Deaf community immediately responded to these claims by posting complaints on their social media pages. Trudy Suggs, an investigative journalist, published two articles on investigating their shady marketing ploys (Suggs,

2015a, 2015b). sComm cofounder and CEO Jason Curry sent out a press release apologizing for the "unapproved posts made by one of our new media staff" (sComm, 2015). Suggs pointed out that Curry made those posts himself, through a video commercial where he made fun of interpreters and people who use interpreters among other social media posts. To this date, Curry and sComm have not continued to engage in open, transparent dialogue with the Deaf community but continue to push UbiDuo 2 as the best way for Deaf and hearing people to communicate with each other.

One app, Cardzilla, developed by a Deaf computer programmer, Tim Kettering, allows people to type on their phones in very large font, so when the phone is shown or handed over, the other person is able to read the text easily. Deaf people often use this app at Starbucks and to order at the window at drive-throughs. The app is marketed to the general public and can be used to communicate across distances or to pass messages silently (Cardzilla, 2020). Hearing nonsigners download this app just like Deaf people do, demonstrating the benefits of universal design.

More and more companies now see the benefit of providing live chats, which is another form of instant messaging, text-based contact forms, chat rooms, and email options on their websites for customers or for intercompany dialogue and discussion. Text can be convenient, fast, saved, and searchable. Some people in the Deaf community find this very convenient for contacting their banks, online stores, and even talking to their coworkers.

Another way technology assists with communication between signers and nonsigners includes speech recognition software and apps. Speech recognition had a rocky start early in the 2000s, with many words spoken that were not recognized in text correctly. Over the years, speech recognition has shown considerable improvement in recognizing words and phrases spoken by different people and immediately showing transcribed text on the smartphone. Originally created for dictation purposes, speech recognition spun off, becoming digital, voice-driven, or voice-activated personal virtual assistants, for instance, finding locations on maps or calling someone on the smartphone without having to press buttons. This feature is very useful for blind consumers but not so much for Deaf people. They would test their speaking skills by trying to say hello and other phrases to their smartphones with hilarious and unexpected results. More and more free voice to text apps came on the market for their target audience: hearing people who did not want to type, but accidentally these apps tapped into another market —Deaf people! Nyle DiMarco, a contestant on *America's Next Top Model*, used a text-to-speech (and vice versa) app in his interactions with other contestants (DiGiondomenico, 2015). Although those apps still have room for improvement (e.g., time lag, robotic voice), they provide some assistance and access to spoken conversations as well as translating text into speech.

What about sign language recognition apps? Originally the technology was developed to recognize gestures and capture motion but then expanded to recognizing ASL signs. Now some companies are experimenting with a two-way communication tool for signers and nonsigners, where sign language is translated into speech and/or text and vice versa. Sign and speech recognition is not entirely accurate and often focuses only on the hands. Deaf communities have been vocal about sign languages not being simply on the hands but also involving specific facial grammar, head movements, and more, which automated recognition machines fail to capture (Erard, 2017).

Motion capture technology is also used to create signing avatars for children's storybook interactive apps, as demonstrated by Motion Light Lab (ML2), a hub under the National Science Foundation's (NSF) funded Visual Language Visual Learning (VL2) Science of Learning center. Motion capture technology tracks lights worn by signers as they sign, using special cameras to capture and track signs. The director of ML2, Melissa Malzkuhn, can be seen in Figure 9–17, wearing the lights on her face and body. One of their first pieces is titled "My Three Animals," a nursery rhyme produced in ASL by an avatar.

There are also apps on the market created by Deaf people like the ASL app and Signily. The ASL App is predominately for those who do not know sign language or are learning sign language. Downloading this app allows the new signer to find signs quickly and use them when with other signers. The menu and functions of the ASL App can be seen in Figure 9–18.

They have different bundles, including signs for the alphabet, numbers, moods, food, countries, wilderness, and more (ASL App, 2015). There are other sign language apps on the market; however, none were developed by Deaf programmers, designers, filmmakers, and signers like those who developed the ASL App.

Signily is a text messaging keyboard entirely in sign language using photos of handshapes and gifs for moving signs such as YES or NO. Nonsigners and sign-

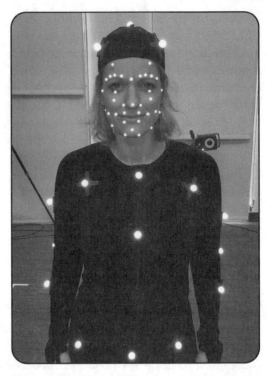

Figure 9–17. The Director of Motion Language Lab (ML2), Melissa Malzkuhn, wearing lights on her face and body for motion capture technology. Used with permission.

ers are able to use this app because there are English translations for each of the handshapes and gifs online. The alphabetic keyboard and images of signs are shown in Figure 9–19.

Again, created and designed by a Deaf team of developers, Signily hopes to have their images and motion images a permanent part of Unicode, which is the computing industry's way to standardize representation of text in most of the world's writing systems. Currently, users of Signily need to type the signs out on their phones, then copy and paste into text, email, or other apps, unlike emojis that are already part of Unicode (Signily, 2015).

Historically, Deaf people have always been excluded from audio-based tours

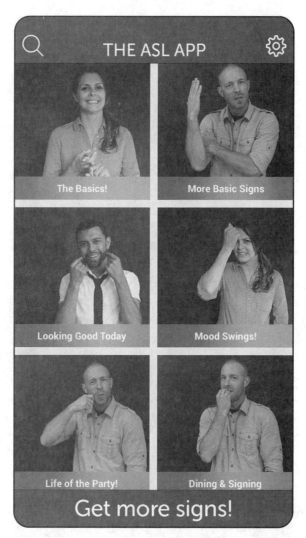

Figure 9–18. The sign language bundles you can purchase in The ASL App. Photo credit: Melissa Malzkuhn. Used with permission.

and guide formats at museums and parks. One relatively new solution to include Deaf people on audio-based tours is to use an augmented reality (AR) platform app. Augmented reality adds sound, video, graphics, or GPS data to your physical real-world environment through the use of a device such as a smartphone. AR was originally created for engineers to build infrastructure using computers rather than actual buildings, but then this technology found its niche in many other fields, including education, gaming, and tourism (AR, 2009). Deaf people were quick to embrace those apps, HP Reveal in particular, to make English-based storybooks bilingual, with an ASL signer popping up next to the image or text. Figure 9–20 shows a student at the California School for the Deaf, Riverside, holding an

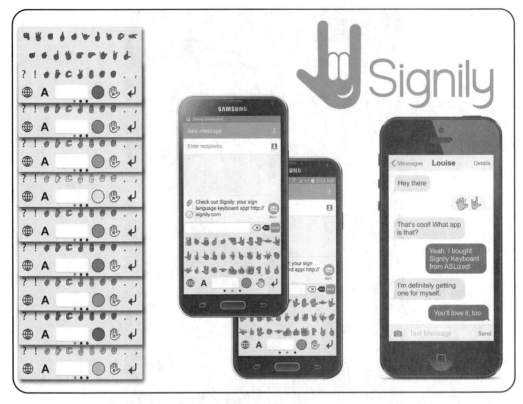

Figure 9–19. The sign language-based keyboard produced by the Deaf team behind Signily. Used with permission: ASLized!

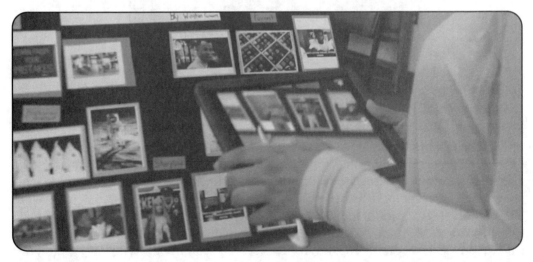

Figure 9–20. HP Reveal in action with California School for the Deaf, Riverside students. Photo courtesy of Alyssa Romano.

iPad and viewing a signer narrating about the photo in front of the iPad.

Other uses include museum guides where icons are posted on the wall, and the person choosing to experience the museum in ASL would bring his or her smartphone up to the icon and watch the signer narrate parts of the tour. At the 2015 national Deaf Interpreters Conference, historic photos of Deaf interpreters were posted and attendees would bring their phones up to the photos to learn about the story behind the photo (Harris, 2015).

A more recent technological innovation involves the use of SignGlasses—glasses that you wear, with the speaker wearing a mic, and a live interpreter showing up on the inside of your glasses! This allows the deaf student to look at their laptop, write down notes, and pour a cylinder into a test tube without having to look for the interpreter—it's already in the glasses itself (Painter, 2018). Figure 9–21 shows a person wearing Sign-Glasses, with an insert showing a closeup look at the glasses, with an interpreter signing on the lens itself.

CONCLUSIONS

Those technologic innovations are attempts at providing equal access to all citizens, particularly Deaf, DeafBlind, and Deaf-Disabled people and signers. Next steps include the ratification of the United Nations proposal, written by and with people with disabilities, titled the *Convention on the Rights of Persons with Disabilities (CRPD)*, protecting the rights of people with disabilities, which has already been ratified by 156 countries in the world, including Canada, China, India, Russia, and all of the countries in Europe and more. To this date, the United States has not yet ratified the CRPD (European Union Agency for Fundamental Rights, 2015; Kanter, 2019). Siegel, in his book, *The Human Right to Language: Communication Access for Deaf Children*, argues that in the U.S. Constitution, the 1st and 14th Amendments should protect all deaf and hard-of-hearing people's right to access language, anywhere and everywhere, as the Constitution states that all citizens have the right to receive and express

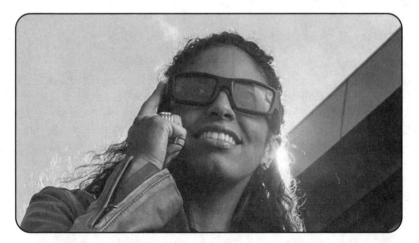

Figure 9–21. SignGlasses with an interpreter on your glasses! Photo courtesy of SignGlasses.

information freely and equally (Siegel, 2008). We are slowly moving toward a more equitable society, where access for all individuals is embraced. In Chapter 12, we will learn about how we can help make this happen through our work with Deaf communities.

REFERENCES

AR. (2009). *Augmented reality.* Retrieved from http://www.vrs.org.uk/augmented-reality/index.html

ASL App. (2015). *Ink & Salt LLC proudly announces: The ASL App.* Retrieved from http://theaslapp.com/news/

ASL Interpreter When? (2015). *When will DC officials have ASL interpreters on TV with them?* Retrieved from https://thewiyatt.wordpre ss.com/2015/02/17/when-will-dc-officials-have-asl-interpreters-on-tv-with-them/

Banks, L. (2019). *Beat smart doorbells for people with hearing loss.* Retrieved from https://www.clearliving.com/hearing/technology/best-smart-doorbells-for-hearing-loss/

Bloodline. (2015). *Part 13.* Los Gatos, CA: Netflix.

Boboltz, S. (2015). In defense of closed captioning, which is entirely underrated. *The Huffington Post.* Retrieved from http://www.huffington post.com/entry/closed-captioning-is-underrated_559d67c7e4b05b1d028f8af5

Camosy, C. (2020). *Coronavirus crisis: The wrong way to decide which patients get hospital care.* Retrieved from https://nypost .com/2020/03/19/coronavirus-crisis-the-wrong-way-to-decide-which-patients-get-hospital-care/

Cardzilla. (2015). *Cardzilla: A fast & simple way to display your messages in large text.* Retrieved from http://www.cardzilla.ws

Caron, C. (2017). *Sign language interpreter warned of 'Pizza' and 'Bear Monster' at Irma briefing.* Retrieved from https://www.ny times.com/2017/09/17/us/sign-language-interpreter-irma.html

Charmatz, M., Hedges-Wright, L., & Ward, M. (2011). *Personal foul: Lack of captioning in football stadiums.* Retrieved from http://scholar .valpo.edu/cgi/viewcontent.cgi?article=1834&context=vulr

Cheek, T. (2015). Lawsuit: Sign-language interpreters fail to communicate. *The Colorado Independent.* Retrieved from http://www.coloradoindependent.com/154149/lawsuit-sign-language-interpreters-fail-tocommunicate

Christian, J. (2014, January 30). How Netflix alienated and insulted its deaf subscribers. *The Week.* Retrieved from http://theweek .com/articles/452181/how-netflix-alienated-insulted-deaf-subscribers

Cohen, A. (2016). *The Supreme Court ruling that led to 70,000 forced sterilizations.* Retrieved from National Public Radio. http://www .npr.com/sections/health-shots/2016/03/07/469478098/the-supremecourt-ruling-that-led-to70-000-forced-sterilizations

Convo. (2015). *History of Convo & VRS.* Retrieved from https://www.convorelay .com/company.html

Cook, A., & Polgar, J. (2014). *Essentials of assistive technology.* St. Louis, MO: Mosby.

Cullen, D. (2014). *DeafBlind organizations file joint statement at FCC.* Retrieved from http://www.doncullen.net/blog/deafblind-orgs-file-joint-statement-fcc/

Davert, S. (2018). *Unique technologies presented at first deaf-blind international conference.* Retrieved from https://www.afb.org/aw/19/6/15089

DBSC. (2015). *Deaf-Blind service center: CF program.* Retrieved from http://seattledbsc .org/cf-program/

DBTT. (2012). *DeafBlind think tank: Video relay service (VRS)—is it really accessible?* Retrieved from http://dbtt.org/video-relay-service-accessible/

DeVinney, J. (2015). *Using your TTY comfortably or how not to panic when the "deaf phone thing rings."* Retrieved from http://www.maine .gov/rehab/dod/using_tty_comfortably .shtml

DiGiondomenico, A. (2015). 'America's Next Top Model' recap: 'The Girl Who Has a

Close Shave.' *Baltimore Sun.* Retrieved from http://www.baltimoresun.com/entertain ment/bthesite/tv-lust/bal-america-s-next-top-model-recap-thegirl-who-has-a-close-shave-20150826-story.html

DiPietro, L., Williams, P., & Kaplan, H. (2007). *Alerting and communicating devices for deaf and hard of hearing people.* Retrieved from https://www.gallaudet.edu/clerc-center/ information-and-resources/info-to-go/ hearing-and-communication-technology/ alerting-devices/alerting-and-comm-dev for-deaf-and-hoh-ppl.html

DOJ. (2014). *Department of justice: Twenty-six charged in nationwide scheme to defraud the FCC's video relay service program.* Retrieved from http://www.justice.gov/ opa/pr/ twenty-six-charged-nationwide-schemedefraud-fcc-s-video-relay-service-program

Erard, M. (2017). *Why sign-language gloves don't help deaf people.* Retrieved from https://www .theatlantic.com/technology/archive/ 2017/11/why-sign-language-gloves-dont-help-deaf-people/545441/

European Union Agency for Fundamental Rights. (2015). *People with disabilities.* Retrieved from http://fra.europa.eu/en/ theme/people-disabilities

FCC. (2020). *Federal communications commission: Telecommunications relay service.* Retrieved from https://www.fcc.gov/consu mers/guides/telecommunications-relay-service-trs

FCC 911. (2008). *Federal communications commission: E911 requirements for IP-enabled service providers.* Retrieved from https:// apps.fcc.gov/edocs_public/attachmatch/ FCC08-78A1.pdf

FCC ASL-Spanish. (2005). *Federal communications commission: ASL-Spanish translation video relay service eligible for compensation from interstate TRS fund.* Retrieved from https://apps.fcc.gov/edocs_public/attach match/DOC-259992A1.pdf

FCC CAAG. (2016). *Federal communications commission: Star VRS letter to close services.* Retrieved from http://apps.fcc.gov/ecfs/ comment/view?id=60001493690

FCC IP Relay. (2015). *Federal communications commission: IP relay service.* Retrieved from https://www.fcc.gov/guides/internet-pro tocol-ip-relay-service

FCC Text 911. (2020). *Text to 911: What you need to know.* Retrieved from https://www.fcc .gov/consumers/guides/what-you-need-know-about-text-911

FEMA Deaf. (2020). *Deaf community outreach.* Retrieved from https://www.fema.gov/ news-release/2020/01/12/deaf-commu nity-outreach

Fleischer, D., & Zames, F. (2001). *The disability rights movement: From charity to confronta-tion.* Philadelphia, PA: Temple University Press.

Ginnerup, S. (2009). *Achieving full participation through universal design.* Strasbourg, France: Council of Europe Publishing.

Gold, S. (2011). *Landmark legislation: Americans With Disabilities Act.* Tarrytown, NY: Marshall Cavendish Benchmark.

Goodland, M. (2016). *Settlement reached in sign-language interpreter case.* Retrieved from http://www.coloradoindependent.com/15 7143/settlement-reached-in-signlanguage-interpreter-case

Graham, B. (1988). *One thing led to the next: The real history of TTYs.* Evanston, IL: Mosquito.

Harrenstien, K. (2009). *Automatic captions in YouTube.* Google Official Blog. Retrieved from http://googleblog.blogspot.com/ 2009/11/automatic-captions-in-youtube .html

Harris, R. (2015, July). *The future of ASL: Reflect, celebrate and dream.* Endnote presentation given at the biannual national ASL Teachers' Association conference, Minneapolis, MN.

Hong, E. (2020). *'Parasite's' win is an awesome test of the one-inch barrier.* Retrieved from https://www.cnn.com/2020/02/10/opin ions/subtitle-barrier-parasite-hong/index .html

Ingraham, C. (2015). *An exploration of how persons with visual and auditory loss use adaptive and assistive technology for daily living and aging-in-place* (Unpublished doctoral dissertation). Lamar University, Beaumont, TX.

Kanter, A. (2019). *Let's try again: Why the United States should ratify the United Nations convention on the rights of people with disabilities.* Retrieved from https://papers.ssrn.com/sol3/papers.cfm?abstract_id=3373259

King, N. (2009). Captioning coming to a theater near you. *Daily Comet.* Retrieved from http://www.dailycomet.com/article/20090504/ARTICLES/905041001?p=2&tc=pg

Kolodny, L. (2014). Spark labs raises $4.9M to help engineers make their devices smart. *Wall Street Journal.* Retrieved from http://blogs.wsj.com/venturecapital/2014/07/08/spark-io-raises-4-9-million-to-help-engineers-make-their-devices-smart/

Laird, G. (2014). *CAAG VRS files to offer VRS for Deaf-Blind consumers!* Retrieved from http://deafnetwork.com/wordpress/blog/2014/11/14/caag-vrs-files-to-offervrs-for-deaf-blind-consumers/

Laird, G. (2015). *First in history: The first Deaf-Blind VRS calls were made with CAAGVRS.* Retrieved from http://deafnetwork.com/wordpress/blog/2015/01/19/first-inhistory-the-first-deafblind-vrs-calls-were-made-with-caagvrs/

Lammle, R. (2013). *A brief history of 7 baby basics.* Mental Floss. Retrieved from http://mentalfloss.com/article/49280/briefhistory-7-baby-basics

Lang, H. (2000). *A phone of our own: The deaf insurrection against Ma Bell.* Washington, DC: Gallaudet University Press.

Malzkuhn, M. (2015, July). *Traversing technology: A deaf designed visual landscape.* Paper presented at the World Federation of the Deaf Congress, Istanbul, Turkey.

McDonald, A. (2015). *Closed captioning at GOP debate actually cat walking on keyboard.* Retrieved from http://www.huffingtonpost.com/entry/gop-debate-closed-captioning_55c3d893e4b0923c12bc4f86

McNeese, T. (2014). *Disability rights movement.* Minneapolis, MN: ABDO.

NAD Communicating. (2020). *Communicating with medical personnel during coronavirus.* Retrieved from https://www.nad.org/2020/03/28/communicating-with-medical-personnel-during-coronavirus/

NAD Coronavirus. (2020). *A message from the NAD about coronavirus.* Retrieved from https://www.nad.org/2020/03/12/coronavirus/

NAD-DSA VRI. (2016). *Minimum standards for video remote interpreting services in medical settings.* Retrieved from https://www.nad.org/about-us/position-statements/minimum-standards-for-video-remote-interpreting-services-in-medical-settings/

NAD Emergency. (2020). *Access to televised emergency information.* Retrieved from https://www.nad.org/resources/emergency-preparedness/access-to-televised-emergency-information/

NAD Hurricane Sandy. (2012). *NAD, state assocs., DHHIG commend NYC, Maryland, and Massachusetts for Hurricane Sandy communication access.* Retrieved from http://nad.org/news/2012/11/nad-state-assocsdhhig-commend-nyc-maryland-and-massachusetts-hurricane-sandy-communica

NAD Movie Captioning. (2006). *Captioned movie access advocacy—timeline.* Retrieved from http://nad.org/issues/technology/movie-captioning/timeline

NAD Movie Technologies. (2006). *Movie captioning technologies.* Retrieved from http://nad.org/issues/technology/movie-captioning/technologies

NAD News. (2014). *NAD news: The battle for accessible housing.* Retrieved from http://nad.org/news/2014/1/battle-accessible housing

NAD News. (2015). *NAD news.* Retrieved from http://nad.org/news

NAD OSU. (2010). *Score for accessibility: OSU to provide in-stadium captioning.* Retrieved from http://nad.org/news/2010/11/score-accessibility-osu-provide-stadium-captions

NAD VRI. (2020). *Video remote interpreting.* Retrieved from https://www.nad.org/resources/technology/video-remote-interpreting/

Napier, J., & Leneham, M. (2011). "It was difficult to manage the communication": Testing the feasibility of video remote signed language interpreting in court. *Journal of Interpretation, 21,* 1–12.

NCI. (2015). *National Captioning Institute: History of closed captioning.* Retrieved from http://www.ncicap.org/about-us/history-of-closed-captioning/

Netflix Agreement. (2012). *Netflix and the National Association of the Deaf reach historic agreement to provide 100% closed captions in On-Demand.* Retrieved from http://nad.org/news/2012/10/netflix-and-national association-deaf-reach-historic-agreement provide-100-closed-capti

Netflix Precedent. (2012). *Landmark precedent in NAD vs. Netflix.* Retrieved from http://nad.org/news/2012/6/landmark-precedent-nad-vs-netflix

Netflix Sued. (2011). *NAD files disability civil rights lawsuit against Netflix.* Retrieved from http://nad.org/news/2011/6/nad-files-disability-civil-rights-lawsuit-against-netflix

New Tech. (2013). *New tech solutions for enjoying a movie with hearing loss.* CapTel. Retrieved from http://www.captel.com/news/speech-to-text-and-captioning/new tech-solutions-for-enjoying-a-movie-with hearing-loss/

NFCA. (2020). *History of freak shows.* Retrieved from https://www.sheffield.ac.uk/nfca/researchandarticles/freakshows

Painter, J. (2018). *Adaptive technology: New tech levels communication field for local deaf and hard of hearing community.* Retrieved from https://www.postregister.com/news/local/adaptive-technology-new-tech-levels-communication-field-for-local-deaf/article_90f19061-1b8a-5374-9d9d-dc187737dcf1.html

Payphone. (2000). *History & invention of the payphone.* California College of the Arts. Retrieved from http://dada.cca.edu/~acompeau/payphone_contents.pdf

Pelka, F. (2012). *What have we done: An oral history of the disability rights movement.* Amherst: University of Massachusetts Press.

Peltz-Strauss, K. (2006). *A new civil right: Telecommunications equality for Deaf and hard of hearing Americans.* Washington, DC: Gallaudet University Press.

Pierpoint, G. (2018). *Nyle DiMarco's tweets spur deaf people to share cinema frustrations.*

Retrieved from https://www.bbc.com/news/disability-43111662

Quinto-Pozos, D., Casanova de Canales, K., & Treviño, R. (2010). Trilingual video relay service (VRS) interpreting in the United States. In R. Locker McKee & J. Davis (Eds.), *Interpreting in multilingual, multicultural contexts* (pp. 28–54). Washington, DC: Gallaudet University Press.

Raum, E. (2008). *The history of the telephone.* Chicago, IL: Heinemann Library.

Robitaille, S. (2001). Movie magic for the hearing impaired. *Bloomberg Business.* Retrieved from http://www.bloomberg.com/bw/stories/2001-10-31/movie-magic-for-the hearing-impaired

Sanders, E. (1964). *Google patents: Receiver amplifier US 3130270A.* Retrieved from http://www.google.com.na/patents/US3130270

Schoepfer-Bochicchio, K. (2013). Sports venues facing more legal battles over captioning. *Athletic Business.* Retrieved from http://www.athleticbusiness.com/contract-law/sports-venues-facing-more-legal-battles over-captioning.html

Schumacher-Rasmussen, E. (2017). *Providing YouTube video captions is an inclusive move for brands.* Retrieved from https://www.streamingmedia.com/Articles/Editorial/Featured-Articles/Providing-YouTube-Video-Captions-Is-an-Inclusive-Move-for-Brands-138530.aspx

sComm. (2015, April 9). *Press release: sComm cofounder and CEO, Jason Curry issues statement regarding communication options for deaf, hard of hearing and hearing.* Retrieved from http://www.scomm.com/jason-curry-issues-statement/

Scott, J. (1987). Deaf confront deadly problem: Unanswered help calls to 911. *Los Angeles Times.* Retrieved from http://articles.latimes.com/1987-02-01/news/mn-308_1_tdds/2

Shapiro, J. (1994). *No pity: People with disabilities forging a new civil rights movement.* New York, NY: Three Rivers Press.

Shulman, S. (2008). *The telephone gambit: Chasing Alexander Graham Bell's secret.* New York, NY: W. W. Norton.

Siegel, L. (2008). *The human right to language: Communication access for deaf children.* Washington, DC: Gallaudet University Press.

Sign1News. (2020). *Board certified and ASL fluent family physician.* Retrieved from https://www.facebook.com/sign1news/photos/a.339810903155900/904295796707405/

Signily. (2015). *Signily: The first sign language keyboard app that comes in different handshapes and colors!* Retrieved from http://signily.com SIPRelay

SIPRelay. (2013). *SIPRelay service permanently ceased on July 31, 2013 at 4 pm MDT.* Retrieved from http://www.siprelay.com

Steinbuch, Y. (2020). *Deaf man from Brooklyn sues Pornhub over lack of closed captioning.* Retrieved from https://nypost.com/2020/01/17/deaf-man-from-brooklyn-sues-pornhub-over-lack-of-closed-captioning/

Suggs, T. (2015a, March 27). *Doing more harm than good.* Retrieved from http://www.trudysuggs.com/doingmoreharmthangood/

Suggs, T. (2015b, July 27). *sComm: An update.* Retrieved from http://www.trudysuggs.com/scomm-an-update/

SVRS. (2019). *Sorenson communications announces ASL interpreting in Texas just got bigger.* Retrieved from https://www.globenewswire.com/news-release/2019/11/01/1939623/0/en/Sorenson-Communications-Announces-ASL-Interpreting-in-Texas-Just-Got-Bigger.html

TDI Milestones. (2015). *TDI—shaping an accessible world: TDI milestones.* Retrieved from https://www.tdiforaccess.org/about_tdi.aspx?key=AboutTDI(History)&select=AboutTDI

Television and Closed Captioning. (2020). *Online closed captioning.* Retrieved from https://www.nad.org/resources/technology/television-and-closed-captioning/online-closed-captioning/

TRS. (2015). *National association of the deaf: Telephone and relay services.* Retrieved from http://nad.org/issues/telephone-and-relay-services/relay-services/tty

Vanderheiden, G. (1996). *Universal design . . . what it is and what it isn't.* Retrieved from http://trace.wisc.edu/docs/whats_ud/whats_ud.htm

Vitac. (2017). *Are you making your stadium accessible to deaf and hard of hearing fans?* Retrieved from https://www.vitac.com/are-you-making-your-stadium-accessible-to-deaf-and-hard-of-hearing-fans/

VRS. (2015). *Video relay service.* Retrieved from https://en.wikipedia.org/wiki/Video_relay_service

Wabash, R. (2019). *61 hilarious closed caption fails.* Retrieved from https://www.nad.org/resources/technology/television-and-closed-captioning/online-closed-captioning/

Wikipedia. (2015). *Rear window captioning system.* Retrieved from https://en.wikipedia.org/wiki/Rear_Window_Captioning_System

Winzer, E. (2009). *From integration to inclusion: A history of special education in the 20th century.* Washington, DC: Gallaudet Press.

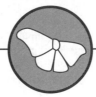

CHAPTER 10

Deaf People and the Legal System: Education, Employment, and Criminal Justice

Two police officers see a student running from the parking lot near cars that have been vandalized. When the police finally overtake him, the student gestures to his ears. The police interpret his hand movements as aggression. After grabbing his arms and handcuffing his wrists behind his back, they escort him to a squad car, then take him to the city jail where he is charged and booked for resisting and assaulting a police officer.

What communication and language accommodations would have to be put in place to protect this Deaf suspect's due

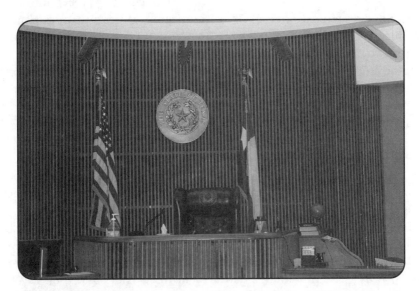

Figure 10–1. Photo of courtroom. Photo courtesy of Jefferson County Courthouse, Beaumont, Texas.

process and constitutional rights? Due process is based on the principle that a citizen has rights and cannot be deprived of life, liberty, or property without appropriate legal procedures and safeguards (LaVigne & Vernon, 2003). Related to Deaf citizens, there are many laws that protect Deaf individuals in education and employment. Laws also exist that shield them from discriminatory treatment by law enforcement when they encounter the police as this opening vignette describes. There are also protections for Deaf individuals when they get caught up in the criminal justice system as a victim of a crime or as an offender. In this chapter, a broad overview is presented of laws in education and employment followed by laws within the criminal justice system. Relevant court cases are highlighted when these laws are broken.

EDUCATION LAWS

Laws in Early Childhood

Legal protections for educational services begin for Deaf, DeafDisabled, and Deaf-Blind infants at birth. These laws have time changing effects for Deaf infants and their families as it provides support, protections, and legal recourse when agencies are discriminatory (Raimondo, 2013).

Early Hearing Detection and Intervention (EDHI) Act

Hospital newborns receive hearing screenings as mandated by Early Hearing Detection and Intervention (EDHI) Act of 2010 (amended in 2012). Depending on these results, states must provide families with audiological services and early childhood

intervention programs (see Chapter 4). The Joint Committee for Infant Hearing (JCIH, 2019) recommends that children be screened by age 1 month, identified by 3 months, and fitted with amplification by 6 months. Further, they suggest the participation of Deaf sign language teachers and mentors in the EDHI early intervention phase (Muse et al., 2013).

Individuals With Disabilities Education Act (IDEA) (Part C)

Part C of the Individuals With Disabilities Education Act (IDEA) also provides services for Deaf babies and toddlers, which can include speech therapy, Deaf mentors, and in-home parent training on how to communicate with their deaf child in order to achieve milestones in language acquisition and literacy (Chapter 4). IDEA was enacted in 1990 and provides children with annual evaluations and resources, including the Individual Family Service Plan (IFSP). The IFSP is developed by an interdisciplinary team and the families and consists of intervention strategies and communication opportunities that support the Deaf child's unique learning needs and strengths.

Even with early newborn infant screening, many Deaf babies and toddlers still fall through the cracks. Follow-up services are often not utilized by families and agencies (Gaffney et al., 2014). Moreover, families often receive misinformation or no information from doctors and audiologists about the importance of sign language and the risks of lack of language exposure, which results in language deprivation (Hall, 2017; Humphries et al., 2016).

To counteract language deprivation, Deaf researchers and their hearing allies have published summaries of linguistic research studies that clear up the misinformation parents typically receive that sign language is detrimental to deaf children's early language growth. These scholarly papers underscore the positive benefits of early exposure to sign language for language and early literacy. They also point to the fact that the lack of language exposure places the child at risk for language learning and the development of thinking and social skills (Andrews, Byrne, & Clark, 2015; Hall, 2017; Humphries et al., 2014, 2018) (see Chapter 4).

Another effort to confront language deprivation is the Deaf-led and Deaf-centric grassroots effort called the Language Equality, and Acquisition for Deaf Kids (LEAD-K) campaign. This movement advocates for language development and accountability by passing legislation called the LEAD-K bill. These state-level bills shift the focus from the needs of the family to the unique language needs of the deaf child. Since 2016, 12 states have adopted a form of the LEAD-K model bill. The goal is that all Deaf and hard-of-hearing children enter kindergarten with age-appropriate language skills. Under the model bill, states must adopt language developmental milestones in ASL and spoken English with children being assessed annually (http://www .lead-k.org/model-legislation-for-states). Each year, states must publicly report the assessment data on the language and literacy progress of their deaf and hard-of-hearing children and compare them to their age peers. If the deaf or hard-of-hearing child does not demonstrate language progress, then the IFSP or Individualized Educational Program (IEP) plans must be revised. One flaw of the LEAD-K legislation is that it does not specifically address the language needs of children who are

DeafDisabled, including those who are DeafBlind (Payne-Tsoupros, 2019).

And still another effort to offset language delay and deprivation is seen in state laws called the Deaf Children's Bill of Rights. According to the National Association of the Deaf website, 16 states have passed a bill of rights for Deaf and hard-of-hearing children. These bills underscore the child's basic rights to communicate freely using any language they choose whether it is spoken, signed, or both. Some states also incorporate the importance of having Deaf peers to socialize with. See the NAD website for details.

Deaf people who have access to and acquire sign language early in life are successful in acquiring developmental milestones. But some Deaf individuals do not succeed. And this is due largely because of the lack of early language exposure. Many of the approximately 96% of Deaf children who are born to hearing families arrive at kindergarten without having full access to languages, signed, spoken, and/ or written. As such, these language barriers later lead to a higher representation of Deaf persons in unemployment lines, in the mental health system, or even in prisons (Lomas, Andrews, & Shaw, 2017; Vernon & Leigh, 2007). Those Deaf individuals who are members of multicultural and DeafDisabled groups are particularly vulnerable to discrimination and lack of services to offset early language deprivation (Lomas et al., 2017).

A compelling case of a Deaf adult who experienced early linguistic deprivation is that of Donald Lang. Lang, a young Black American, grew up in poverty in the Chicago projects. At age 20, he was charged with two accounts of murder. The judge recommended that Lowell J. Myers, a white deaf attorney, represent Lang in court. Myers communicated with his Deaf client using gestures, drawings, and pictures (Tidyman, 1974). Lang could not talk, read lips, read, write, or understand sign language. With limited language exposure at home and little formal schooling, he was deprived of access to basic concepts and to world knowledge. He used gestures and vocalizations to communicate. Lang was unable to defend himself and participate in court proceedings because of how society prevented him from gaining access to languages early in life, in spoken, signed, or written language.

Laws With School-Age Deaf Children

IDEA (Part B)

Part B of IDEA provides goals, services, and annual evaluations with measurable outcomes for Deaf children and youth from age 3 to 21 years. Under IDEA, the student, guardian(s), and teachers participate in developing the IEP. The law also incorporates goals and services for youth (ages 14 to 22 years) who transition into vocational, postsecondary education or the workplace (see Chapter 4).

IDEA (Part A)

Part A of IDEA mandates free and appropriate public education (FAPE) and placement in the least restrictive environment (LRE) based on the students' strengths and needs. The acronyms FAPE and LRE have become controversial. Since their original inclusion in the Education of All Handicapped Children's Act (1975), a special education law that predated IDEA, some interpret FAPE and LRE as meaning Deaf children should be educated alongside hearing children in public schools. Others

claim that the LRE is not the public school where communication and linguistic access is severely restricted but rather Deaf schools where Deaf students will have full access to signing Deaf peers and teachers who provide direct access and instruction using signing (Tucker, 2010/2011). See Figure 10–2 for Child First Logo.

> The Child First Campaign is a movement that challenges schools' interpretations of the IEP and the LRE. James E. Tucker (2010), Superintendent of the Maryland School for the Deaf and a Deaf Leader in the Child First Campaign, proposes that Deaf children benefit from learning with their Deaf peers through the shared language of ASL and a shared Deaf culture and that the individual needs of the Deaf child should be considered foremost, hence the title "Child First."

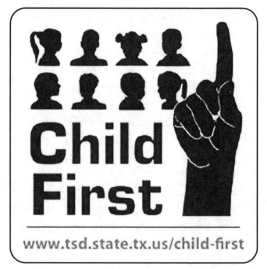

www.tsd.state.tx.us/child-first

Figure 10–2. Logo of the Child First Campaign. Used with permission of the Conference of Educational Administrators of Schools and Programs for the Deaf.

American With Disabilities Act (ADA)

If the guardian decides to place their Deaf child in a private school, the child becomes eligible for "service plans" covered by Title II of the Americans With Disabilities Act (ADA). This law requires that state and local governments ensure access for Deaf students to programs at schools, after school, summer camps, sports teams, and community events. At these sites, Deaf students should be provided with auxiliary aids such as interpreters, real-time computer-aided transcription services (CART), closed captions on TV, and videophones. And when Deaf children and youth go to a museum, park, or zoo, or any other facility open to the public, accommodations must be provided under ADA, Title III (Raimondo, 2010, 2013).

Section 504 of the Rehabilitation Act of 1973

Likewise, Section 504 of the Rehabilitation Act of 1973 protects Deaf children and youth as it applies to school systems and public or private educational agencies that receive federal financial assistance, including free lunch programs (Rosenbaum et al., 2016). These cases show how the courts have interpreted FAPE and LRE when challenged by families of Deaf, DeafBlind, and DeafDisabled children.

The first case in special education that reached the Supreme Court was *Hendrick Hudson Central School District v. Rowley* (458 U.S. 176) (1982). Amy Rowley was a white Deaf child mainstreamed in the first grade at a public school. Her parents, who were also white Deaf, requested a sign language interpreter for their daughter in her classroom. However, during the IEP meeting, the parents' request was denied. Throughout the school year, Amy performed well academically so the school district did not believe she needed an interpreter to succeed. Amy's parents took the case to the federal district court, claiming that denial of an ASL interpreter was a violation of FAPE. The courts initially sided with the Rowley family. They declared that even though Amy was passing each year without an interpreter, she could realize even more of her academic potential with an interpreter. However, the Supreme Court disagreed and said that the school district only had to provide basic education, which it was doing, without the interpreter. Amy's parents and her attorney disagreed and argued that for Amy to receive full access to communication and language throughout the school day, she needed a sign language interpreter (Smith, 1996).

> Discuss the communication and activities that Amy might have missed out on in her first-grade classroom, in the cafeteria, and on the playground without an interpreter.

To somewhat resolve the controversial interpretations of FAPE and LRE, due in part to the advocacy of the National Association for the Deaf (NAD) and other deaf education organizations, special factor requirements were added to the IDEA in 1997 (IDEA, Part B, Section 614(d)(3)(B)(iv)). The IEP teams are now required to consider the Deaf child's language and communication needs. They must also provide opportunities for direct instruction by the teachers and communication with peers and professional personnel in the child's preferred language and communication mode (Tucker, 2010/2011).

Another case in 2000, involving disputes over FAPE, LRE, and *F.M. & L.G. v.*

Barbour County was analyzed by Easter-brooks, Lytle, Sheets, and Crook (2004). In this case, two Black Deaf youth were enrolled in a special education classes for students with multiple disabilities. Their teachers did not have preparation in deaf education teaching practices or skills in sign language. Consequently, the Deaf youth could not learn language, communicate with others beyond gestures, and, more pointedly, and could not access the curriculum. The students never were exposed to sign language in the classroom because the teachers could not sign. According to IDEA, the teens were denied FAPE and LRE. After the school district failed to respond to the request for due process, a civil suit was filed for violation of IDEA, Section 504 of the Rehabilitation Act of 1973, Title II of the ADA, and the 14th Amendment of the Constitution. Easterbrooks and her colleagues (2004) claimed that these youth were victims of language deprivation, which negatively influenced their future educational outcomes and employment. The Deaf youth were awarded compensatory damages of a $2.5 million settlement as allowed by the Handicapped Children's Protection Act of 1986 (see Easterbrooks et al., 2004, for detailed discussion of the case).

In *The Human Right to Language: Communication Access for Deaf Children*, the Deaf special education attorney Larry Siegel (2008) argued that the 1st and the 14th Amendments to the Constitution protect Deaf children's rights to access and development of communication and language. Discuss how these amendments can protect Deaf youth from the risk of language deprivation.

In still another classroom case, *S.F. v. McKinney Independent School District*, a white DeafDisabled child on the autism spectrum was placed in a self-contained classroom with hearing disabled children. The Deaf child received instruction from a special education teacher who did not sign and another teacher who only had minimal sign skills. The courts determined that a deaf education classroom with Deaf peers was the most appropriate and least restrictive environment (LRE) for this child (*S.F. v. McKinney Independent School District*, 2012).

In still another case, a 4-year-old hard-of-hearing child with Down syndrome of Mexican American heritage was labeled by the school district only as "hearing impaired and speech impaired" and not by his primary diagnosis of Down syndrome. He was enrolled in a preschool program for children with disabilities. The child's home communication was ASL. However, at school, the boy only received 45 minutes per week of sign instruction by a teacher with minimal sign skills. The parents requested a teacher with fluent ASL skills. During a due process hearing, the hearing officer overruled the parents and determined that the special education placement with the teacher who knew minimal sign language met the criterion for an appropriate education. Eventually, an expert in Down syndrome evaluated the boy. She attributed his social and academic success to the mother and family's early use of ASL in the home. Still the school district refused to provide a competent signing teacher or aide. After years of litigation, the courts continued to rule in favor of the school district; however, the case was eventually mediated and the family received compensation. Today, the youth is in the 10th grade and learning independent living skills. To increase his access to social skills and world knowledge, his family founded a community theater group for individuals with special needs. Now their son has an outlet where he can learn acting and other theater production skills and socialize with a community of signing peers (Leah Chapa, personal communication, November 4, 2019). See Figure 10–3 for a photo of this youth in costume to the right of his mother.

Every Student Succeeds Act (ESSA)

Another law, *Every Student Succeeds Act* (ESSA, 2015) replaced the *No Child Left Behind Act* (NCLB, 2001), an unpopular law that required states to set up strict testing accountability systems. The goals of NCLB were to ensure that every child would be reading and performing in math on grade level by 2014. Like *NCLB, ESSA* is the law for K–12 public education in the U.S. Unlike *NCLB, ESSA* gives states more flexibility in determining academic standards, annual testing, and school accountability. ESSA takes into consideration students from economically disadvantaged homes, students of color, students in special education and those who do not have full access to English language skills. *ESSA* also requires that states allow parents to get involved in the accountability process for schools.

Laws in Foster Care Placements

IDEA, ADA, and Section 504

Foster care placements also fall under IDEA, ADA, and Section 504 protections. Deaf, DeafBlind, DeafDisabled, and DeafBlind youth who have limited language are often the victims of sexual and physical

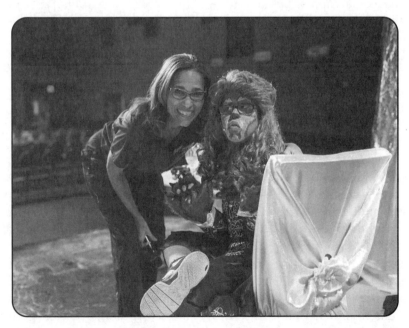

Figure 10–3. Community theater provides this teenager who is hard of hearing with Down syndrome opportunities to socialize with other signing youth with disabilities. Photo courtesy of Leah Chapa.

abuse, neglect, and emotional mistreatment because they do not have the language to report the offense to authorities. As a result of this abuse, they are removed from their biological homes and placed in foster care (Lomas et al., 2017). These children need therapeutic foster homes where foster caregivers are trained to meet Deaf youths' psychological as well as communication needs. Because foster care falls under state agencies, the Child Protective Services (CPS), Title II of the ADA applies. This law requires that accommodations must be provided for communication and language access. Because CPS receives federal funds, Section 504 applies as well. Here is a case about a youth in foster care.

Rose (pseudonym), a DeafDisabled 16-year-old white female, had a history of physical abuse and neglect from her mother and sexual abuse from her father. She was tested in the mildly challenged range in intellectual capabilities and diagnosed with bipolar disorder, depression, and attention-deficit/hyperactivity disorder (ADHD). No one in her biological home or foster homes used sign language. To communicate, Rose used a blend of ASL, signed English, home gestures, and spoken English. She was functionally illiterate, reading at the 2.8 reading grade level. The young teen was removed from her abusive biological home and repeated foster home placements with families who did not know sign language. Because of Rose's outbursts due to frustration with her caretakers not being competent enough to understand her, she was placed in a residential treatment center for hearing youth with behavioral disorders. The employees at this facility did not have specialized training in working with DeafDisabled youth. A noncertified

interpreter was employed during class hours. No interpreter was provided for out-of-school activities or for counseling on a regular basis. Under IDEA, she was not receiving FAPE and LRE in the classroom, nor were the other four Deaf youth who were at the facility. Since the facility received federal funds, Title II of the ADA would apply, as does Section 504 of the Rehabilitation Act. The court ordered that Rose be removed from this facility and sent to a residential facility that had trained professionals and staff to work with the educational and psychiatric needs of Deaf and hard-of-hearing youth.

> The National Association for the Deaf (NAD) has provided the foster care system with guidelines for providing cultural and linguistic access to services for Deaf children and youth. See the NAD's position paper on Foster Care online.

Laws in Juvenile Justice Facility Placements

IDEA, ADA, and Section 504

Another type of placement for Deaf youth is the Juvenile justice facility. Within these facilities are programs that are required under IDEA, ADA, and Section 504 to provide access to communication, language, and appropriate services. Youth are placed here because they committed unlawful violent crimes involving physical and sexual assault, property crimes such as car theft, drug-related offenses, or even homicide. The aims of these facilities are to educate, rehabilitate, and encourage youth to make positive changes in their lives (Masters et al., 2012).

Within juvenile justice facilities, Deaf youth need communication and language access beyond the classroom as they must attend drug/violence/sex abuse counseling sessions, participate in after-school activities, communicate with correctional officers, and integrate with hearing youth in the cafeteria and during after school and dormitory activities. In one case, Roberto and George (pseudonyms) were the only Deaf juveniles in the facility with more than 200 hearing juveniles convicted of felonies, having been sent there by the courts for rehabilitation. Roberto was a 16-year old youth of Mexican American heritage. He had little communication with his family. At a young age, he was diagnosed with ADHD. He reported that he had hallucinations of seeing people who wanted to kill him. Based on this behavior, he was on suicide watch. Academically, Roberto read at the 1.7 reading grade level and had minimal ASL skills. Roberto's offenses included theft, possession of weapons at school, fighting, drug and alcohol use, attempted burglary of a car, attempted sexual assault, and indecency with a child. Roberto's mother reported that a teacher sexually assaulted her son when he was young but there was no follow-up counseling for him. Roberto reported he did not know why he was at the facility.

His roommate George was a white Deaf 14-year-old with average intelligence and a history of oppositional and defiant behavior, probably due to lifelong lack of language exposure. He read at the 4.2 reading grade level and had some basic sign language skills. George, like Roberto, was a repeat offender of sexual assault of children. His mother noted that a teacher sexually assaulted her son when he was younger. George refused to go to counseling, probably because the counselor was not linguistically or culturally adept, and thus the judge placed him in this facility.

Both Roberto and George were enrolled in high school classes at the facility with hearing students. They had a sign language interpreter in their classes. In addition, a certified teacher of the deaf met with them for 45 minutes per week. There were no videophones in school or in the dormitories for them to contact their families. They were not provided with sign language interpreters in their sex offender counseling sessions, nor were interpreters provided for after school, during mealtimes, or for activities in the dormitories at night. Consequently, they had no access to communication and language during these times when the correctional officers often provided behavioral correction to them and other students. Neither youth could read the rules that were found in the Juvenile Corrections Handbook as it was written at the 11th-grade reading level. The facility did not provide an interpreter for the youth to understand the handbook. As a result, the youth experienced difficulty following the rules of the facility and lost many privileges for infractions they did not know about (Andrews, 2013).

Overall, within the facility, the Deaf youth were denied full access to education and correctional and psychiatric treatment, and thus ADA and Section 504 were violated (Lomas et al., 2017). Juvenile cases such as these pose a challenge to the court system. On one hand, if they are released, they may not be ready to integrate in society. Considering the youths' linguistic deprivation, while they are incarcerated in these facilities, they are constantly deprived of accessible treatment for their psychological and rehabilitation needs (Andrews, 2013).

EMPLOYMENT

Laws exist to protect the rights of Deaf, DeafBlind, and DeafDisabled individuals. These laws also provide services to these persons after they finish high school and transition into adulthood.

Social Security Act

The Social Security Act (U.S. Congress, 1934), enacted in 1935, provides a system of paid retirement benefits to workers. Disability benefits were added in 1956. The Social Security Administration (SSA) administers programs such as the Social Security Supplemental Income (SSI) and the Social Security Disability Insurance (SSDI) programs for Deaf, DeafBlind, and DeafDisabled, as well as individuals with disabilities. SSI provides financial support based on family income for disabled individuals from birth to adulthood and is provided prior to the Deaf person having a work history. If the Deaf person does not work full-time anymore (e.g., laid off) and because they were paid Social Security those years they worked full-time, they are now eligible for SSDI.

Rehabilitation Act of 1973

The Rehabilitation Act, enacted in 1973, was the first law protecting Deaf, Deaf-Blind, and DeafDisabled individuals (Raimondo, 2010, 2013). This act provides support for vocational rehabilitation services. It includes a set of rules focused on rights, advocacy, and protections for Deaf, DeafBlind, and DeafDisabled as well as persons with other disabilities. Vocational Rehabilitative (VR) services begin at age 14 during the Deaf youth's preemployment stage. Here the VR counselor provides job coaching to find summer employment. Together, they develop the Individual Work Plan for Employment (IPE), a document that is reviewed and amended annually. The IPE contains employment goals, with a listing of services agreed on by both parties (https://www.nad.org/resources/employment-and-vocational-rehabilitation/vocational-rehabilitation/).

> Search the Internet and find out what specific services are provided on the IPE for Deaf and DeafDisabled youth.

Americans With Disabilities Act (ADA)

The ADA is a civil rights law that protects and prohibits discrimination against individuals with disabilities at schools (see section above), during employment, with transportation, and in all private and public places that are open to society at large. Because institutions of learning, places of employment, and community events are neither accessible nor constructed using tenets of universal design, oftentimes accommodations need to be made for professionals and individuals who are Deaf, DeafDisabled, DeafBlind, or a combination of these disabilities.

The aim of the law is to ensure that people with disabilities have the same rights and opportunities as other citizens. The ADA gives protections of civil rights to persons with disabilities similar to those provided to individuals on the basis of race, color, sex, national origin, age, and religion. The ADA guarantees fairness, equity, and equal opportunity in private and public accommodations, employment, transportation, state and local government services, and telecommunications. There are five sections in the ADA. Title I guarantees equal employment opportunities. Title II forbids discrimination on the basis of disability in state and local government services. Public accommodations is the topic of Title III, which prohibits discrimination at public and commercial facilities. Title IV relates to telecommunications and requires telephone and Internet companies to provide a nationwide system of interstate and intrastate telecommunications relay services that allows Deaf, DeafDisabled, and DeafBlind persons to communicate over the telephone. It also mandates that federally funded service announcements be closed captioned. This service is regulated by the Federal Communication Commission. The last one, Title V, is an all-inclusive section that covers impact on insurance providers and benefits, as well as prohibition against retaliation and coercion, illegal use of drugs, and attorney's fees (Rosenblum, Charmatz, Patkin, Phillips, & Jackson, 2015).

Both ADA and Section 504 provide protection for Deaf, DeafBlind, and DeafDisabled workers. Those who are licensed drivers have experienced discrimination. Even though studies show that Deaf drivers have safe driving records (Hamilton, 2015), they have still faced repeated discrimination in jobs related to driving post office vehicles, semitruck trailers, school vans, and United Parcel Service (UPS)

vehicles. Challenging lawsuits with subsequent settlements to these cases have resulted in the removal of the ban on Deaf drivers and accessibility to promotions and technology for Deaf workers (see *Rizzo v. Children's World Learning Center*, 1999; *Bates v. United Parcel Service, Inc.*, 2007; *Bruce Hubbard et al., v. Patrick R. Donahue*, 2013). These cases also addressed other discriminatory practices such as the denial of promotions. Deaf workers are also not provided with sign language interpreters, vibrating and texting devices, and safety training programs (Dewey, 2016). In 2013, the U.S. Department of Transportation provided exemptions for the hearing tests for Deaf drivers and recognized their safe driving records, thereby giving them the right to drive large trucks (Dewey, 2016).

Today, Deaf individuals are using Uber and Lyft taxi services because of the ease of contacting a driver, providing the location, and paying for the service all online. This Deaf consumer can then control most of the transaction and communication prior to getting into the car. Companies such as Uber have provided its drivers with tips on how to communicate with Deaf and DeafDisabled customers (Lyft, 2018).

Brenda Palmigiano and her Deaf colleagues secured a Commercial Driver's License (CDL) from the Federal Motor Carrier Safety Administration (FMCSA) at the Department of Transportation (DOT). In 2011, with the NAD's help, she founded the Deaf Trucker United group. How does this Deaf-led group protect the rights of other Deaf drivers?

HIGHER EDUCATION

Deaf adults entering higher education may face bias in professional examinations, lack of accommodations such as sign language interpreters and tutors at universities, and discrimination in practicum and internships and faculty promotion procedures (Smith & Andrews, 2015) (Figure 10–4).

Deaf persons involved in these cases are protected under the ADA, Section 504 of the Rehabilitation Act, and other state statutes. These case studies provide examples.

ADA and 504 Protections

The case *Deaf teachers v. the Texas Education Agency and the State Board of Educa-* *tion* never went to trial. But a hearing on test bias resulted in changes in the Texas Education Code (TEC) 13.050. This action led to the exemption of Deaf persons from biased teacher proficiency tests. As a result of this change in the law, more individuals who are Deaf could become certified as teachers in Texas (Smith & Andrews, 2015).

Another law, Title III of the ADA, provides Deaf, DeafBlind, and DeafDisabled students with accommodations during professional examinations and test preparation courses, continuing education courses, and other examinations. In 1996, the Department of Justice (DOJ) issued the consent order (*United States of America v. Robin Singh Educational Services, Inc.*, 2006) with Testmasters, a LSAT preparation company. This company failed to provide accommodations for its

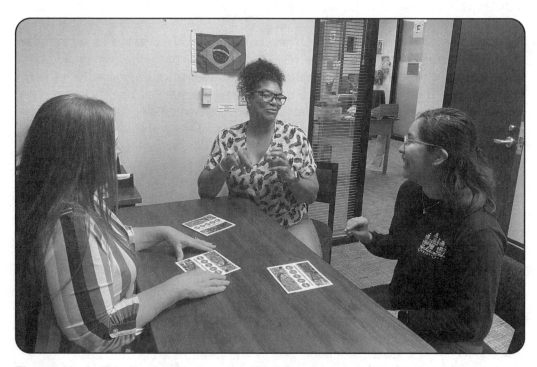

Figure 10–4. This Deaf student supported by her sign language interpreter discusses accommodations she will need for her college classes.

LSAT preparation course for Deaf test takers. DOJ also entered a settlement agreement (*Settlement Agreement Between U.S. and National Board of Medical Examiners*, 2011). This agreement ensured that Deaf students have accommodations during medical licensing examinations (Rosenblum et al., 2016).

Accommodations were also in question with this next case, *Camenisch v. University of Texas* (1980). A district court issued an injunction requiring the university to provide and pay for sign language interpreters for a Deaf white man, Walter Camenisch, who had been denied when he was enrolled in graduate coursework at the University of Texas. In still another case, *Argenyi v. Creighton University*, a white Deaf student attending a private medical school requested interpreting and captioning. He was awarded these accommodations due to this court case (Rosenblum et al., 2016).

Other cases in higher education involve discrimination on the job and during internships. Dr. Michael Collier, a white Deaf professional, was hired in a tenured faculty position. Subsequently, he was fired without any mentoring or remediation plan. Dr. Collier never had any contact with the department chair and was placed under the supervision of a nontenured professor. A lawsuit was filed, *Michael L. Collier, Ph.D., v. Texas Tech University* (2011), and the jury awarded him a settlement. In still another discriminatory case, Nadelle Grantham, a white woman, was expelled from a teacher-education program during her last semester because she was Deaf. Even though she passed all of her coursework, the dean and faculty of the College of Education did not believe she could teach and supervise children during her student-teaching internship. The lawsuit, *Grantham v. Moffett* (1998), resulted in a verdict supporting Grantham.

> Click on the NAD website and find Howard Rosenblum, Esquire, the Chief Executive Officer of the NAD. He describes how Deaf persons can utilize the power of the ADA by registering a complaint in order to document and report on discrimination they faced on the job or in the community.

JUSTICE SYSTEM

Family, Education, and Language Factors

Because of family, education, and language factors, Deaf persons often are denied fair treatment within the justice system. A small minority of Deaf persons who commit crimes have childhood histories of lack of language exposure and learning in the home. They were subjected to poor education during the school years because the curriculum was not made accessible to them. They were never taught about civics or their constitutional rights. When they reached adulthood, they were not provided with the tools to defend themselves in court (Lomas et al., 2017). Such early language deprivation and barriers in accessing schooling (among other factors) can lead to a condition in adulthood called "linguistic incompetence." Due to familial and societal factors, this means that individuals were never given the opportunity to develop fundamental communication skills in ASL and English. They were never given opportunities to develop concepts, background, and world knowledge. Specifically, they were often not even made aware of by teachers so they could develop knowledge about the legal system and how to operate within it (Glickman & Hall, 2019; LaVigne & Vernon, 2003). These Deaf individuals may know some basic ASL and English skills to discuss bodily functions, routine activities, food, and objects, but they do not know enough ASL to understand abstract and complex legal information through an interpreter. Hearing persons who are illiterate and have knowledge gaps about legal issues can seek help by asking questions to those around them (i.e., police, lawyers, criminal justice officials), whereas Deaf individuals are vulnerable to not obtaining their basic rights due to factors beyond their control (LaVigne & Vernon, 2003; Vernon & Andrews, 2011). What laws protect Deaf individuals?

Section 504 and ADA Protections

Specific laws such as Section 504 of the Rehabilitation Act of 1973 and the ADA (amended in 2008) prohibit discrimination against Deaf, DeafBlind, and DeafDisabled individuals within the justice system. For communication to be effective with most Deaf individuals, sign language interpreters are required throughout the justice system, including with law enforcement, in the courtroom, and with prison and jail officials. These laws also cover equal access to programs and services within jails and prisons, including educational, rehabilitative, medical, psychiatric, and psychological assessments and therapy. Further, under ADA (Title IV, Telecommunications), Telecommunications Relay Service (TRS) was established to facilitate communication between hearing and Deaf callers with no cost to TRS

users (Raimondo, 2013). TRS uses operators, called communication assistants (CAs), to facilitate telephone calls between Deaf, DeafBlind, and DeafDisabled persons and other individuals.

DeafBlind individuals often do not have equal access to TRS services to make calls. Deaf and DeafBlind consumer groups such as the American Association of the DeafBlind, Telecommunications for the Deaf and Hard of Hearing, National Association for the Deaf, and others support a form of DeafBlind Relay Service (DBRS). These relay services provide the ability for many DeafBlind persons to communicate by telephone. They will need communication assistants to assist them to call and to interpret conversations among themselves and with others. Because the DeafBlind community is diverse and uses a variety of communication methods, they should have a choice of DBRSs to choose from and should not be limited to one form of DBRS offered by one TRS provider (http://aadb.org/information/DBRS/dbrs_comment01.html).

The Bill of Rights and the 14th Amendment

Other laws for Deaf, DeafBlind, and DeafDisabled citizens consist of protections under the Constitution's Bill of Rights and the 14th Amendment (Leigh & Andrews, 2017). The first 10 amendments to the U.S. Constitution guarantee rights and liberties to citizens such as freedom of speech, press, and religion and limit the power of the government. They put in place rules and procedures for due process. The 14th Amendment prohibits the state from denying any citizen life, liberty, or property with due process of law or to deny any person equal protection of the law.

How do the Bill of Rights and the 14th Amendment relate to Deaf, DeafDisabled, and DeafBlind citizens?

The 1st Amendment provides them with freedom of speech. The 4th Amendment shields them from unreasonable searches and taking of belongings. The 5th Amendment provides protection from self-incrimination and the right to remain silent when questioned by police or detectives. The 6th Amendment provides the right to have an attorney, a speedy and public trial, and a trial by jury; to present a defense; and to confront the accuser and witnesses. And the 14th Amendment provides the right to due process ensuring suspects and defendants have safeguards when encountering officials throughout the criminal justice system (Andrews, Vernon, & LaVigne, 2006, 2007). Tragically, these rights have been denied to Deaf, DeafDisabled, and DeafBlind citizens as the many cases illustrate below. This situation is somewhat improving with advocacy of the organizations as the National Association for the Deaf and other agencies have educated law enforcement, attorneys, judges, and criminal justice officials about how society more often than not has denied many of them equity in legal matters even when they are victims of crimes.

Victims of Crimes

Crime victims, the targets of illegal actions of others, often suffer physical, sexual, mental, or emotional harm; death or economic loss; or a combination of these injuries (Masters et al., 2017). As victims of crimes, Deaf, DeafBlind, and DeafDisabled people are often victimized twice, first by the crime and then by the criminal justice system that fails to respond to

them (Vernon & Miller, 2005). During the time period from 2009 to 2015, the U.S. Department of Justice, Bureau of Justice Statistics (2017) reported that crimes of violence are more likely to be committed against persons with multiple disabilities from multiethnic backgrounds compared to crimes committed against able-bodied white persons. Take this example of Jack, a victim of domestic assault.

Jack (pseudonym), a white Deaf immigrant man from Eastern Europe, was confronted by his landlady in the kitchen. When he refused to pay rent, in anger, she threw a chair at him. As he was backed against the wall, Jack reached for a kitchen knife to ward off this attack. Another housemate in the room called 911. During the call, the police dispatcher discovered that Deaf people resided in the house. But she failed to follow department policy requiring that a sign language interpreter be sent to the scene. When the police arrived, they only listened to the landlady's story. She was hard of hearing and had understandable speech. Jack, being Deaf and fluent in sign language, was ignored. He was handcuffed behind his back, preventing him from using his hands to communicate. He was taken to the police station, where he was booked for assault. Several days later, he posted bail and subsequently met with an attorney who provided a sign language interpreter. The assault charges were dropped. Jack later filed a class-action lawsuit with other Deaf plaintiffs with similar stories against the police department for not providing interpreters during the arrest and booking stages.

Like Jack, other Deaf persons are frequently victims of crimes. In a study that investigated crimes against Deaf college students, Barrows (2008) surveyed 71 hearing college students and 118 Deaf and hard-of-hearing college students, all between the ages of 18 and 24 years. The Deaf students (44%) recounted repeated victimization compared to 35% of hearing students, confirming a higher rate of vulnerability related to sexual and violent victimizations. Furthermore, Barrows found that persons who are Deaf more often than not knew their offenders and they were more likely to be hearing.

After an assault, many Deaf victims may not know whom to turn to for assistance. Victims' assistance agencies may lack accessibility (Chapter 7). As a result, victim assistance organizations may not see crime victims, not because they don't exist but because crimes often go unreported (Barrows, 2008). To address this situation, Deaf-led organizations have set up organizations to address the issue of violence, as described in this box.

> The Deaf Abused Women's Network (DAWN) aims to reduce abuse and promote accountability in the Deaf community in the District of Colombia metropolitan area. DAWN provides a 24-hour hotline for Deaf and DeafDisabled persons who are experiencing domestic violence, sexual violence, trafficking, and stalking. See what services are offered in other states.

Prevalence and Types of Crimes

The U.S. prison population numbers nearly 2.2 million (BJS, 2017). Within these facilities, multiple sources indicate an overrepresentation of Deaf and hard-of-hearing individuals who are incarcerated in county jails and state and federal prisons and can be as high as 30% (Talia Lewis, personal communication, August 15, 2019; Miller, 2001). Studies show that individuals who are Deaf commit the same types of crimes as found in the hearing population. These crimes include the following: homicide, rape, assault, arson, child molestation (pedophilia), child pornography, online solicitation of minors for sexual encounters, car theft, check forgery, theft, larceny, and burglary (Miller, 2001). In a sample of 97 Deaf individuals who were incarcerated in the Estelle Unit at Huntsville State Prison in Texas, 64% of the Deaf inmates had been convicted of violent crimes compared to 49% of the general hearing population. Sexual offenders made up 32.3% of the Deaf individuals compared to only 12.3% of the hearing prison population. Within the Deaf population, murder was committed by 10%, assault by 9%, robbery by 7%, and child injury by 3% (Miller, 2001).

Homicide

Deaf individuals who murder pose safety issues for society if they are released. On the other hand, it is difficult, if not impossible, to give them a fair trial and ensure their constitutional rights if they are linguistically incompetent as the text box below shows.

Psychologists who have studied Deaf individuals who murder have emphasized how biological, environmental, and social factors converge to create violent behaviors (Vernon, Steinberg, & Montoya, 1999). Similar to the three examples in the textbox, a clinical study of 28 Deaf murderers indicated that a significant number of them were linguistically incompetent and could not comprehend

Daphne Annette Wright is a white Deaf woman who was convicted of premeditated murder, felony murder, and aggravated kidnapping (*State of South Dakota v. Daphne Annette Wright*, 2009). She had difficulty understanding the sign language interpreter during her trial. Donald Lang, a Black Deaf man who was charged with having killed two women in Chicago in 1965 and 1971, could not be convicted as he was unable to read or write and did not know speechreading or sign language (Tidyman, 1974). And Patrick McCullough, a white Deaf man with a history of psychiatric diagnoses, killed three persons and himself (Vernon & Vernon, 2010). What challenges did the courts have in providing these Deaf individuals with due process?

the charges against them or participate in their own defense. Moreover, the majority had medical or psychodiagnostic evidence of cognitive challenges associated with them being linguistically deprived. Consequently, the linguistic deprivation early in life reinforced the possibility of violent behaviors. Moreover, half of them had been diagnosed with antisocial personality disorder, which has been linked to criminal histories, and almost 65% were addicted to alcohol and drugs (Vernon et al., 1999).

Sexual Offending Crimes

Crimes related to sexual offending consist of pedophilia, rape, sexual assault, downloading child pornography, and texting in a chat room to solicit sexual encounters.

Pedophilia refers to a sexual preference for young children found mostly in men (American Psychiatric Association, 2013). Pedophilia is believed to be a medical condition. Still, the public responds with strong disgust toward pedophiles (Vernon & Rich, 1997). As such, the legal system has responded with harsh, punitive legislation such as the Adam Walsh Child Protection and Safety Act (AWA, 2006), establishing a national sex offenders' registry law and limitations on where they can live and mingle with society, along with increased sentences.

Two studies on pedophiles who are Deaf were conducted with 14 cases in one (Miller & Vernon, 2003) and 22 cases in the other (Vernon & Rich, 1997). Similarly to murderers, pedophiles who are Deaf were found to have high rates of neurological impairment, illiteracy, poor communication skills, inferior education, and psychiatric illness (Vernon & Miller, 2003). Seventeen of the males were illiterate or read below the 2.9 reading grade level. Most of the individuals in the two studies had criminal records that also involved assault, burglary, arson, and car theft (Miller & Vernon, 2003).

Downloading child pornography is a deviant sexual behavior found among sex offenders. One young white DeafDisabled man with Usher syndrome had sufficient functional vision to enroll in a computer maintenance classes at a community college. He had a 2.8 reading grade level, so while he could not read his textbooks, he followed class lectures with a sign language interpreter. The FBI arrested him for downloading child pornography on his home computer. A second young white man who was DeafDisabled with cognitive disabilities and a second-grade reading level lived rent free in an apartment complex where he was a handyman and caretaker. His older sister assisted him with food shopping, laundry, and bill paying. The young man was charged with soliciting sex in a chat room with a minor and was arrested during a sting operation (Andrews, 2013). The third case was a hard-of-hearing white man in his 50s with mild cognitive disabilities. He lived semi-independently with help from a sister and was employed as a janitor for 30 years at a city court. The FBI charged him with downloading child pornography on his home computer (*USA v. Thomas Heyer*, 2011).

All three men were socially isolated who spent most of their free time on the computer. They depended on their families socially and economically. All had additional disabilities and low reading levels. Two had minimal sign proficiency, and the hard-of-hearing man did not use sign at all. The courts dismissed two of the defendants as linguistically incompetent because in a competency hearing, it was determined that they were not able to participate in their defense. However, in the third case, the hard-of-hearing individual was denied the motion of dismissal for linguistic incompetence and later was sentenced to prison. With these cases, the judges and prosecuting attorneys assumed that if the Deaf person in question lived independently (with support) and graduated from high school at the 12th grade, then they are literate and capable of understanding and participating in their defense. However, these three men only received certificates of attendance in special education classes, which meant they did not meet the requirements for an equivalent 12th-grade diploma similar to a hearing youth who graduates from an academic track. The judge

and prosecuting attorneys also assumed that even with this special education, the three men who read below the 3rd-grade level could navigate the Internet for pornography. However, the argument was made that navigating the Internet to find child pornography does not take a high degree of computer literacy. It can be done using icons and pictures without any text literacy. Moreover, texting and chat room conversations are far simpler than legal language found in the courtroom and do not require high levels of literacy. These three men were linguistically incompetent when answering the arresting detective's questions. They did not have the language skills to understand their attorneys or to stand trial. When charged with the sex offense, they did not understand the consequences of pleading guilty and the rules and requirements for registering as a sex offender. For example, being a registered sex offender impacts where they live and their job prospects. They cannot live near a school (and schools are everywhere!). They cannot work where there are children (e.g., McDonald's). They cannot live with their families if their family members have children. If they go to prison, most prisons are designed for hearing sex offenders, with staff having no knowledge of Deaf culture or Deaf ways of teaching and learning. And even though the facility may provide sign language interpreters, this accommodation is not enough for the linguistically incompetent individuals who are Deaf (Glickman, Lemere, & Smith, 2013; Vernon, 2010). Few prisons have programs that specialize in treating sex offenders who are Deaf. Prisons have been challenged by court cases to review their access to interpreters, videophones, and correctional plans for Deaf individuals who are incarcerated for criminal offenses (*United States v. Thomas Heyer*, 2015; *VanValkenburg v. Oregon Department of Corrections*, 2016).

The Criminal Justice Process

The criminal justice process is even difficult for educated Deaf individuals. In one study college, Deaf students report that they have difficulty in understanding concepts as presented in the Miranda warning and waiver (Seaborn, Andrews, & Martin, 2010). In other study college, Deaf students recounted they had difficulty understanding concepts such as acquittal, plea-bargaining, and the roles and responsibilities of police, prosecutors, and judges (Barrows, 2008). And still in another study, Deaf college students conveyed they had difficulty comprehending the polygraph questionnaire (Roth, Bentley-Sassaman, & Lizor, 2017). For the estimated 20% to 30% of Deaf persons in the total Deaf population who are uneducated and linguistically incompetent, obstacles within the criminal justice system are unbelievably high (LaVigne & Vernon, 2003). These obstacles start immediately during the arrest and continue with the booking to incarceration to probation and parole as discussed below (Miller, 2001; Vernon, 2010; Vernon & Miller, 2005).

Barriers at the Arrest

Barriers begin with the law enforcement officials who are typically not trained in how to recognize and communicate with a Deaf individual, as seen in our first case study in this chapter. A sign language interpreter should have been contacted as soon as the officers realized they do not know sign language or how to communicate with the Deaf youth. A young Deaf college student could try to rely on written notes for simple commands (i.e., name, address, etc.). But under such an emotionally charged interaction with civil liberties at stake, a sign language interpreter is necessary to ensure that effective communication is provided and takes place (Vernon & Andrews, 2011).

Visit these websites to find out more about the legal aspects for Deaf suspects and defendants; David Greenburg's blog "Deaf in Prison," Civil Rights Education and Enforcement Center (CREEC), the National Association for the Deaf (NAD) position papers, and fact sheets on the websites for Helping Advance the Rights of Deaf Communities (HEARD) and the Civil Liberties Union's National Prison (ACLU) Project.

Booking, Medical/Psychological Intake, and Orientation

The situation becomes even more traumatic for the Deaf person who has been arrested. To be booked into jail or prison is an emotional, frustrating, and even terrorizing experience for Deaf individuals, particularly if there is no sign language interpreter available (Vernon, 2010). For one, the Deaf individual has no idea what lies ahead. While some parts of the booking process are easy to understand such as fingerprinting, being handed a change of clothes, and following the officer's gesture to a change room, other aspects have strong visual components, such as the fingerprinting station (Figures 10–5 and 10–6).

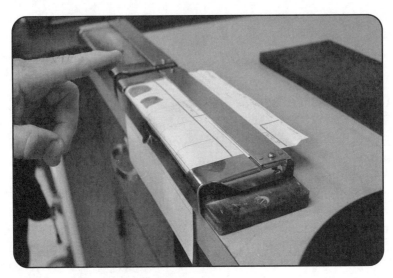

Figure 10–5. Traditional paper and ink fingerprinting station in jail. Photo courtesy of Jefferson County Jail.

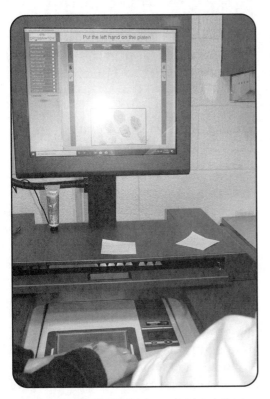

Figure 10–6. Digital computerized fingerprinting station in jail that takes the prints, and stores and manages the data. Photo courtesy of Jefferson County Jail.

However, other directions by jail officials are not so easy to understand. For example, when meeting with a medical officer or counselor without a sign language interpreter, Deaf individuals may not be able to provide accurate information. Asking them to read medical and psychological questionnaires is challenging because the vocabulary written on these forms is higher than third grade level (Andrews, 2011; LaVigne & Vernon, 2003). And for those with struggles in reading, written communication is also not effective for discussing serious medical issues such as diabetes, heart conditions, allergies needing medications, or mental health issues such as depression and suicide. When procedures for providing interpreters are denied, the consequences can be tragic, as illustrated in this next case.

A white Deaf man was not provided an interpreter during the medical intake, even though the official made note that he was Deaf on the report. ASL was his primary language, and school records showed he read at the second-grade reading level. When booked in jail, he could neither lipread the officer nor read the intake document. He was moved around to another jail. In his last jail placement, when his cellmate left, he committed suicide by hanging (*Ulibarri v. City & County of Denver*, 2012).

Another case relates to Abreham Zemedagedehu, a Deaf man who was homeless. Born in Ethiopia, Mr. Z. grew up using Ethiopian Sign Language. He came to the United States, became a U.S. citizen, and learned ASL and learned only some basic English. Mr. Z. was falsely accused of stealing an iPad by another man who was also Deaf. Mr. Z. was arrested and incarcerated in a jail in Virginia for 6 weeks and never provided with an interpreter. He was made to sign medical forms he could not read and undergo medical treatment (tuberculosis shot), which he did not know he needed. After the shot, he experienced an allergic reaction to the injection. Mr. Z. did not know why he was in jail and what the charges were until he was arraigned and provided a court interpreter. His public defender encouraged Mr. Z. to plead guilty to a lesser misdemeanor charge in exchange for time served. After the other Deaf man confessed he found his iPad, the charges were dropped. A lawsuit was filed against the sheriff's office because it failed to provide a sign language interpreter for him while he was in jail. A settlement of $250,000 was provided to Mr. Z. Furthermore, the sheriff's office must take steps to comply with ADA, which includes appointing an ADA coordinator and ensuring that auxiliary aids and services are provided such as sign language interpreters (https://www.nbcwashington.com/news/local/arlington-co-sheriffs-office-settles-claim-for-deaf-inmate/2074443/).

These stories of Deaf persons who are arrested and incarcerated without interpreters are common and occur frequently. But the barriers are even greater when the Deaf defendants enter the courtroom.

Barriers at Trial

Such obstacles include obtaining the services of sign language interpreters. They also mean being able to read court transcripts (most are written above the seventh-grade reading level), as well as being able to communicate with one's attorney.

It is unethical to use family and friends as interpreters in any situation, especially when it involves the police and the legal system. Sign language interpreters who have legal certification must undergo years of professional training that includes cultural, cognitive, and linguistic knowledge along with highly technical skills in producing and comprehending legal discourse. Interpreters must be certified and follow a strict code of ethics that includes confidentiality and knowledge of state laws regarding sign language interpretation. The lawyer must provide his or her own interpreter for a Deaf client. The courts provide the interpreters for the trial proceedings, including the witnesses (Mather, 2009).

For Deaf defendants who are linguistically deprived, the use of a DI (Deaf Interpreter) or a CDI (Certified Deaf Interpreter) with legal and court training and background is crucial (see description in Chapter 12). DIs can help them gain access to information in the courtroom. They have special linguistic knowledge of distinctive ASL signs, phrases, and usages understood by Deaf individuals. Here is some of the commonly used interpreting sequence. First, the hearing interpreter translates the judge or lawyer's spoken language into what is considered English-influenced ASL for the Deaf interpreter. Viewing this and using their expert knowledge, the DI then attempts to remove as much of the English-influenced component and includes more structurally appropriate and accessible sign language for the Deaf defendant (Leigh & Andrews, 2017).

The effect of having a team of four interpreters (e.g., two hearing interpreters and two DIs) in the courtroom may initially seem chaotic by many judges, prosecuting attorneys, and juries. Why so many interpreters, they may ask? Attorneys must explain the need for the complex legal language to be broken down into simpler concepts using the professional expertise of DIs. Moreover, judges, prosecutors, and juries need information about Deaf cultural knowledge in order to understand the linguistic incompetence of Deaf defendants who are accused of a crime.

In prior competency hearings or meetings with prosecutors and defense attorneys, even after these explanations about Deaf defendants and linguistic incompetence, the judge may approve the use of DIs and rule that the trial must go on. This happened in the *State of Texas v. Carl Doyle* (2011). In this case, the DIs were pivotal in providing Mr. Doyle as close to a fair trial that could happen given his linguistic incompetence.

Mr. Doyle, a Black American who is DeafBlind and has diabetes, lived at home and received insulin three times a day from a home health agency. As a DeafDisabled person, he lived independently with a wide support system of family, social, and medical agencies that provided him with daily and weekly services. He did not drive and his deteriorating vision has prevented his use of his bicycle.

Mr. Doyle was accused and charged with assaulting a home health nurse at his residence. He had no previous criminal history or encounters with law enforcement or the criminal justice system. Mr. Doyle's attorney was granted DI interpreters for the trial since his client, age 55, did not use speech or speechreading and had minimal sign language skills. A linguistic and literacy evaluation revealed that Mr. Doyle read at the first-grade level and used home signs, pointing, and gestures to communicate. Even though he had only a few years of formal education, he held a job as a janitor for 17 years at a hospital. Now retired, he lived in a home that he paid for with his savings managed with the assistance of his cousin. When Mr. Doyle took the stand, even with the team of DI interpreters, the prosecutor quickly realized Mr. Doyle's difficulty in answering his questions. But with his limited gestures (translated by DIs), he was able to communicate his side of the story that the accusing home health nurse abruptly shook him from a nap and physically grabbed and pushed him into the kitchen to get his insulin shot. He relayed how he raised his arms and pushed her away to defend himself from her. Mr. Doyle was reported by his accuser to yell and shout at her and grab her jacket to smell it. She interpreted these behaviors as part of the assault. It was explained to judge and jury that as a DeafBlind person, Mr. Doyle was using his remaining vision, touch, and olfactory (smell) senses to understand his environment, not to attack the nurse. Not being familiar with Deaf voices, the accuser commented on Mr. Doyle's loud screams, which she considered threatening. However, being Deaf, Mr. Doyle does not hear his voice in order to be able to monitor it. His screams emphasized his frustration about being pushed and shoved by the accuser. The assistance of the DIs and the explanations about Deaf and DeafBlind cultural behaviors all supported the efforts of Mr. Doyle's defense lawyer, who convinced the jury to acquit him (*State of Texas v. Carl Doyle*, 2011).

Barriers in Jail or Prison

Jails or prisons can be lonely, isolating, and even terrorizing for Deaf individuals. They are confined physically and cannot communicate with other individuals who are incarcerated or with the jail officials (Figure 10–7).

Many individuals who are Deaf do not know why they are in jail, nor do they know how long they will be incarcerated (Miller, 2001). Many do not have the reading skills to read or watch captioned TV.

TTY devices may be available, but many of their hearing families don't own them. Videophones often are not available. While in jail, Deaf individuals can be subject to assault and rape by other inmates. They have no one to turn to for protection because they cannot communicate with anyone around them. They don't understand the jail routines because they did not have full access during the orientation, nor can they read the inmate handbook (Vernon, 2010). Inmate handbooks are written at the 11th-grade reading level or above, so very few can read them. Hearing inmates who are illiterate can ask other inmates or correctional officers about the prison rules, but Deaf individuals do not have this access unless they have a skilled sign language interpreter who can translate this document for them (Andrews, 2011).

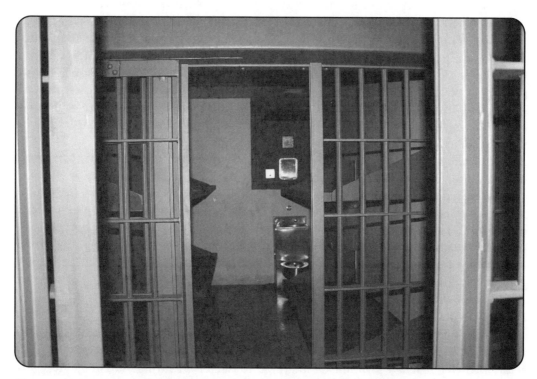

Figure 10–7. Jails can be small, crowded, confined spaces that limit movement and activities for long hours of the day. Photo courtesy of Jefferson County Jail.

In one case, a Deaf man was incarcerated in an Oregon prison for 14 years, during which he was not provided with sign language interpreters on a regular basis. Consequently, he filed a federal lawsuit against the department of corrections in Oregon under the ADA for not providing him with effective communication while in prison. As an alternative, he was asked by the prison officials to ask fellow inmates to interpret for him. Neither did these unqualified hearing inmates keep the information they supposedly interpreted confidential. This created a safety risk for the Deaf individual, making him vulnerable to humiliation and beatings from fellow inmates. In one incident, a miscommunication resulted in him being placed in solitary confinement. Furthermore, throughout his incarceration, he was not provided with qualified sign language interpreters so he could not participate in educational, rehabilitative, counseling, and volunteer programs. As a result, he lost 14 years of learning. Given his profile as utilizing ASL as his primary language, a qualified sign language interpreter should be provided at all critical meetings such as the prison intake, medical and psychological intake and evaluation, and prison orientation; during all disciplinary hearings; and for counseling, education, rehabilitative, and volunteer programs. In addition, a videophone should have been provided for him just like a telephone being provided to a hearing person incarcerated at the same prison. Also, documents that he must read and sign as well as medical forms and educational materials must be translated for him using a qualified sign language interpreter. A lawsuit was filed and a large settlement was reached for the Deaf man (*VanValkenburg v. Oregon Department of Corrections*, 2016).

This situation of Deaf persons not having access to communication through interpreters as well as through videophones in prison is widespread, as indicated by class-action suits throughout the country. The U.S. District Court for the Eastern District of Michigan has approved a settlement in a class-action lawsuit brought on by the Michigan Protection & Advocacy Service (MPASS) for about 200 Deaf and hard-of-hearing persons who are incarcerated in prisons throughout the Michigan Department of Corrections (MDOC). These Deaf persons did not have access to telephones or visual alerting devices for fires, and they did not have access to sign language interpreters for disciplinary hearings. As part of the settlement, the MDOC must provide videophones and necessary auxiliary aids, including sign language interpreters, as well as ensure that they can participate in prison programs. MDOC staff are to receive proper training in how to identify and interact with persons who are Deaf. Furthermore, appropriate policies and procedures are to be put in place by MDOC officials so that these areas are addressed and accounted for (Ankney, 2019).

Search the Internet for other class-action suits filed and settled in other states related to rights and services for Deaf, DeafDisabled, and Deaf-Blind persons who are incarcerated.

Barriers in Probation and Parole

After release from prison, Deaf individuals may have difficulty integrating back into society, finding housing, and getting a job. More often than not, the sexual offender and court-mandated substance abuse programs are not accessible unless an interpreter is provided. Even with the interpreter, many Deaf persons who are linguistically incompetent do not understand the regulations for probation and parole. When they unknowingly break the rules, they find themselves back in jail, as in this case.

Jerome (pseudonym), a Black Deaf-Disabled man, was not provided with a sign language interpreter consistently throughout his arrest, booking, incarceration, plea-bargaining, and parole. Jerome became Deaf at 2 years of age. He also had cognitive disabilities, heart problems, and asthma. Jerome was raised in an oral mainstreamed public school and learned sign language when he was older. Thus, he had minimal sign language skills for basic communication. In the first event that sent him to jail, Jerome reported that he refused to give his girlfriend $2,000 that she demanded. After this, the woman allegedly lied to the police and told them that Jerome inappropriately touched her young daughter. Jerome was arrested and booked in jail without a sign language interpreter. His first attorney provided him with an interpreter a few times. She urged him to sign a plea bargain to get him released from jail. Jerome did not understand that the plea bargain entailed admission of guilt and having to register as a sex offender for 10 years with restrictions on where he lived and moved around in his city. Because he wanted to get out of jail, he signed the plea-bargain form. After his release, his parole officer initially did not provide him with a sign language interpreter. In a series of miscommunications with his parole officer, Jerome failed to register as a sex offender. Consequently, he was jailed for a second felony. His family secured a second attorney, who convinced the judge of Jerome's

linguistic incompetence. He was released from jail upon the condition that he fulfilled his parole obligations. This time, his parole officer provided a sign language interpreter for his meetings.

Because the criminal justice system is not equipped to work with persons like Jerome, his case is similar to many other cases. Because of poor educational practices they have had to endure, Deaf individuals who become suspects and defendants of crimes often do not have the language to defend themselves in hearings or trials. They are forced to sign documents and waivers such as Miranda and the plea-bargain without understanding them. They do not know why they are incarcerated. When discharged, they do not understand how to follow the regulations of their probation and parole requirements (Vernon, 2010).

CONCLUSIONS

In this chapter, we reviewed the laws that protect Deaf individuals in education, employment, and the criminal justice system. Throughout, we note how Deaf professionals have functioned as change agents in their roles as lawyers, CEOs, interpreters, and grassroot advocates who assisted in the passing of laws and in their support of Deaf clients in due process hearings, in investigations and pleadings, and through the pretrial, trial, settlement, and appeal processes (Rosenblum et al., 2016; Smith, 1996; Tidyman, 1976). Despite advocacy attempts and protective laws for early communication and language access for Deaf individuals, language deprivation still frequently occurs in childhood. This is partially due to families and a deaf educational system that does not provide quality exposure to sign language and English so that language competence can be obtained. To reduce the likelihood of linguistic incompetence, early sign language access with appropriate early childhood education is necessary as soon as possible after birth. That, combined with providing education to the criminal justice system officials on the rights and protections for Deaf citizens, is paramount in protecting the constitutional rights of every Deaf citizen.

REFERENCES

Adam Walsh Child Protection and Safety Act, 42 U.S.C. § 16901. (2006).

American Psychiatric Association. (2013). *Diagnostic and statistical manual of mental disorders* (5th ed.). Arlington, VA: Author.

American With Disabilities Act of 1990, Pub. L. No. 101-336 § 2, 104 Stat. 328. (1991).

Andrews, J. (2011). Deaf inmates: Cultural and linguistic challenges and comprehending the Inmate Handbook. *Corrections Compendium*, 36(1), 1-6, 14–16.

Andrews, J. F. (2013). *Deaf juvenile and youth sex offenders*. Unpublished manuscript.

Andrews, J. F., Byrne, A., & Clark, M. D. (2015). Deaf scholars on reading: A historical review of 40 years of dissertation research (1973–2013): Implications for research and practice. *American Annals of the Deaf, 159*(5), 393–418.

Andrews, J. F., Vernon, M., & LaVigne, M. (2006, May). The deaf suspect/defendant and the Bill of Rights. *RID Views*, pp. 7–10.

Andrews, J. F., Vernon, M., & LaVigne, M. (2007, Summer). The Bill of Rights, due process, and the deaf suspect/defendant. *Journal of Interpretation*, pp. 9–38.

Ankney, D. (2019, July 3). Michigan: Settlement in class-action suit by prisoners with hearing disabilities. *Prison Legal News*, 30(7), 60.

Argenyi, v. Creighton University, 703 F. 3rd 441. (8th Circuit 2013).

Barrows, L. (2008). *Criminal victimization of the deaf*. New York, NY: LFB Scholarly Publishing.

Bates v. United Parcel Service, Inc., 511 F.3rd 974, 995. (9th Cir. 2007).

Bruce Hubbard, et al., v. Patrick R. Donahue, Postmaster General, United States Postal Services, Civil Case No. 03-1062 (RJL), 958 F. Supp. 2d 116. (2013).

Bureau of Justice Statistics, National Prisoner Statistics, 1978–2017; and U.S. Census Bureau, U.S. Department of Justice, Office of Justice Programs, Bureau of Justice Statistics. https://www.bjs.gov/content/pub/pdf/p17.pdf

Camenisch v. University of Texas, 616 F.2d 127. (5th Cir. 1980).

Dewey, J. (2016). Flail v. Bolger. In G. Gertz & P. Boudreault (Eds.), *The Sage deaf studies encyclopedia* (pp. 420–421). Thousand Oaks, CA: Sage.

Easterbrooks, S., Lytle, L., Sheets, P., & Crook, B. (2004). Ignoring free, appropriate, public education, a costly mistake: The case of F.M. & L.G. versus Barbour County. *Journal of Deaf Studies and Deaf Education, 9*(2), 219–227.

Education of All Handicapped Children's Act (EAHC), Pub. L. 94-142. (1975).

Every Student Succeeds Act of 2015, Pub. L. No. 114-95 § 114 Stat. 1177. (2015–2016).

Gaffney, M., Eichwald, J., Gaffney, C., Alam, S., & Centers for Disease Control and Prevention. (2014). Early hearing detection and intervention among infants—Hearing screening and follow-up survey, United States, 2005–2006 and 2009–2010. *Morbidity and Mortality Weekly Report (MMWR) Surveillance Summary, 63*(2), 20–26.

Glickman, N., & Hall, W. (2019). *Language deprivation and deaf mental health*. New York, NY: Routledge.

Glickman, N. S., Lemere, S., & Smith, C. M. (2013). Engaging deaf persons with language and learning challenges and sexual offending behaviors in sex offender-oriented mental health treatment. *Journal of the American Deafness & Rehabilitation Association (JADARA), 47*(2), 168–203.

Grantham v. Moffett, 101 F.3d 698. (5th Cir. 1998).

Hall, W. C. (2017). What you don't know can hurt you: The risk of language deprivation by impairing sign language development in deaf children. *Maternal and Child Health Journal, 21*(5), 961–965.

Hamilton, P. T. (2015). *Communicating through distraction: A study of deaf drivers and their communication style in a driving environment* (Unpublished master's thesis). Rochester Institute of Technology, Rochester, NY.

Handicapped Children's Protection Act (HCPA), Pub. L. 99-372. (1986).

Hendrick Hudson Central School District v. Rowley (458 U.S. 176). (1982).

Humphries, T., Kushalnagar, P., Mathur, G., Napoli, D. J., Padden, C., Pollard, R., . . . Smith, S. (2014). What medical education can do to ensure robust language development in deaf children. *Medical Science Educator, 24*(4), 409–419.

Humphries, T., Kushalnagar, P., Mathur, G., Napoli, D. J., Padden, C., Rathmann, C., & Smith, S. (2016). Avoiding linguistic neglect of deaf children. *Social Service Review, 90*(4), 589–619.

Humphries, T., Kushalnagar, P., Mathur, G., Napoli, D. J., Rathmann, C., & Smith, S. (2018). Support for parents of deaf children: Common questions and informed, evidence-based answers. *International Journal of Pediatric Otorhinolaryngology, 118*, 134–142.

Individuals With Disabilities Education Act, Pub. L. 101-476, 20 U.S.C. § 1401 et seq. (1990).

Joint Committee on Infant Hearing. (2019). Principles and guidelines for early hearing detection and intervention programs: Position statement: *Journal of Early Hearing Detection and Intervention, 4*(2), 1–44.

LaVigne, M., & Vernon, M. (2003). An interpreter is not enough: Deafness, language and due process. *Wisconsin Law Review, 844*, 843–936.

Leigh, I., & Andrews, J. F. (2017). *Deaf people and society: Psychological, sociological, and educational perspectives* (2nd ed.). New York, NY: Routledge.

Lomas, G., Andrews, J., & Shaw, P. (2017). Deaf and hard of hearing students. In J. Kauffman, D. Hallahan, & P. Pullen (Eds.), *The handbook of special education* (2nd ed., pp. 338–357). New York, NY: Routledge.

Lyft: Hard of Hearing Driving Feature. (2018). Retrieved from https://help.lyft.com/hc/en-us/articles/115012927627-Hard-of-hearing-driver-feature

Masters, R. E., Way, L. B., Gerstenfeld, P. B., Muscat, B. T., Hooper, M., Dussich, J. P., . . . & Skrapec, C. A. (2012). *CJ: Realities and challenges*. New York, NY: McGraw-Hill Higher Education.

Mather, C. (2009). Modifying instruction in the deaf interpreting model. *International Journal of Interpreter Education, 1*, 68–76.

Michael L. Collier, Ph.D., v. Texas Tech University, No. 2008-545,781. (Lubbock County District Court, 99th, TX, 2011).

Miller, K. (2001). *Forensic issues of deaf offenders* (Unpublished doctoral dissertation). Lamar University, Beaumont, TX.

Miller, K., & Vernon, M. (2003). Deaf sex offenders in a prison population. *Journal of Deaf Studies and Deaf Education, 8*(3), 357–362.

Muse, C., Harrison, J., Yoshinaga-Itano, C., Grimes, A., Brookhouser, P. E., Epstein, S., . . . Martin, P. (2013). Supplement to the JCIH 2007 position statement: Principles and guidelines for early intervention after confirmation that a child is deaf or hard of hearing. *Pediatrics, 131*(4), e1324–e1349.

No Child Left Behind Act of 2001, P.L. 107-110, 20 U.S.C. § 6319. (2002).

Payne-Tsoupros, C. (2019). Lessons from the Lead-K Campaign for Language Equality for Deaf and Hard of Hearing Children. *Loyola University Chicago Law Journal, 51*(1), 107–159.

Raimondo, B. (2010). Legal advocacy for deaf and hard of hearing children in education. In M. Marschark & P. Spencer (Eds.), *The Oxford handbook of deaf studies, language, and education* (pp. 31–40). New York, NY: Oxford University Press.

Raimondo, B. (2013). It's the law! A review of the laws that provide Americans with access for all. *Odyssey: New Directions in Deaf Education, 14*, 4–8.

Rehabilitation Act, Section 504, Pub. L. 93-412, 29 U.S.C. § 701 et seq. (1973).

Rizzo v. Children's World Learning Center, 173 F.3rd 254. (5th Cir. 1999).

Rosenblum, H., Charmatz, M., Patkin, D., Phillips, A., & Jackson, C. (2015). *Legal rights: The guide for deaf and hard of hearing people.* Silver Spring, MD: National Association for the Deaf.

Roth, K., Bentley-Sassaman, J., & Lizor, K. (2017). Whether or not ASL interpreters are needed to administer polygraph examinations on deaf individuals. *Polygraph, 46*(2), 146–171.

Seaborn, B., Andrews, J. F., & Martin, G. (2010). Deaf adults and the comprehension of Miranda. *Journal of Forensic Psychology Practice, 10*(2), 107–132.

Settlement Agreement Between U.S. and National Board of Medical Examiners, DJ# 202-16-181. (February 23, 2011).

S.F. v. McKinney Independent School District, No. 4:10-CV-323-RAS-DDB, 2012 U.S. Dist. LEXIS 29584. (E.D. Tex. 2012).

Siegel, L. (2008). *The human right to language: Communication access for deaf children.* Washington, DC: Gallaudet University Press.

Smith, D. H., & Andrews, J. F. (2015). Deaf and hard of hearing faculty in higher education: Enhancing access, equity, policy, and practice. *Disability & Society, 30*(10), 1521–1536.

Smith, R. C. (1996). *A case about Amy.* Philadelphia, PA: Temple University Press.

State of South Dakota, Plaintiff and Appellee, v. Daphne Annette Wright, Defendant and Appellant, No. 25531. (2009).

State of Texas v. Carl Doyle, Cause Number 07-00504, in the Criminal District Court of Jefferson County Texas. (April 27, 2011).

Tidyman, E. (1974). *Dummy.* Boston, MA: Little, Brown Co.

Tucker, J. (2010/2011). Child first campaign. *The Maryland Bulletin, 12. CXXXI(2), 3.*

Ulibarri v. City & County of Denver, No. 07-CV-1814-ODS. (D. Colo. 2012).

United States of America v. Robin Singh Educational Services, Inc., d/b/a Testmasters, No. CV06-3466 ABC. (C.D. Cal. June 21, 2006).

United States v. Thomas Heyer, Docket No.: 5:08-HC-2183-BO, Commitment Case to evaluate progress of Sexual Offenders Program at Butner Prison, Raleigh, NC, Office of Federal Public Defender, Raleigh, N.C. (2015).

USA v. Thomas Heyer, No. 5:08-HC-2183-BO in the US District Court or the Eastern District of North Carolina Western Division (court hearing). (2011).

U.S. Congress. (1934) *United States Code: Social Security Act, 42 U.S.C. §§ 301- Suppl. 4 1934.* [Periodical] Retrieved from the Library of Congress, https://www.loc.gov/item/uscode1934-005042007/

U.S. Department of Justice. (2017). Bureau of Justice Statistics, crime against persons with disabilities, 2009–2015 statistical tables. Retrieved from https://www.bjs.gov/content/pub/pdf/capd0913st.pdf

VanValkenburg v. Oregon Department of Corrections, Case No 3:14-cv-00916-BR. (2016).

Vernon, M. (2010). The horror of being deaf and in prison. *American Annals of the Deaf, 155*(3), 311–321.

Vernon, M., & Andrews, J. F. (2011). Basic legal issues in handling cases of defendants who are Deaf. *The Champion, XXXV*(2), 30–37.

Vernon, M., & Leigh, I. W. (2007). Mental health services for people who are deaf. *American Annals of the Deaf, 152*(4), 374–381.

Vernon, M., & Miller, K. (2005). Obstacles faced by deaf people in the criminal justice system. *American Annals of the Deaf, 150*(3), 283–291.

Vernon, M., & Rich, S. (1997). Pedophilia and deafness. *American Annals of the Deaf, 142*(4), 300–311.

Vernon, M., Steinberg, A. G., & Montoya, L. A. (1999). Deaf murderers: Clinical and forensic issues. *Behavioral Sciences & the Law, 17*(4), 495–516.

Vernon, M., & Vernon, M. (2010). *Deadly charm.* Washington, DC: Gallaudet University Press.

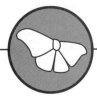

CHAPTER 11

Arts, Literature, and Media

Culture is heavily rooted in customs, traditions, values, and norms passed on from generation to generation by a community of people. The culture and communities of Deaf people are no different. Many of those traditions and norms include artifacts, which are often ways for members of the culture to create ways to document and share their experiences or to influence cultural values and norms. The arts, literature, and media are vital components of Deaf culture because of their expressive power and historical significance (Nomeland & Nomeland, 2012). The arts are not limited to visual (and tactile) arts, which are usually objects such as drawings, paintings, ceramics, sculptures, and 3D printing, but also include performing arts (theater, dance and music), literature (poetry, novels, short stories, and epics), and media arts (print media, photography, and cinematography).

Hearing people may not be aware that Deaf communities have all those types of arts and more. This chapter is in no way a comprehensive review or collection of art, literature, and media in the Deaf-World, both historical and contemporary artists and artwork. Rather, selected art, litera-

ture, and media products by Deaf artists will be highlighted. To continue your exploration of Deaf cultural art, literature, and media, check the references at the end of this chapter and resources on the companion website for this book. Here we start our journey into the arts.

ARTS

The arts created by Deaf people possibly date far back to even before the United States became a country, very likely starting with Deaf Indigenous Americans who produced different types of art and performances (Holcomb, 2013; McKay-Cody, 2019). The Deaf-World has always had deep roots in the arts, with many artistic contributions revolving around the Deaf experience, culture, and language. Similarly, there are many Deaf artists who produce general art that is not rooted in Deaf culture. Some say that what separates Deaf artists from hearing artists is the increase in Deaf people's extraordinary ability to sense shades of sight and touch that are not usually as available to people who hear (Durr, 1999; Lane, 2004).

Sonnenstrahl (2002), a Deaf retired art professor, published a scholarly book titled *Deaf Artists in America: Colonial to Contemporary*, which recognizes hundreds of Deaf artists and their work, including sculptors, porcelain artists, woodcut printmakers, painters, photographers, wildlife artists, landscape artists, portrait painters, drypoint etchers, silhouettists, primitive folk artists, potters, and many more. More recently, the definition of art and artist has expanded to become more inclusive of many more ways to express art, such as digital artists, animators, fashion designers, sound artists, makeup artists, graphic designers, cinematographers, and culinary (food) artists!

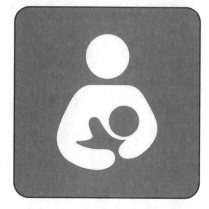

Figure 11–1. International Breastfeeding Symbol designed by Matt Daigle. Image courtesy of Matt and Kay Daigle.

Visual and Tactile Arts

Several prominent Deaf artists stand out in this artistic realm. One is Regina Olson Hughes (1895–1993), who was a scientific botanical illustrator for the U.S. Department of Agriculture from 1925 to 1969. She retired in 1969 and continued as a freelance illustrator for the Smithsonian Institution, Department of Botany, producing thousands of illustrations that were featured in museums, art galleries, and many official publications. An orchid plant was named in her honor, *Hughesia reginae* (Hughes, 2015).

Another example is that of Matt Daigle, a cartoonist, designer, and illustrator who submitted a logo for a breastfeeding symbol contest hosted by *Mothering* magazine in 2006. Matt Daigle's submission won amid 500 entries and is now an international breastfeeding symbol. Figure 11–1 shows Daigle's winning submission, a blue background with white figure depicting an adult cradling a baby (IBFS, 2105).

Deaf artist Christine Sun Kim, who holds a master's degree in Fine Arts and a master's degree in Sound Arts, specializes in "unorthodox, defiant art," with the aim to "perceive sound without considering social norms," in other words, "unlearning sound etiquette" (Weisblum, 2015, p. 1). In 2013, Christine was named a TED fellow, and her work was shown at the MoMA (Museum of Modern Art) exhibit *Soundings* in 2013 and again in 2015 at the *Greater New York* exhibit held in the MoMA's affiliate, PS1, among many other locations, including Massachusetts Institute of Technology (MIT) List Visual Arts Center in 2020. She has served as artist in residence at numerous institutions and was named 2015 Media Lab Director's Fellow at Massachusetts Institute of Technology (Weisblum, 2015) and 2018 Artist in Residency at Crisp-Ellert Art Museum at Flagler College. Figure 11–2 shows Christine Sun Kim signing the ASL sign for DAY, with purple paint in an arc above her head showing the motion of the sign for DAY.

Douglas Tilden (1860–1935), a world-famous artist, is also recognized as the

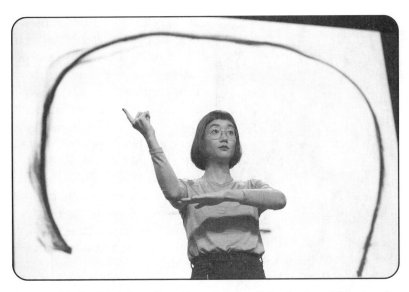

Figure 11–2. Christine Sun Kim, Deaf artist, signing ASL sign for DAY. Photo credit: Ryan Lash. Used with permission.

first California-born sculptor to receive recognition outside of the United States. His sculptures are considered to be the greatest legacy of public art in the San Francisco Bay Area, and he is known as "the first great sculptor of the West" (Albronda, 1994, p. 138). *The Mechanics Monument*, produced in 1900, is located in San Francisco, California, and featured in Figure 11–3. President Theodore Roosevelt stood by this very sculpture to give a passionate speech about trading with other countries in 1903 (Anderson, 2013).

An emerging artist in the Deaf art scene is *NIOVISION*, which is owned by Natasha Ofili. Natasha is a Deaf writer, fashion artist and designer, actress, and creative artist. She was recently featured in Netflix's *The Politician* and Amazon Prime's *Undone* (Jean-Philippe, 2019). Natasha is pictured in Figure 11–4 wearing her art.

There are so many Deaf artists out there that a chapter, or even a book, cannot cover them all.

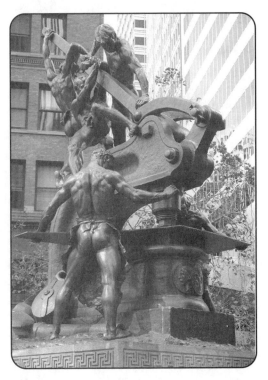

Figure 11–3. Mechanics Monument (1901), sculpture by Douglas Tilden, located in San Francisco. Photo courtesy of Wikimedia Commons.

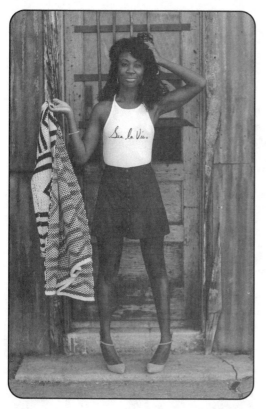

Figure 11–4. Natasha Ofili of NIOVISION, fashion artist and blogger, modeling her design. Photo credit: Ali Mojahedi. Used with permission of Natasha Ofili.

2012). Other disenfranchised communities such as the Deaf, Latinx, Indigenous, Black, LGBTQIA, and Disabled communities often communicate their resistance to the majority culture as well as culturally affirming experiences through art (Durr, 2006). Like those communities, there are two types of De'VIA: resistance and affirmative art. Resistance art grew from Deaf people's experiences with oppressive, marginalizing, and patronizing practices by hearing people. Durr (2006) produced a table identifying themes of resistance and affirmative De'VIA art (Table 11–1).

Classic examples of resistance art come from the mother of De'VIA, Betty Miller, EdD, who drew *Ameslan Prohibited* in 1972, showing hands that are handcuffed and fingers chopped off in pieces, representing the many years of physical abuse deaf children have experienced at deaf schools that prohibited sign language. Another classic example of resistance art is *Family Dog*, drawn by Susan Dupor, which depicts family members sitting on a couch with blurred faces and

De'VIA

Some Deaf artists specialize in creating artwork rooted in Deaf culture. This is called De'VIA. In 1989, *The Deaf Way*, an international conference, brought Deaf people from all over the world to Washington, DC. Deaf artists convened prior to the conference and proposed a new term for artwork produced by Deaf people: De'VIA. The term De'VIA represents *Deaf View/Image Art*. Deaf artists wanted a way to differentiate their unique work that often expresses cultural Deaf experience from the general artwork done by Deaf artists (Nomeland & Nomeland,

Table 9–1. Themes Within Resistance and Affirmative De'VIA Art

Resistance De'VIA	Affirmative De'VIA
Audism	Empowerment
Oralism	ASL
Mainstreaming	Affiliation
Cochlear implants	Acculturation
Identity confusion	Acceptance
Eugenics	Deafhood

Source: From Durr (2006, p. 169). Used with permission.

the deaf child on the floor, panting, as if the deaf child is a dog. This represents many deaf children's experiences growing up in hearing families. The deaf child, like a dog, has a home and is loved but is not truly a part of the family conversation. Another contemporary example of resistance art, shown in Figure 11–5, comes from Deaf artist Maureen Klusza, who created *The Greatest Irony: Deaf Baby, Hearing Baby* in 2007.

The story behind this piece of significant artwork originated from Amy Cohen Efron's groundbreaking *The Greatest Irony* video publication in March 2007. Efron argued the incredible irony of preventing deaf babies from learning to sign because their speech would be harmed in the process, contrasted with the wildly popular *Baby Signs* movement for hearing babies to learn sign language (Efron, 2007). The video publication by Efron inspired Ray-chelle Harris to share her vision with Deaf artist Maureen Klusza about having two babies, one deaf and one hearing, sitting side by side, one with their hands tied and the other one signing. By the next day, Klusza came up with a radical, mind-blowing drawing that became the nationwide symbol of the Deaf community's fight for deaf babies to have access to sign language from birth—an example of De'VIA resistance art.

In a different vein, affirmative art is about confirming Deaf culture and sign language (Durr, 2006). Ann Silver, a Deaf pop artist, transforms ordinary household items and road signs into De'VIA affirmative artwork. Among many of her classic works include *Deaf Identity Crayons: Then & Now* (1999), *One Way/Deaf Way* (1996), and her more recent work with Jim Van Manen, *Deaf Pride No. 2* (2013), as shown in Figure 11–6.

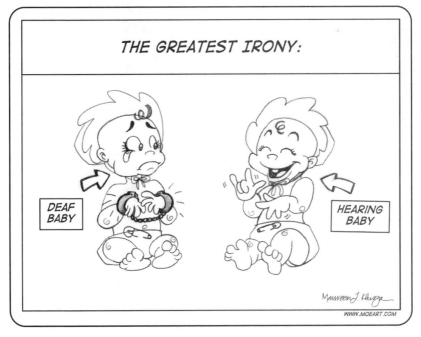

Figure 11–5. *The Greatest Irony* by Maureen Klusza. Artwork courtesy of MoeArt.com.

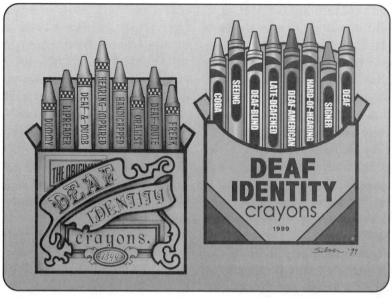

A

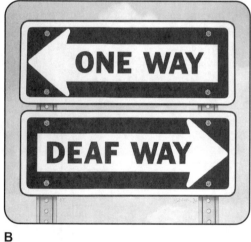

B

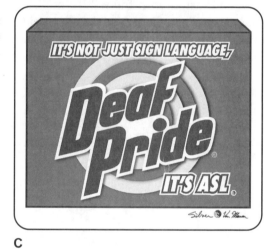

C

Figure 11–6. A. *DEAF IDENTITY CRAYONS: Then & Now.* © 1999, Ann Silver. Image courtesy of Ann Silver. **B.** *ONE WAY/DEAF WAY.* © 1996, Ann Silver. Image courtesy of Ann Silver. **C.** *DEAF PRIDE, No. 2.* © 2013, Ann Silver and Jim VanManen. Image copyright and courtesy of SilverMoonBrand.com.

Despite being widely acclaimed in the Deaf community as an artist, Silver points out, "I still face audism on all levels, especially art funding. Museums and galleries still have not embraced Deaf Art on a major scale." (deaffriendly, 2013, p. 1)

Another Deaf cartoonist, Shawn Richardson, has produced a variety of De'VIA affirmative art in the past decade. One

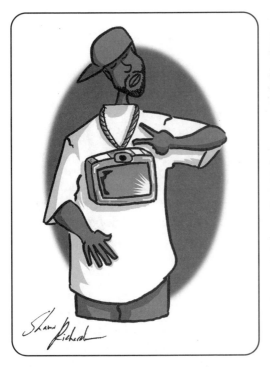

Figure 11–7. *Bling-Bling Videophone Necklace* by Shawn Richardson. Used with permission.

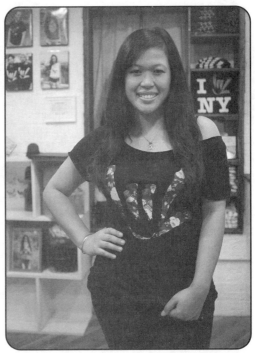

Figure 11–8. Deaf fashion designer and store owner, Mara Ladines, modeling her product in her store in New York City. Photo courtesy of *ByMara*.

example is shown in Figure 11–7, *Bling-Bling Videophone Necklace*, where a "hip-hop urban guy" is shown wearing a heavy gold chain necklace attached to a wireless videophone on his chest (Richardson, 2008, p. 1).

Deaf artist and fashion designer Mara Ladines and her store ByMara, established in Los Angeles in 2008 with only two products, now sells over 100 products nationwide. The brand includes two specialized collections, I.L.Y. and the Mara Ladines Collection, and is now also featured at her flagship store in Brooklyn, New York (Jejeune, 2019). In Figure 11–8, Mara is wearing her I.L.Y. design and logo for ByMara.

Mara elaborates, "The logo is about spreading positive love vibes . . . and sup-

porting the Deaf and signing communities" (Jejeune, 2019).

Matt Daigle (mentioned earlier) and his comic strip, co-created with his wife, Kay Daigle, *That Deaf Guy*, are popular in classes and workshops studying Deaf culture and ASL. Matt and Kay's comics are predominately affirmative art, with some resistance art, embedded in humor. Their affirmative art is portrayed through their comic series focused on *The Benefits of Being Profoundly Deaf*. One comic strip under that series is depicted in Figure 11–9, with a neighbor mowing grass early in the morning, waking up hearing neighbors and his hearing wife, but not *The Deaf Guy*, who is still blissfully sleeping.

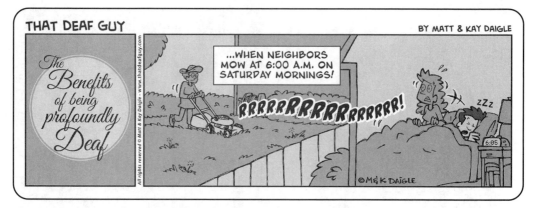

Figure 11–9. *The Benefits of Being Profoundly Deaf: Early Morning Mowing.* Image courtesy of Matt and Kay Daigle.

PERFORMING ARTS

Like visual arts, performing arts has a long history in Deaf culture. It is very likely that the original inhabitants of what is now the United States had Deaf people who created performances with their sign language(s). When home video camera recording devices became more affordable and widespread in the late 1970s, this meant more and more Deaf performing arts events could be documented and preserved over time.

Deaf Theater

Theatrical events in the Deaf communities are popular and cherished. Current research documentation regarding Deaf theater in the United States goes as far back to 1817, although the authors are confident Deaf theater existed before 1817 among indigenous Deaf Americans. In 1817, the first public Deaf school was established in Hartford, Connecticut, now called the American School for the Deaf (ASD). ASD is considered the "mother

school," graduating many educators who contributed to the establishment of many new Deaf schools all over the United States and eventually in the establishment of Gallaudet University in 1964 (ASD History, 2015, p. 1). Deaf students at ASD would perform roles from original scripts written by Deaf people, often including storytelling and poetry. Those events would occur in the dormitories during the weekends when students who lived far from the school usually could not go home (Nomeland & Nomeland, 2012). The performances were often in a small room with a raised platform so everyone could see the performance clearly; this provided a closer connection between the audience and the performances (Holcomb, 2013).

In the 1950s, Deaf schools started integrating school plays and performances as part of the academic experience, with large productions including auditions and backstage work held once a year. These school performances spilled over into the Deaf clubs as well as Gallaudet theater productions and formal academic courses in drama (Lane, Hoffmeister, & Bahan, 1996).

In 1967, the National Theater of the Deaf (NTD) was established with federal funding from the Department of Health, Education and Welfare (NTD, 2015). Its goal was to push for departure from regular, spoken performances, where hearing people would perform speaking roles on the stage, and sign language interpreters would sit below the stage and interpret into sign language for deaf attendees. Instead, performances would use Deaf actors on the stage and hearing actors/readers in the background, so both Deaf and hearing audience members could appreciate the play equally (Nomeland & Nomeland, 2012). NTD is the oldest existing touring company in the United States, having performed in all 50 states in the United States and 33 countries internationally. NTD was and continues to be instrumental in spreading awareness about sign languages, removing stigma and stereotypes from sign languages and Deaf people, and promoting Deaf cultural pride among Deaf communities of the world (NTD, 2015). Figure 11–10 depicts a recent NTD performance.

Shortly after the NTD was established, six theatrical groups for deaf children were also established. These include the Little Theater of the Deaf, established in Hartford, Connecticut, in 1967; the International Center on Deafness and the Arts, set up in 1973; Imagination State, set up in 1979; Seattle Children's Theater with a Deaf youth drama program, established in 1993; and Wheelock Family Theater, PAH!'s Deaf youth theater, established in 1994. Although these deaf children's theaters are no longer performing

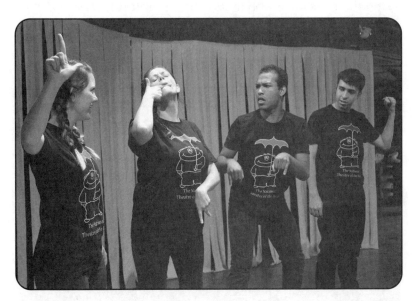

Figure 11–10. National Theatre of the Deaf actors performing "Dog VS. Dog" using the full American Sign Language alphabet. Left to right: Caitlin Hemmer with "L," Chrissy Cogswell with "K" and "L," Chris Joseph with "I" and "J," and Chris Ogren with "J." Photo taken at the Barn at the O'Neill Theater Center, 2014–2015. Photo by A. Vincent Scarano, courtesy of the National Theatre of the Deaf.

due to lack of funding, they played a special role in spreading ASL to young deaf and hearing audiences as well. They also provided inspiration, imagination, and positive ASL and Deaf culture exposure (Kilpatrick, 2007).

NTD's success and inspiration for many also led to the establishment of many smaller, regional theater groups and one-person shows. In California, Deaf West Theater (DWT), the first professional regional sign language theater in the western half of the United States, was founded in 1991. The theater has 90 seats and subwoofers (loudspeakers designed to reproduce very low-bass frequencies, which emit vibrations that can be felt) under the seats, particularly important for Deaf attendees as vibrations of the sounds on stage can be felt through the flooring and seats, including music beats and sound effects. DWT productions have won more

than 80 different awards, and two of DWT's performances have appeared on Broadway, *Big River* in 2003 and *Spring Awakening* in 2015 (DWT, 2015). *Spring Awakening* includes Deaf characters signing on the stage along with their hearing counterparts who are voicing the lines (Hockenberry, 2015). *Spring Awakening* came with quite a number of accessibility breakthroughs: *Spring Awakening* was the first time Broadway had a wheelchair performer. *Spring Awakening* was the first time Broadway provided interpreting for DeafBlind patrons (Spring, n.d.). Part of the *Spring Awakening* cast performing on Broadway is shown in Figure 11–11.

In 2016, the National Endowment for the Arts awarded Gallaudet University a $25,000 grant to put together DeafBlind protactile experts in developing, documenting, and creating DeafBlind Theater using protactile. *Romeo and Juliet* was the

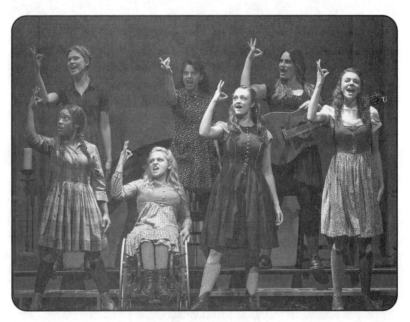

Figure 11–11. Cast of *Spring Awakening* in action. Photo courtesy of Joan Marcus, 2015.

first script the team worked on. Their goal was to challenge typical theater norms, which are more exclusionary and prohibitive for DeafBlind patrons. Examples of exclusionary theater practices include having a separation between the elevated stage and the rows of fixed chairs, taking away the opportunity to include tactile experiences. Instead, DeafBlind Protactile Theater Institute (PTTI) created theater the DeafBlind way, "where attendees and actors interact" (Bradbury et al., 2019, p. 86). Theatergoers, in essence, have roles within the play itself (e.g., as emotional, weeping attendees at Romeo and Juliet's funerals). Actors at the funeral could use several different types of theatrical models such as "the mingle," where actors would mingle with each attendee, sharing their costumes and lines tactilely, and in no set order. Another approach would be the "conveyor belt," where each attendee would experience a succession of actors going through them. Other senses would be activated such as hot-tempered and violent Tybalt reeking of beer, Juliet radiating the peony scent (which evokes youth), and lavender for the Nurse, associated with older women. The actors built the set incorporating tactile cues (e.g., rugs, railings, tables) so that all actors would know exactly where they were on the stage as they performed their roles. Instead of swords, which are more visual and require distance between actors and attendees, and contradictory toward DeafBlind culture, the actors brainstormed equivalent replacements such as brass knuckles or a small dagger that is retractable so the knife itself would go inside the hilt when stabbed. Protactile theater challenges our understanding of theater and the sighted bias inherent in theatrical productions (Bradbury et al., 2019).

Search for "Protactile Romeo and Julie" on the web. You'll find a YouTube video explaining the entire process, including captions and image descriptions. What do you think? Would you attend a protactile theater showing? Should regular mainstream theater look into adopting more features from protactile theater to make their performance more accessible for everyone?

Many Deaf actors transition between the stage and film sets, leading us to explore the presence of Deaf, DeafBlind, and DeafDisabled people in television and movies.

Deaf in Television and Movies

Many people are familiar with Deaf actress Marlee Matlin, the youngest Oscar winner for Best Actress for her 1986 role in the film, *Children of a Lesser God*, at 21 years old. As the youngest winner of the Best Actress Academy Award since 1987, she continues to hold the record for over three decades! In comparison, Jennifer Lawrence is the second youngest winner and has held the record since only 2013 (List, n.d.). However, many other Deaf actors came before Marlee and helped pave the way for Deaf actors. Bernard Bragg joined the acting circuit after meeting and then traveling with the world-famous mime Marcel Marceau in 1956, which then led to Bragg cofounding the National Theater of the Deaf (NTD) in 1967. That same year, NBC featured Bragg along with seven other Deaf actors in the very first televised show of deaf and hearing actors conversing fully in ASL, which was immediately and heavily criticized by the Alexander Graham Bell Association for the Deaf and Hard of Hearing based on the inappropriate use of sign language (Bragg, 2015). Phyllis Frelich was the original leading actress for the Broadway production of *Children of a Lesser God*; she won the 1980 Tony Award for Best Actress. She also won an Emmy Award for her role in *Love Is Never Silent* and appeared in multiple TV series such as *CSI*, *ER*, and *LA Law*.

Linda Bove is another Deaf actress whose recurring role as Linda, the Librarian, on the *Sesame Street* TV series from 1971 to 2003, including five *Sesame Street* TV movies, also paved the way for other Deaf actors. She, along with her husband, Ed Waterstreet, were among the founders of the Deaf West Theater Company. Other Deaf actors include Howie Seago, best known for his role in *Star Trek: The Next Generation*, and Darrell Utley, who starred in *Days of Our Lives* and *Beverly Hills, 90210*.

Contemporary Deaf actors include Shoshannah Stern, who performed in *This Close* and *Grey's Anatomy*; Michelle Banks in *Soul Food*, *Girlfriends*, and *Strong Medicine*; Russell Harvard in *CSI: NY*, *Fargo*, *Switched at Birth*, and *Fringe*; Sean Berdy in *Switched at Birth* and *The Society*; CJ Jones in *Baby Driver* and *Avatar 2*; Deanne Bray in *CSI*, *Law & Order*, *The L Word*, *Heroes*, and *Grey's Anatomy*, as well as playing the main character in *Sue Thomas: F.B.Eye*; Lauren Ridloff in *The Walking Dead* and *The Eternals*; Millicent Simmonds in *Wonderstruck*, *A Quiet Place*, and *A Quiet Place II*; and Treshelle Edmond in *House M.D.* and *Glee*. CJ Jones with *Avatar* director, James Cameron, and a plastic head model of Neytiri are pictured in Figure 11–12A. In addition, Lauren Ridloff in *The Walking Dead* is pictured in Figure 11–12B.

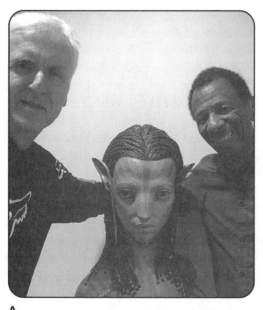
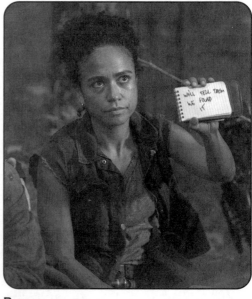

A

B

Figure 11–12. A. CJ Jones with James Cameron, director of the movie *Avatar*, and a plastic head model of Neytiri. Photo courtesy of CJ Jones. **B.** Lauren Ridloff in *The Walking Dead*, Episode 1005, writing on a paper pad to communicate. Photo Credit: Jace Downs/AMC, © 2019 AMC Film Holdings LLC. All Rights Reserved

Today, unenlightened casting directors still cast ignorant, nonsigning hearing people in Deaf, signing roles, expecting them to quickly learn how to wave their hands around and look like they're Deaf. This is an example of hearing people taking advantage of Deaf people, a cultural and linguistic minority. This is also called "cultural appropriation," when one from the majority culture and language takes features or traditions from marginalized groups, usually for money and/or fame. This "cultural appropriation" is not limited to taking advantage of Deaf people; it also happens to women, Black people, LGBT communities, Asians, and many more marginalized groups.

At the 2015 Oscars, #OscarsSoWhite trended after April Reign posted that hashtag on Twitter after seeing that no people of color were nominated. The trending hashtag led to more scrutiny regarding the voting, nomination, and award process for Oscar winners. After some research, it showed that the Oscar voters were 94% white, were 77% male, and had a median age of 62. More specifically, the Oscars' executive branch was 98% white. Of the 43-member board of governors, six were women, with only one as the sole woman of color (Horn, Sperling, & Smith, 2012). In addition, notice how those statistics and discussions often exclude people with disabilities and LGBT representation. Want to guess how many of the Oscar voters are Deaf? None. Factor those facts in, and now you know why people of marginalized groups struggle with representation in TV and movies.

In 2015, Catalina Sandino Moreno, a hearing woman with no experience with the Deaf or signing communities, played the main role of a Deaf mother in a movie titled *Medeas*. After Moreno completed an interview with *New York Daily*

> How would you feel if someone who is not a member of your culture was picked to impersonate your language and culture in an acting role? To learn more about this terrible practice and the devastating impact this had on marginalized groups for centuries, search the terms "blackface" and "yellowface." To learn more, check out the hashtags: #OscarsSoWhite #HollywoodSoWhite #DeafTalent #Cultural Appropriation #WhiteWashedOUT #DisabledAndCute #Hollywood MustDoBetter #DisabilityTooWhite #GetYourBellyOut #CripTheVote #TheBarriersWeFace #AbleismExists #ActuallyAutistic #InvisibleIllness #ShitHearingPeopleSay.

News, the news spread in the Deaf community about her role (Callis, 2015). The Deaf community quickly responded in an uproar, and then the #DeafTalent hashtag started trending on January 31, 2015, for 49 straight days, with many actors and activists affirming support for spreading awareness about casting Deaf people in Deaf roles. The goal of this campaign is to push casting directors to cast Deaf actors for Deaf roles (Callis, 2017; Young, 2015). Casting authentic Deaf people in Deaf, signing roles has resulted in multiple awards and nominations, such as *A Quiet Place* and *Baby Driver*. Films that featured increased diversity both behind the camera and in the front of camera, such as *Black Panther*, *Crazy Rich Asians*, *Coco*, *Get Out*, and *Parasite*, "drove a multicultural gold rush at the box office" (Ugwu, 2020, p. 1). Based on the results of those wildly successful movies, it is clear people want authenticity.

Deaf in Game and Reality Shows

Although not considered professional actors or acting (although that has been disputed), Deaf people have participated in a variety of game and reality shows ranging from dancing to modeling, fighting, cooking, designing, and more on television shows such as the *Amazing Race* (Luke Adams), *America's Next Top Model* (Nyle DiMarco), *American Gladiators* (Shelley Beattie, also known as Siren), *Celebrity Apprentice* (Marlee Matlin), *Chopped* (Kurt Ramborger), *Dancing With the Stars* (Marlee Matlin), *Extreme Makeover* (Phil Janes; Larry and Judy Vardon; Oregon School for the Deaf), *Janet Dickinson Modeling Agency* (Martin Ritchie), *Jimmy Kimmel Show* (JoAnn Benfield), *Let's Make a Deal* (Candace Hodgson), *Project Runway* (Justin LeBlanc), *Survivor* (Christy Smith; Nina Poersch), *The Price Is Right* (Kristine Hall), *Tyra Banks Show* (Floyd McClain), *Ultimate Fighter* (Matt Hamill), and *Work of Art* (Leon Lim).

Although this list is far from comprehensive, members of the Deaf community have noticed more and more Deaf representation in game and reality shows, Broadway performances, TV shows, and movies. It is important to recognize that the majority of those Deaf actors are white, sighted, straight, and abled. There are many diverse members of the Deaf community interested in being cast for movies, television shows, plays, and game and reality shows. Diverse theatrical talent in the Deaf community is underutilized and not recognized in theatrical companies and TV productions.

Deaf Music and Dancing

You may be surprised to learn that a breakout Broadway show with over five Deaf actors, titled *Spring Awakening*, is actually a musical. You may ask, Deaf people and music? And dancing? Yes! There is culturally Deaf music and dancing, which does not require the ability to hear.

Deaf music often integrates visual and tactile rhythmic elements. And similar to the art of De'VIA, music is often essential in communicating a political message, serving as a tool of resistance, and promoting cultural pride and identity (Loeffler, 2014). Neuroimaging studies of Deaf people's brains show that when Deaf persons feel music through vibrations, this stimulates the same area of the brain where hearing people hear music. Loeffler (2014) points out that "hearing is not a prerequisite for appreciating music" (p. 442).

Percussion songs are a beloved, traditional type of Deaf music. These songs incorporate a visual and tactile beat with the performance of songs and often use a drum. Many of those songs follow a "one, two, one-two-three" rhythm, with the audience participating by clapping along (Loeffler, 2014, p. 447). Gallaudet University's Bison Song tradition is shown in Figure 11–13, where two singers clap and sing the song in ASL, following the beats of the drummer (also pictured), and the audience claps along.

As you can see, dance and music are an integral part of Deaf culture. There are many historical milestones with regard to dance and music. In 1955, the Gallaudet Dance Company was founded (GDC, 2015). The National Deaf Dance Theater (NDDT) was established in 1988. The Wild Zappers, founded in 1989, combines ASL, music, and dance to promote cultural and educational awareness of sign language and Deaf people. There are deaf jazz singers (Mandy Harvey), deaf bands (Beethoven's Nightmare), opera singers (Janine Roebuck), and solo percussionists

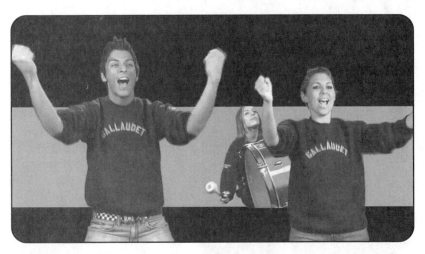

Figure 11–13. Bison Song team 2009 featuring Cesar Ayala, Emily Jo Nochese, and drummer Vanessa Scarna. Photo courtesy of Summer Crider Loeffler.

(Dame Evelyn Glennie) (Lammle, 2010). There are also deaf rappers and groups, such as Prinz-D, Warren "Wawa" Snipe, DJ Supalee, Sho'Roc, Signmark, Matt Maxey, and Sean Forbes (Peisner, 2013). Prinz-D is shown rapping and entertaining his audience in Figure 11–14.

What about musicals and concerts done in spoken languages? Often they are interpreted for Deaf, DeafBlind, and DeafDisabled audience members who request an interpreter in advance. Deaf stage interpreters study, analyze, translate, and memorize the lyrics in ASL and study the movement and expressions of the singer(s) (Adam, Aro, Druetta, Dunne, & Klintberg, 2014). They stand on the stage, looking down subtly at a hearing interpreter sitting, giving cues as to when the song begins and where in the song the singer is. The hearing interpreter also interprets any additional lyric changes, spoken dialogue by the singer, or event announcer to the Deaf interpreter on stage. The Deaf interpreter then renders the message, more authentically, to the audience (Adam et al., 2014; Wilde,

2015). Deaf interpreter JoAnn Benfield is pictured in Figure 11–15 signing a song at the Austin City Limits (ACL) festival in 2015. Notice the light blue circle above JoAnn depicting two hands? That is the symbol for interpreting, easily seen from the distance, so Deaf attendees can find and move closer to the Deaf interpreter.

A common practice that is of concern to the Deaf community is when hearing people sign songs in what they think is ASL, achieving some popularity online, for monetary gain or to increase followers. The practice of gaining fame and/or making money from sign language that is rendered incorrectly is not ethical and is often considered cultural and language appropriation (Maler, 2013; Torrance, 2014; Whitworth, 2014; Zola, 2015). Cultural and language appropriation happens when elements of language or culture are taken from a minority culture and used by members of the majority culture, often associated with portraying themselves as seeming charitable and sweet by helping disabled people or minority groups, possibly used to gain fame, earn revenue, find

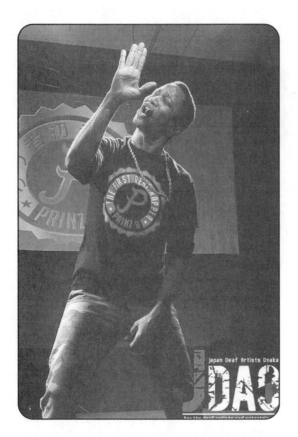

Figure 11–14. Prinz-D The First Deaf Rapper is shown performing in Osaka, Japan. Photo courtesy of Team Prinz, http://www.prinzd.com

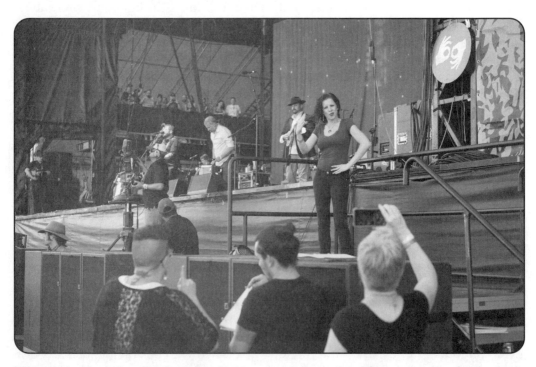

Figure 11–15. JoAnn Benfield, Deaf interpreter, interpreting ASL music lyrics for the audience. Photo courtesy of JoAnn Benfield.

job opportunities, or increase their social media presence by having more followers (Hill, 2008).

Hearing people learning sign language often think it is fun to translate songs written in English to ASL, often with good intentions, but they do not realize that this practice is offensive. Although they mean well, hearing amateurs signing songs are found on YouTube, and their links often have more viewers than actual Deaf signing professionals and their professionally translated ASL songs (Zola, 2015). Often the hearing signers or interpreters, signing songs, are more there for hearing people's enjoyment and awe, rather than to provide actual, authentic access for Deaf audiences. This is a good example of what is termed inspiration porn, where people with disabilities or instruments needed for their access (e.g., walking cane or sign language) are objectified and made into something that makes hearing audiences feel good about themselves (Grushkin, 2014, 2015). Westfall (2015) adds that opportunities, paid or not, to translate songs from English to ASL are often given to hearing people who sign, while numerous expert Deaf actors and performers are frequently and inadvertently overlooked. A recent example of language and cultural appropriation was when Jimmy Kimmel hosted a "rap battle," where people on stage translated Wiz Khalifa's song as he performed "Black and Yellow." Of the three white women on stage, two were hearing (Okrent, 2014; Zola, 2015). Why weren't professional Black Deaf rappers, who spent years studying and performing their craft, invited?

Another example of language and cultural appropriation is when Brian Guendling, a hearing ASL student at Texas State University, decided to put on the First Sign Language Concert Ever by performing "Uptown Funk" at a bar (Patterson, 2015). He posted the video footage of his performance on YouTube, and within 3 days, there were over 65,000 views (a few months later, his video had over 228,000 views), and he woke up to over 200 messages, as well as many media and interview requests, and had many articles about him published in prominent news outlets such as CBS Sports and *Sports Illustrated* (Rodriguez, 2015). In 2020, Guendling revised his YouTube video description:

Looking back, I was a little uneducated about deaf culture when I made this video (fixing this now in 2020). My intentions of this video were to provide more entertainment and maybe inspire a hearing person to learn ASL. (Guendling, 2020, p. 1)

Contrast this with a popular Deaf ASL song translator in the Deaf community, Rosa Lee Timm, a professional Deaf performance artist honing her craft for over two decades. Her very popular live solo performances for the Deaf community all over the United States are always sold out. She has approximately 12,000 subscribers for her YouTube page, and none of her professionally produced ASL song translations have reached the numbers ASL student Brian Guendling reached in 3 days. Pictured in Figure 11–16 is Rosa Lee signing a translation of "What's Love Got to Do With It?" by Tina Turner.

Things become more murky when it comes to hearing professional sign language interpreters whose interpretation of songs at a concert becomes viral because hearing nonsigners used their phones to upload a video of the interpreter signing what they thought was "epic" and "a true inspiration" (Zola, 2015, p. 1).

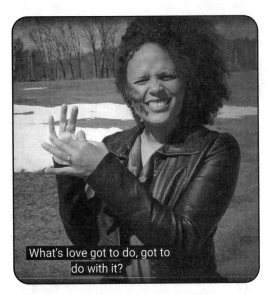

Figure 11–16. Rosa Lee Timm, Deaf performance artist, translating a Tina Turner song, "What's Love Got to Do With It?" into ASL. Used with permission.

The first problem here is that hearing nonsigners are exoticizing and trivializing something that is actually providing access for Deaf people. Don't. Second, those videos are shared on social media incessantly by nonsigners, essentially making this "inspiration porn" (as discussed in Chapter 2). Again, don't.

Things become worse when the media become involved and contact the viral interpreter to ask questions. If the interpreter answers their questions (and technically participates in an interview), this is a gross violation of interpreting ethics. One rule of interpreting ethics is to always facilitate interpretation between parties involving nonsigners and Deaf signers, so the interpreter should not be answering questions about their work. Additionally, completed interpreting work is always confidential; hence, the interpreter should not be discussing (or answering

questions) about specific experiences with previous interpreting jobs. Professional interpreting ethics require the interpreter to always refer all questions to the Deaf community and Deaf people. Registry of Interpreters for the Deaf (RID) states, "Performance interpreting is not a vehicle for interpreters to become performers, but rather a vehicle for the target audience members to enjoy the performance event" (RID Performing Arts, 2014, p. 2). Interpreters can support the media and the Deaf community in developing a direct, authentic relationship. The interpreter is there to facilitate communication between nonsigning entities and Deaf, DeafBlind, and DeafDisabled people. The professional interpreter knows to always put the spotlight on Deaf people and the Deaf community and allow them to answer questions posed by the media regarding the viral interpretation.

Sadly, some interpreters have the gall to post photos, gifs, or videos of themselves signing on their social media accounts. This, again, is a serious violation of professional interpreting ethics and certainly can be reported to the interpreter's certifying agency. Some unethical interpreters develop contracts with organizations calling their work "performance art" and call themselves "performance artist" in order to avoid getting caught on not following professional interpreting ethics. Those unethical interpreters have argued that they are not essentially interpreting but adding their own style to their interpretation of the performance, and therefore it is okay to (1) advertise their work as performance artists, (2) do TEDx Talks, (3) accept interviewing requests from the media, (4) promote their work on social media, and more. Those disingenuous interpreters-performance artists are literally stealing the spotlight from sign language and Deaf communities of the world, or as Zola (2015) says, "appropriation at the hands, literally, of the hearing" (p. 1). To prevent this type of violence toward Deaf communities, ensure all performances are interpreted by Deaf interpreters, with the Deaf interpreter on stage and the hearing interpreter on the floor, facing the Deaf interpreter, and out of sight.

> Explore the meaning of an ally. Norma Morán, a Deaf Latina, noted that there is no such thing as an ally but, instead, acts of allyship. What are examples of acts of allyship that you have done with marginalized communities?

> Check the videos produced by Deaf Action Center (DAC) Interpreting on Facebook (@DACInterpreting), particularly the two videos, *Best Practices: Confidentiality* and *Best Practices: Conduct and Respect for Consumers*. What do you think?

Sign language came from Deaf people, who share their language with hearing people freely and in abundance. How might Deaf people feel when hearing people take credit in using sign language that belongs to Deaf people and Deaf communities? Many Deaf community members feel this way: Hearing people who learn sign language can certainly embrace the role of an ally. It is also strongly recommended that they keep their often sadly butchered, signed songs to the confines of their shower stall and work to ensure that the spotlight is kept on Deaf artists and performers when it comes to expressing ASL translated songs in their culture and language (Efron, 2014). This issue points to how the Deaf community is uncomfortable with hearing persons' misuse of their language and lack of linguistic respect for ASL.

LITERATURE

You are probably familiar with the rich English literature tradition in the United States. Your caregivers may have told you stories such as Sumi's *First Day of School Ever* by Soyung Pak and sang you nursery rhymes from Mother Goose. When you arrived at school, you may have read books by famous authors such as Ezra Jack Keats's *The Snowy Day*. In middle school, you may have read *Anne Frank: The Diary of a Young Girl* and, in high school, Alice Walker's *The Color Purple* and William Shakespeare's poems and plays. English literature in the United States includes both oral and written literature.

Literature in the Deaf Community

Like English literature in the United States, the Deaf community has a rich history of literature. Most people think literature can only be written. That is not the case. Literature can be passed from generation to generation through speaking and singing, just like written literature. Likewise, literature in ASL and other sign languages is also passed from generation to generation through sign language. People often consider written literature to be superior to oral (which includes spoken and signed languages) literature. That, too, is not true. Often, when oral stories are transcribed into written language or translated to another written language, part of the message is lost. The story is not the same. Also, to someone outside of the culture, stories from that culture can be difficult to understand, "because understanding the story means also understanding the complexity of the culture itself" (Nomeland & Nomeland, 2012, p. 141).

Most of the documented and commonly recognized literature in the Deaf communities in the United States is in either ASL or English. ASL literature includes works of art that are composed in ASL and play on the linguistic structure of ASL in the genres of poetry, narratives, and drama by Deaf authors (Byrne, 2013). Deaf literature includes works of art that are written in English and utilize the linguistic structure of English for artistic effect in the genres of poetry, narratives, and drama by Deaf authors (Holcomb, 2013). Literature in the U.S. Deaf community (and parts of Canada), especially in ASL, is essential in creating a strong cultural identity, reflecting resistance against the majority culture, affirming Deaf culture, and creating a sense of belonging for Deaf people (Bahan, 2006).

Regardless, it is important to realize and recognize that deep-seated systemic racism and other forms of -isms practiced by white Deaf communities have erased, ignored, and suppressed the preservation and documentation of Black ASL literature in the Black Deaf communities (McCaskill, Lucas, Bayley & Hill, 2011). Things are slowly changing. Gallaudet University offered the first Black ASL literature course in the spring of 2020. White Deaf people have much work to do in unpacking and restoring Deaf communities' collective understanding of valuable and suppressed literary pieces, stories,

and performances by Black Deaf, Asian Deaf, Indigenous Deaf, DeafDisabled, LGBT Deaf people, and more—over time.

ASL Literature

ASL literature is primarily oral literature, in sign language, passed on by generations of mostly white, sighted, abled Deaf people in the United States and most parts of Canada. The majority of the languages spoken throughout the world do not have a written form, yet those languages also have rich oral traditions that are preserved through cultural activities. The stories and poems that were performed, spoken, or signed originated in oral literature before some of them were eventually written down (Byrne, 2013). Although ASL does not yet have a written system used widely by the Deaf community, ASL does have a rich reservoir of storytelling, poetry, drama, humor, and folklore, which have been passed down from generation to generation at white Deaf schools, clubs, and festivals. Oral or signed literature thrives and materializes with appreciative audiences. These audiences would often be at festivals, campgrounds, reunions, sporting tournaments and competitions, timberfests, and Deaf expos (Holcomb, 2013). Live audiences are not the only way to keep ASL literature thriving, and more recently, online ASL literature submissions are gaining in popularity, diversity, and accessibility.

With film recording technology available during the past hundred years, fortunately, some of those stories have been recorded, preserving sign language over time, similar to the preservation of written literature on paper or digitally (Byrne, 2013; Peters, 2000). The very first films made in America were silent films of a race horse, an outdoor dance, and a locomotive arriving at a train station (1878, 1888, and 1895, respectively). The very first movie with actual *language* expressed was of a Deaf woman signing (not singing!) "The Star-Spangled Banner" in 1902. This recording was made by Thomas Edison, a famous deaf inventor who invented not only the electric light bulb but also the motion picture camera. By 1913, 18 ASL presentations and performances were filmed and preserved by the National Association of the Deaf (Padden & Humphries, 2005). The former president of the NAD at that time, George Veditz, was recorded in 1913 signing a presentation titled *Preservation of Sign Language*:

> As long as we have Deaf on earth, we will have signs. And as long as we have our films, we can preserve our beautiful signs in their old purity. I hope we all will love and guard our beautiful sign language as the noblest gift God has given to Deaf people. (NADvlogs, 2010)

Veditz signed that phrase near the end of his presentation, as seen from 13:26 to 14:36 in the video of his presentation (NADvlogs, 2010). In the 1930s, privileged white, sighted, and abled Deaf people at Deaf clubs were filmed performing stories, poetry, and skits (Padden & Humphries, 2005). From that time onward, ASL literature has continued to be recorded. Nowadays, recorded ASL literature products are uploaded regularly, on a daily basis, by Deaf people from various backgrounds and walks of life.

Products of ASL literature range from stories to poetry, legends, riddles, folklore, jokes, and many more. ASL literature also includes fairytales, expositions, English to ASL translations, personal anecdotes, sign play, percussion songs, rap, fables, tall tales, epics, humorous stories, and visual vernacular, formerly called mimery

(Bahan, 2006; Byrne, 2013). Exploring a specific genre in ASL literature opens up a whole new set of characteristics and patterns, such as the ASL poetry genre, which has many subdivisions, including handshape rhyming (using numbers, specific handshapes, closed/open handshapes, and so on), movement rhyming, location rhyming, palm orientation rhyming, nonmanual signal rhyming, and handedness rhyming (Bahan, 2006; Byrne, 2013). Many new explorations into ASL literature include ASL fingertutting, where storytellers integrate intricate movements and shapes with fingers, similar to Egyptian hieroglyphics, with ASL signs (Witteborg, 2015). Some new artistic explorations involve film work and special effect editing, including distorting or enhancing handshapes and movement such as Ian Sanborn's fascinating rendition of a rooster, aptly titled *Rooster* (Katz-Hernandez, 2013; Sanborn, 2014).

Andrew Byrne, a nationally known and prolific Deaf ASL storyteller, did a scholarly study on ASL literature, surveying experts in ASL literature and their perspective of essential features that characterizes ASL literature (2013). He writes that the essential features of successful ASL literature pieces include (1) using sign language to narrate (as opposed to written/oral forms of expression); (2) the narrator knowing the audience and working well with the audience; (3) the narrator having a distinctive storytelling style, almost like a signature; (4) the narrator being competent in weaving cadence in the story (e.g., rhythmic flow); (5) the narrator incorporating rhyme and rhythm through the use of handshape, movement, or location of signs; (6) the narrator following the pattern established in the genre; (7) the story revolving around oppression and/or celebration of Deaf culture; and (8) the use of particular literary devices to smuggle in representation of oppression (Byrne, 2013).

Common resilience themes associated with being a marginalized culture appear in ASL literature, often revolving around typical Deaf themes, such as the discovery and development of a Deaf identity, ridiculing ignorant hearing people, using self-deprecating humor intended to exaggerate stereotypes, and the leverage of being Deaf or knowing sign language (Holcomb, 2013; Martin, 2011).

The discovery and development of a Deaf identity is a source of pride for the Deaf community—almost like a deaf person being reborn Deaf and welcomed into the Deaf community, and many stories like this are told and passed on among Deaf people (Leigh, 2009; Nomeland & Nomeland, 2012).

The second theme revolves around Deaf people who compete and come out on top over hearing people. More often than not, certain hearing people engage in oppressive actions or create obstacles for Deaf people. When Deaf people succeed in the end, beating out ignorant hearing people, those kinds of stories make Deaf people feel good but also function as a collaborative, cohesive survival tool for Deaf people who encounter similar situations (Holcomb, 2013).

Raychelle's father, Ray, was dropped off by his parents at the Florida School for the Deaf and Blind in the fall of 1944, when he was 7 years old, since the family lived more than 200 miles away. His hearing parents spoke with a supervisor, who told them to wait and leave when Ray was distracted so he would not become upset when they tried to say goodbye. They disappeared when Ray was distracted by another Deaf student who showed his World War II model plane. He missed his parents and his family dearly, but he also slowly realized he was also being born into another beloved family—his Deaf school, Deaf culture, and sign language, which would become his home too. And planes and flying became a lifelong passion for Ray as well!

A Russian, a Cuban, and a Deaf person are on a train. The Russian throws half a bottle of vodka out of the window. The Cuban and Deaf person ask why. The Russian says, "Oh, in my country, we have plenty of vodka." Later, the Cuban throws a cigar that was smoked only halfway out of the window. The Russian and the Deaf person ask why. The Cuban says, "Oh, in my country, we have plenty of cigars." Later, a hearing person walks down the aisle, and the Deaf person throws the hearing person out of the window. The Cuban and the Russian ask why. The Deaf person says, "Oh, in my world, we have plenty of hearing people" (Holcomb, 2013, pp. 165–166).

There are also stories that include self-deprecating humor intended to exaggerate stereotypes, disguised as a critique of the majority and their discriminatory practices, such as:

There's a good reason why I've never made much of my life. Every time opportunity knocked, I was in the shower with my hearing aid (or cochlear implant) on the sink. (Nomeland & Nomeland, 2012, p. 147)

This joke implicitly points out the absurdity of, and subtly criticizes, the stereotype that Deaf people are lazy and apathetic. As elaborated in Chapter 8, Deaf people often encounter discrimination when seeking employment—or even while working.

A classic story involves Deaf newlyweds who, after a busy and exciting wedding day, arrived at their honeymoon suite. The wife winked at the husband and said she needed to go to the bathroom and would be out shortly. The husband chuckled, undressed, and went under the covers, waiting for his wife. Suddenly, one of her high heels flew out the bathroom door. Then the other heel came flying by. Then her dress sailed past. Next came her bra. And her undies. The husband smirked, anticipating an exciting surprise performance from his wife. Then a bathroom rug went flying. A brush bounced off the floor. Next came the soap. The husband, puzzled, jumped out of bed and approached the bathroom only to find his wife shouting in sign language, "What took you so long?! We're out of toilet paper!"

This narration focuses on the daily frustrations of Deaf people, integrated with self-deprecating humor. Hearing people cannot tell stories like this, because they would be making fun of Deaf people and their experience, deeply disrespecting Deaf people and their lived experiences. Only members of the Deaf community culture are allowed to engage in self-deprecating humor about being deaf for different reasons, including group solidarity, cultural pride, and unity.

Why do you think hearing people are not allowed to make fun of Deaf people's daily challenges in being Deaf? Why is it okay for Deaf people to make fun of themselves? Can you think of other situations that may be similar in principle?

Also, there are many stories that revolve around being Deaf and/or knowing sign language as leverage, such as the widely known and embraced Motel joke. A Deaf couple checks into their motel room, and both go to bed. The husband wakes up with a headache and asks his partner to retrieve aspirin from the glove compartment. The partner, groggy, leaves the room, retrieves the aspirin, and then realizes he has forgotten their room number. The motel office is closed for the night. He decides to press the car horn and holds it down while the motel rooms in front of him start to light up, one by one. After a few minutes, all of the motel rooms' lights are on, except one. He now knows which room is his, and off he goes to his room (Nomeland & Nomeland, 2012).

Although the examples of ASL literature translated to English examples listed here are humorous and brief, there are many more deeply moving, profound, and insightful literary pieces in ASL that cannot be translated to English without losing some of their meanings. The ASL literature performances by Ben Bahan, Michelle Banks, Bernard Bragg, Patrick Graybill, Monique Holt, CJ Jones, Ella Mae Lentz, Nathie Marbury, Dorothy

Miles, Debbie Rennie, Rosa Lee Timm, Clayton Valli, and many more are not to be missed. Pictured in Figure 11–17 is Dr. Nathie Marbury performing one of her many poems.

In sum, one way to gain a better understanding of the Deaf experience and multiple Deaf lives is to absorb and appreciate the stories and poetry shared with you by Deaf people themselves.

Deaf Literature: English

Although ASL literature focuses on literature in sign language by Deaf people in the United States and parts of Canada (Byrne, 2013), Deaf literature focuses on literature in English written by Deaf people in the United States and parts of Canada (Holcomb, 2013). However, some people argue that since there is no "hearing" literature, there is no "Deaf" literature (Byrne, 2013). Additionally, some may wonder why there is Deaf literature in written English, as written English isn't the primary or

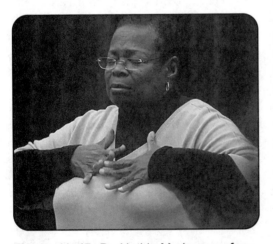

Figure 11–17. Dr. Nathie Marbury performing one of her many ASL poems. Photo courtesy of Alberta Stewart and Norma L. Holt, Nathie's daughters.

preferred language for many Deaf people. English is not as valued in Deaf culture as ASL is among Deaf people, often due to many traumatic experiences growing up in schools with red marks splashed across their written submissions due to language deprivation early in life, as elaborated in Chapters 4 and 5 (Lane et al., 1996). Not only that, the differences in teaching English between hearing students (emphasis on appreciating and creating literature) and deaf students (emphasis on grammar rules and rules of speech) have negatively impacted many deaf students' views of English. The emphasis on rules of grammar and speech has been shown to do more harm than good in the acquisition of English and does not improve the perception of written English by Deaf people (Wood & Wood, 1997). For more about Deaf people and English literacy, see Chapter 4.

Even with negative experiences with English, there are countless exceptional literature products in English written by Deaf people. That in itself is a clear indication that many Deaf people in the United States tend to be somewhat bilingual in ASL and English (and possibly more languages) as well as being bicultural and/or multicultural (Brueggemann, 1995). Since Deaf people are bilingual (possibly multilingual) and bi/multicultural, they are capable of expressing themselves in different languages, including the language of the majority, English, incorporating elements of their cultures in their writing, hence the rationale for calling their written work "Deaf Literature" (Holcomb, 2013).

There are two types of Deaf literature, much like Deaf art and De'VIA. There are written English publications by Deaf authors that have nothing to do with Deaf culture or sign language, and there are written English publications by Deaf authors that revolve around their Deaf experience among other, equally important lived experiences such as being Deaf and Gay, Black DeafBlind PanQueer, and/or a DeafDisabled Woman, for example (Holcomb, 2013). There are over 500 documented magazines, newspapers, journals, and other publications by Deaf people (Holcomb, 2013). Publications in regular intervals such as weekly or monthly publications are called periodicals. Notable historical achievements in Deaf periodicals range from Deaf proprietors of newspapers and having the longest running educational journal documenting the achievements of Deaf people.

> Can you imagine running a publication, editing and publishing in your second or third language, none of which you can fully access in their spoken forms?

In 1837, Levi Bacus, a graduate of the American School for the Deaf, became the first Deaf editor of a weekly newspaper syndication in upstate New York, and the banner of the newspaper under his helm was in fingerspelling (Gannon, 1981). In 1847, the *American Annals of the Deaf* was established and is the oldest continually publishing educational journal in the United States (Gannon, 1981). Many different publications have come and gone over the years, with some being schoolwide publications, some regional/statewide publications, and some national publications, such as *Deaf Mute's Journal, Silent World, The Silent Worker, The American Deaf Citizen, The Silent Cavalier, The Silent News,* and many more. It is also important to acknowledge that those pub-

lications reflect systematic racism, sexism, ableism, and more at that time in history—most of those writers were white, male, sighted, and abled. This bias was representative of the times when white males dominated the writing, editing, and production of deaf publications.

Since 1849, in print shops at Deaf schools in the United States, there was a proliferation of school newspapers called the "Little Paper Family." These publications became the main source of communication and source of identity and pride for the Deaf community. The articles were written by deaf men who provided events, information, jokes, and alumni news. These writers also wrote vehemently against oralism practices as well as defended the rights of deaf teachers who were being replaced by hearing teachers, and they wrote about other issues important to Deaf people. Deaf students read those newspapers for entertainment, information, and as models of written composition (Reed, 1993).

In September 1948, the National Association of the Deaf (NAD) started publishing *The Silent Worker* newspaper. Sixteen years later, in 1964, the name of the publication changed to *The DEAF American*. Fifteen years later, in 1979, the name once again changed to *The NAD Broadcaster*. The latest change came in 2001, with the current name being *NADmag*. For over 65 years, NAD members have enjoyed reading NAD publications. Figure 11–18 shows a collage of *NADmag* magazine covers over the years.

Paper-based publications currently active include *NADmag* and *Deaf Life*. Some publications transitioned from being paper based to online or originated completely online, some bilingually in ASL and English, including *The Buff and Blue* and *Bison TV Productions* (Gallaudet

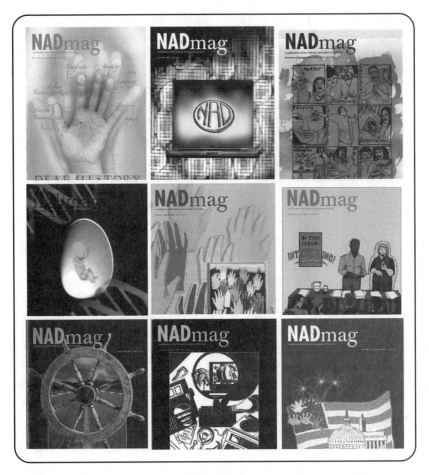

Figure 11–18. A collage of *NADmag* magazine covers over the years. Photo courtesy of the National Association of the Deaf.

University student newspaper) and *Deaf Digest*. A DeafBlind editor, John Lee Clark, ran *The Tactile Mind Literary Magazine and Weekly* e-zine for a few years. *KissFist*, which disseminated online magazines from 2008 to 2014 by Child of Deaf Adult (CODA) editor Frank Gallimore, with his Deaf sister, Rosa Lee Timm, also an editor, with a total of 12 issues, is pictured in Figure 11–19.

Deaf people publish books too, including anthologies, science fiction, novels, poetry, autobiographies, poetry, and many more. According to the books currently carried by the Gallaudet University Press and Harris Communications, there are approximately 150 books written by Deaf authors currently on the market. James Nack was the very first Deaf author to publish a book in the United States, in 1827, titled *The Legend of the Rocks: And Other Poems*, which consists of over 60 poems written when he was between 14 and 17 years old (Krentz, 2000). Although most publications revolve around Deaf culture and sign language, like Deaf art,

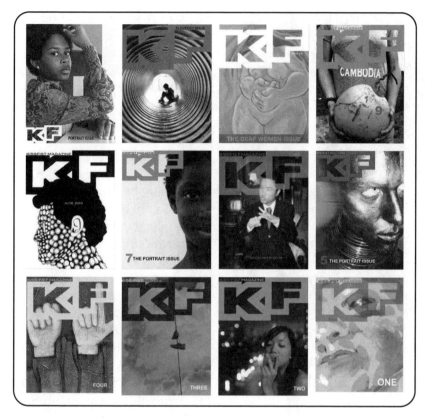

Figure 11–19. The 12 covers of Issues 1 through 12 of *KissFist*, a Deaf magazine. Photo courtesy of KISSFIST Magazine.

there are Deaf people writing pieces that have nothing to do with Deaf culture or sign language, such as Connie Briscoe's best-selling publications *Sisters and Lovers* (1994), shown in Figure 11–20, and *Big Girls Don't Cry* (1996).

Catherine "Kitty" Fischer published an autobiography with Cathryn Carroll titled *Orchid of the Bayou: A Deaf Woman Faces Blindness* in 2001. A prolific Deaf Gay writer, Raymond Luczak has published books revolving around Deaf and gay themes, such as *Eyes of Desire: A Deaf Gay & Lesbian Reader* (1993), *Assembly Required: Notes From a Deaf Gay Life* (2009), and *Whispers of a Savage Sort: And Other*

Plays About the Deaf American Experience (2009). There are Deaf publishing houses, including Savory Words and Handwave Publications.

To appreciate more published written English (and other written languages) literature pieces by diverse Deaf, hard-of-hearing, and DeafBlind people of different backgrounds and experiences, it is important for all children to have full, natural access to sign language from birth and full access to the written majority language of the country from birth in order to become fully bilingual (and even multilingual) adults (Cummins, 2006; NAD Bilingual Position, 2015).

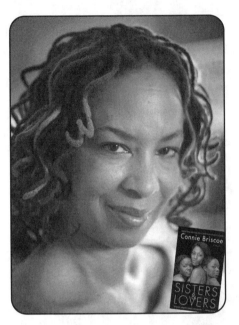

Figure 11–20. Deaf bestselling author Connie Briscoe, with the cover of one of her books, *Sisters & Lovers*. Photo credit: Chris Hartlove. Used with permission.

Online ASL and Deaf Literature

Thanks to one of the inventors of the Internet, Vinton Cerf, a hard-of-hearing man, more and more Deaf people are finding the online platform the perfect place to share their literary works in both ASL and English to a much more broad and diverse audience and with immediate feedback. There are many Deaf bloggers and vloggers (people who blog with videos instead of the printed word). There are also multiple sites that serve as repositories, exhibiting many contributions by Deaf people in a centralized place. The majority of the contributions may not satisfy the definition of "literary" works; however, there are many gems in the rough.

The more professionally done (as in editing, high-definition filming, some including captions) ASL videos by Deaf people often can be found at *ASLized*, the *Daily Moth*, *Deaf Studies Digital Journal (DSDJ)*, *Deaf Newspaper*, *Deaf News Today*, *Deaf Studies Digital Journal*, *DPAN. tv*, *Journal of American Sign Language and Literature (JASLL)*, *Melmira* with Melissa Yingst, *Real People*, Seek the World, Sign-1News, TEDxIslay, and TEDxGallaudet. *The Daily Moth* with Alex Abenchuchan, particularly the Deaf Bing section, shows videos sent by Deaf people that analyze differences between Deaf and hearing cultures. Sign1News is the first Deaf news organization that is affiliated with CNN to share current events with the masses in ASL. Figure 11–21 is a photo of the three anchors for Sign1News, Jethro Wooddall, Candace Jones, and Crystal Cousineau.

Trudy Suggs, a Deaf writer and publisher, who also owns T. S. Writing Services, regularly posts ASL and English articles on her blog. She is well known for her meticulous investigative reporting of fraud by hearing and/or deaf people within the Deaf community, in particular, the Saturn commercial that featured a "Deaf" driver, who originally lied that she was deaf but eventually was exposed to be actually hearing.

Members of the Intersectional Souls Project created a powerfully stunning and passionate poetry showcase titled *The Nathie ASL Soul Project* in Austin, Texas, on January 28, 2015. Black Deaf women translated into ASL and performed Dr. Nathie Marbury's written English poems in ASL. Nary a dry eye was in the audience. A collage of photos of the poets is shown in Figure 11–22.

For the more casual and homegrown atmosphere, you can visit *ASL THAT!* and many other ASL-related public groups on Facebook, DeafVideo.tv, DeafRead. com, and AllDeaf.com. You can also find many emerging amateur or professional

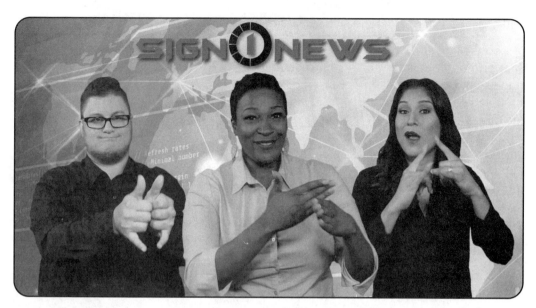

Figure 11–21. A photo of three anchors for Sign1News, from left to right, Jethro Wooddall, Candace Jones, and Crystal Cousineau. Used with permission.

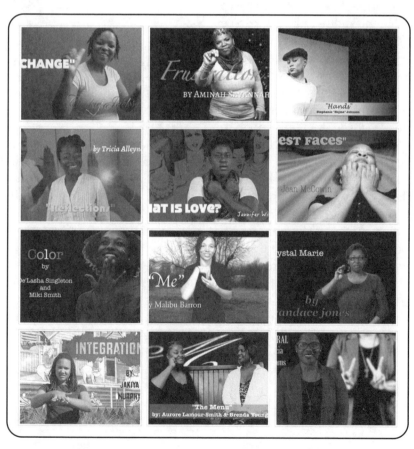

Figure 11–22. A collage of poets in *The Nathie ASL Soul Project*. Photo courtesy of the *Intersectional Souls Project*.

Deaf photographers, performers, artists, models, and comedians on social media through their Instagram, Twitter, Vine, and YouTube accounts such as *The Harold Foxx Show*, *Eyes on the Road* with John Maucere, *DO DO* with Daniel Durant, *Flip Side Show*, and *The RiRi Show*. On Facebook, Queen Foreverrr, a Black Deaf female entertainer, is very popular in the Deaf community, with over 50,000 likes. Her themes revolve around Deaf and hearing cultures, such as a character exploding in Deaf road rage only to find out the other driver also understands ASL! *Deafies in Drag* has a Facebook page with 220,000 likes. Latinx Deaf drag queens with the stage names of Selena Minogue and Casavina act in brief comedic video skits. One video had a Deaf son calling his mother using VRS (see Chapter 9 for an explanation of VRS). The son becomes distracted and ends up talking to a friend off camera. The VRS interpreter does not realize the son is talking to someone off camera and continues to interpret what the Deaf son is saying, much to the mother's despair. The comedic duo in *Deafies in Drag* can be seen in Figure 11–23.

Although Deaf humor is a strong theme in Deaf cultural literature, there are also many very powerful literary works out there. Maya Angelou's "Phenomenal Woman" poem was brilliantly translated and signed in ASL by 32 different phenomenal Black Deaf Womxn on the Black Deaf Village YouTube channel. The online landscape has certainly opened up many opportunities for Deaf people from all walks of life to experiment, play with, and share their literary contributions in ASL, English, and more.

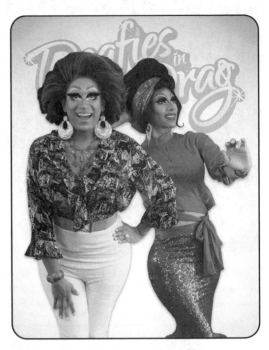

Figure 11–23. Selena Minogue and Casvina, Latinx Deaf drag queens, pose in front of the *Deafies in Drag* logo. Photo courtesy of *Deafies in Drag*.

growing very fast in popularity among Deaf people and Deaf communities. Media arts include photography, cinematography, and other types of digital arts such as comics and cartoons. More and more new types of art revolving around the use of technology include digital art, computer graphics, computer animation, background and set artists, computer robotics, and 3D printing. As you can see, there is tremendous overlap among the arts, especially visual arts, performing arts, and media arts.

Deaf Images: Digital Arts and Photography

Are photographs taken by Deaf people any different from photographs taken by hearing people? Dalit Avnon, says yes—"The

MEDIA

With the advent of accessible and reasonably priced technology, media arts are identifying marks of many deaf and hard-of-hearing artists are the use of bold and contrasting colors, contrasting textures and emphasis on facial features, especially eyes, mouth, ears and hands" (McKinsey, 2014, p. 1). She explains that Deaf photography is enhanced because Deaf photographers "use their eyes not just to see, but also to listen" (McKinsey, 2014, p. 1). Some say that it's an advantage to be a Deaf photographer when working in crowds (such as weddings and concerts) as photographers are often interrupted by people wanting to ask questions about their profession, often giving unwanted advice or direction for photographers, and taking them away from valuable photography opportunities. When interrupted, Deaf photographers can simply sign back, "I'm Deaf" with a smile and immediately return their focus on their work with very little or no time wasted—leaving the surprised, speechless hearing person behind.

There are quite a number of Deaf photographers! Maggie Lee Sayre, a Kentucky School for the Deaf graduate, had hundreds of her photos of Tennessee river culture published in a book in 1995 (Sayre & Rankin, 1995). Her photography work was recognized at a festival of American Folklife on the National Mall in Washington, DC. The now defunct *Deaf Mosiac* television show featured her in an episode, and she was selected as a Person of the Week on *ABC Evening News* in 1995 (Berke, 2012). Tate Tullier, a Deaf professional photographer, has had his photos published in modeling magazines and displayed at an art gallery (Berke, 2012). Michael Pimentel, a Deaf professional sports photographer, works as a team photographer for University of California, Berkeley athletics, International Sports Images and Allstate Sugar Bowl, Major League Soccer's San Jose Earthquakes, and more. His photos have appeared in *Sports Illustrated*, *ESPN*, and the *San Francisco Chronicle* (Pimentel, 2015). Brendon Borellini, a DeafBlind photographer, feels the subject and the environment with his senses, such as smelling the ocean, the mist on his face from the breeze, or the crinkle of leaves beneath his feet. He takes photographs by placing the back of the camera on his forehead and then prints out his photographs using a 3D topographic printer so he can feel the texture of the photos he takes (Krassenstein, 2014). Amelia Hamilton, a Deaf photographer, popular for her friendly and charismatic approach, calls herself a "visual storyteller and designer" (Hamilton, 2020, p. 1). Michael Samaripa, a professional Deaf photographer with clients ranging from local businesses to national and global nonprofit companies for commercial and marketing work, also teaches photography, focusing on lighting techniques, composition skills, location, and scouting discussions and retouching (Samaripa, 2015).

Deaf graphic designers create images integrating text, art, and design techniques, using computers and technology. Matt Daigle, Ann Silver, and Shawn Richardson, mentioned earlier in this chapter, are Deaf artists who incorporate the use of text, art, and design principles in their work. More Deaf graphic artists include Lauren Benedict, Bilal Chinoy, Hoon Jeong, and Robyn Girard. Kaori Takeuchi, while studying for her Deaf Studies master's thesis at Gallaudet University, created a new genre—ASL Manga, which incorporates the visual language of a Japanese artistic practice with ASL (Takeuchi, 2012). In Figure 11–24, Takeuchi is standing by a life-sized banner of her work, which features many different Deaf signers signing Gallaudet and a central figure signing THAT.

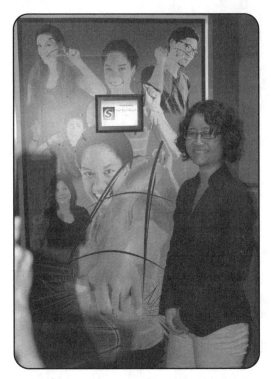

Figure 11–24. Kaori Takeuchi stands beside a life-sized ASL Manga publication, with signers signing GALLAUDET and the person in middle signing THAT. Used with permission.

Some graphic designers are also animators who create multiple images, known as frames, which give an illusion of movement. You can see the work of Gino Giudice, a Deaf animator, in the *Charlotte's Web* movie, and the following 1965 to 1978 TV series: *The Flintstones, Josie and the Pussycats,* and *Scooby Doo, Where Are You!* (Giudice, 2015). He was a background artist in the Hanna-Barbera Animation Department in Hollywood (Bug, 2007). Mark Fisher, a Deaf animator and filmmaker, won the Best Animation category out of 350 entries at the Atlantic City Film Festival in 2001. Fisher was involved as an animator for Universal's *The Land Before Time,* Disney's *The Little Mermaid*

and *The Prince and the Pauper,* and Warner Bros' *Thumbelina* and *The King and I* movies, along with the *King of the Hill* TV series, from 1992 to 1999 (Suggs, 2001). Other Deaf animators include James Merry of the United Kingdom, who has a master's degree in Animation from the Royal College of Art. Braam Jordaan of South Africa created visual effects and animation for BMW, Mitsubishi, World Wildlife Fund, and American Eagle TV commercials (Jordaan, 2015). Jordaan is best known in the Deaf community as the director, producer, writer, and animator for *The Rubbish Monster,* an animated movie and storybook. Another Deaf motion designer and animator, Robyn Girard, has had her work featured by *PBS Newshour, Make Magazine,* and South by Southwest (SXSW). Figure 11–25 depicts Robyn in her own animated footage teasing about how hearing people cannot eat and talk at the same time, while Deaf people can.

Transitioning from frozen images to an animated series of images, we now move on to motion-based filming and cinematography in the next section.

Deaf Motion: Cinema and Film

As mentioned earlier in this chapter, one of the very first film footage with language was of a Deaf woman signing "The Star-Spangled Banner." This film was taken by the inventor of the motion picture, Thomas Edison, a deaf man. It was not until amateur filming equipment became more affordable that "an explosion in the production of films by Deaf filmmakers" came on the scene (Christie, Durr, & Wilkins, 2006, p. 91).

How are Deaf cinema and film different from mainstream cinematography and digital arts? Hearing filmmakers use

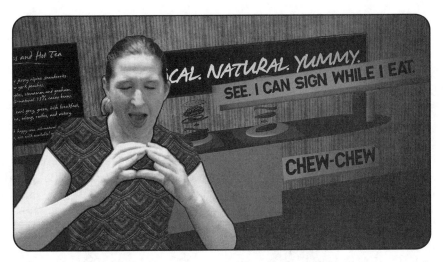

Figure 11–25. Robyn Girard, a Deaf animator, narrates in her own animated video about how Deaf people can eat and talk at the same time. Used with permission.

sound and music to build up (or down) climatic periods in their footage, trigger emotions, and make scene changes. How do Deaf filmmakers evoke emotion and transitions in their filmed work? Like De'VIA, there are particular visual aesthetics that are typically associated with Deaf cinematography. There are many identified techniques, including visual rhythm (patterns of camera and editing techniques), visual representation of sound (e.g., a closeup of a spoon tapping a dish), visual representation of hearing people (e.g., footage of hearing people talking without sound), deaf views of deaf self (e.g., an extreme closeup of an ear mold being slowly pulled out of an ear, a metaphor for freedom), and emphasizing story elements such as foreshadowing and climatic film moments such as emphasis on eye contact between actors (Christie et al., 2006).

Wayne Betts Jr., a Deaf filmmaker and the originator of the term *Deaf lens* (mentioned in Chapter 7), explains a few unique Deaf cinematic principles that came to him as he worked to detach himself from the regular script and filming style of hearing filmmakers (Betts, 2010). He mentions a few differences in his TEDx publication: (1) His scripts originate in ASL (rather than written English). (2) His filming style is constant, is fluid, and follows the natural movement of Deaf people and Deaf eyes, rather than the choppy back-and-forth editing between two speaking people. (3) Betts incorporates text on the screen next to the actors, rather than on bottom of the screen, fixed and disconnected from the story on the screen. (4) Betts has also come up with ways to include on-screen narration (rather than voiceover) by superimposing several footages at once of the narrator and of the actual scenes. Incorporating those principles and shooting with Deaf lens allow viewers a brief glimpse of how to see the world through Deaf eyes. He closed his presentation by saying, "I think the cinematic value of sign language is far more richer than cinema itself. ASL goes far and beyond that." (Betts, 2010)

There are many different Deaf film festivals all over the world, celebrating Deaf filmmakers and their work: UK Deaf Focus Film Festival, Swedish Deaf Film Festival, Festival Clin D'Oeil, Deaf Maine Film Festival, Florida Deaf Film Festival, California Deaf Film Festival, Chicago Institute for Moving Image Festival, and Deaf Rochester Film Festival (Christie et al., 2006).

Gallaudet University hosted the first international Deaf film festival, WORLDEAF Cinema Festival in 2010, selecting more than 170 films produced by over 130 Deaf filmmakers from over 30 countries. Jane Norman, the chair of the event, explained, "Deaf people have a special affinity for filmmaking—it's a 'visual thing,' and we are a 'visual-centric' people. We want to tell our stories in our way while at the same time provide opportunities for our people to succeed in mainstream media." (Puente, 2010, p. 1) Dr. Alan Hurwitz, the president of Gallaudet University at that time, added,

> Filmmaking allows us to preserve our language in ways that cannot be achieved through books, photographs or other art forms. Like sign language, 'film language' involves much more than the spoken words of a script. An actor's facial expression and deliberate body movements, which are also essential elements for communicating in sign language, are critical in conveying the full meaning of a movie line or scene. (Puente, 2010, p. 1)

An explosion in Deaf films and Deaf film festivals can only mean an explosion in the number of professional Deaf filmmakers and Deaf people who work with films in many different capacities, such as director, producer, editor, screenwriter, special effects, set designer, and makeup artist. Accomplished contemporary Deaf filmmakers include Bim Ajadi, Bellamie Bachleda, Wayne Betts Jr., Jules Dameron, Susan Dupor, Bradley Gantt, Jay Kowalczyk, Leon Mian Sheng Lim, Melissa Malzkuhn, Adrean Mangiardi, Brent Macpherson, Louis Neethling, Ruan du Plessis, Andres Otalara, Zilvinas Paludnevicius, Storm Smith, Mark Wood, and many more. Featured in Figure 11–26 is professional Deaf filmmaker Storm Smith with the cover of four of her films.

Many of them taught or are teaching at Deaf Film Camp for young Deaf teens in Rochester, New York, ensuring that the next generation of Deaf filmmakers will

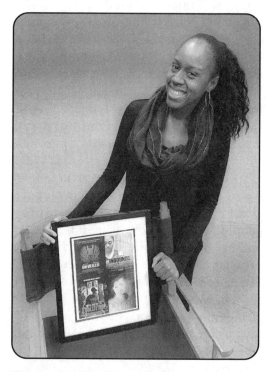

Figure 11–26. Storm Smith, a Deaf filmmaker, stands with the cover of four of her film productions. Courtesy of Thunderography Films.

receive a much earlier introduction to filmmaking. Watch out for the next generation of Deaf filmmakers!

CONCLUSION

It is often argued that sign languages, requiring the use of the face, body, and more, often evoke much more than written and spoken literature can. Jean-Jacques Rousseau, in his writings on the *Origin of Language* in 1754, was quoted as saying,

> Although the language of gesture and spoken language are equally natural, still the first is easier and depends less upon conventions. For more things affect our eyes than our ears. Also, visual forms are more varied than sounds, and more expressive, saying more in less time. (Bauman, Nelson, & Rose, 2006, p. xv)

The amazing artistic, literary, and media contributions by Deaf people of different lived experiences have opened up many new ways of seeing, creating, and experiencing the world through Deaf art, literature, and media. Cohn (1986) proclaimed, "I do not believe it is coincidence that what deaf people DO with language is what hearing poets try to MAKE their language do" (p. 263). Continue appreciating, experiencing, and blowing your mind with all the gifts sign language gives us.

REFERENCES

Adam, R., Aro, M., Druetta, J., Dunne, S., & Klintberg, J. (2014). Deaf interpreters: An introduction. In R. Adam, C. Stone, S. Collins, & M. Metzger (Eds.), *Deaf interpreters at work: International insights* (pp. 1–18). Washington, DC: Gallaudet University Press.

Albronda, M. (1994). *Douglas Tilden: The man and his legacy.* Seattle, WA: Emerald Point Press.

Anderson, R. C. (2013). *The history of the Mechanics Monument: Nude, well-muscled and hardworking.* Retrieved from http://www.rchristiananderson.org/mechanics monument/

ASD History. (2015). *This is where it all began.* Retrieved from http://www.asd1817.org/page.cfm?p=1160

Bahan, B. (2006). Face-to-face tradition in the American deaf community: Dynamics of the teller, the tale, and the audience. In H. Bauman, J. Nelson, & H. Rose (Eds.), *Signing the body poetic: Essays on American Sign Language literature* (pp. 21–50). Berkeley: University of California Press.

Bauman, H., Nelson, J., & Rose, H. (Eds.). (2006). *Signing the body poetic: Essays on American Sign Language literature.* Berkeley: University of California Press.

Berke, J. (2012). *Deaf photographers.* Retrieved from http://deafness.about.com/od/deaf people/a/deaf_photographers.htm

Betts, W. (2010). *TEDxIslay: Deaf lens.* Retrieved from https://youtu.be/ocbyS9-3jjM

Bragg, B. (2015). *Life and works of Bernard Bragg: Act two—All the world's a stage.* Retrieved from http://bernardbragg.com/biography/2/

Bradbury, J., Clark, J. L., Grossman, R., Herbers, J., Magliocchino, V., Norman, J., . . . Van Der Mark, L. (2019). ProTactile Shakespeare: Inclusive theater by/for the DeafBlind. *Shakespeare Studies, 47,* 81–15.

Brueggemann, B. (1995). The coming out of Deaf culture and ASL: An exploration into visual rhetoric and literacy. *Rhetoric Review, 13,* 409-420.

Bug. (2007). *Deaf cartoon artist in "Flintstone," "The Pebbles and Bamm-Bamm."* Retrieved from https://fookembug.wordpress.com/2007/08/14/deaf-cartoon-artist-in-flintstone-the-pebbles-and-bamm-bamm/

Byrne, A. (2013). *American Sign Language (ASL) literacy and ASL literature: A critical appraisal* (Unpublished doctoral dissertation). University of Toronto, Toronto, Canada.

Callis, L. (2015). *Let's see more #DeafTalent in Hollywood.* Retrieved from http://www.huffingtonpost.com/lydia-l-callis/lets-seemore-deaftalent-_b_6690324.html

Callis, L. (2017). *The rise of #DeafTalent.* Retrieved from https://www.huffpost.com/entry/the-rise-of-deaftalent_b_58cc25e1e4b0537abd957054

Carroll, C., & Fischer, C. (2001). *Orchid of the bayou: A deaf woman faces blindness.* Washington, DC: Gallaudet University Press.

Christie, K., Durr, P., & Wilkins, D. (2006). *Close-up: Contemporary deaf filmmakers.* Retrieved from http://scholarworks.rit.edu/other/597/

Cohn, J. (1986). The new deaf poetics: Visible poetry. *Sign Language Studies, 52,* 263–277.

Cummins, J. (2006). *The relationship between American Sign Language proficiency and English academic development: A review of the research.* Retrieved from www.gallaudet.edu/documents/cummins_asl-eng.pdf

deaffriendly. (2013). *Ann Silver: Don't (just) call her the crayon lady.* Retrieved from http://deaffriendly.com/articles/ann-silver-dontjust-call-her-the-crayon-lady/

Durr, P. (1999). Deconstructing the forced assimilation of deaf people via De'VIA resistance and affirmation art. *Visual Anthropology Review, Society for Visual Anthropology, 15,* 47–68.

Durr, P. (2006). De'VIA: Investigating deaf visual art. In B. Eldredge, D. Stringham & M. Wilding-Diaz (Eds.), *Proceedings from Deaf Studies today!* (Vol. 2). Orem: Utah Valley State College.

DWT. (2015). *Deaf West Theater.* Retrieved from http://www.deafwest.org

Efron, A. (2007). The greatest irony. *Deaf World as Eye See It.* Published March 17, 2007. No longer available online. Information retrieved directly from author.

Efron, A. (2014). *Singalongs—Bastardization or authenticity of ASL music artistry.* Retrieved from http://www.deafeyeseeit.com/2014/09/07/signalongs/

Gannon, J. (1981). *Deaf heritage: A narrative history of deaf America.* Silver Spring, MD: National Association of the Deaf.

GDC. (2015). *Gallaudet Dance Company.* Retrieved from http://www.gallaudet.edu/act/gallaudet-dance-company.html

Giudice, G. (2015). *Gino Giudice: Animation Department.* Retrieved from http://www.imdb.com/name/nm0321271/

Grushkin, D. (2014). *Who are they really signing for?* Retrieved from https://www.youtube.com/watch?v=5xhU3i3gllY

Grushkin, D. (2015). *What do deaf people think of the "performance" of the sign-language translator in Sia's video below?* Retrieved from https://www.quora.com/What-do-Deaf-people-think-of-the-performance-of-the-sign-language-translator-in-Sias-video-below

Guendling, B. (2020). *College football players perform ASL concert- Uptown Funk (Mark Ronson).* Retrieved from https://www.youtube.com/watch?v=Ql3oJsG-gEg

Hamilton, A. (2020). *Amelia Hamilton: About me.* Retrieved from https://www.ameliakhamilton.com/info

Hill, J. (2008). *Linguistic appropriation: The history of white racism is embedded in American English, in the everyday language of white racism.* Oxford, UK: Wiley-Blackwell.

Hockenberry, J. (2015). *Transcription: Broadway in song, in sign language, and on wheels.* Retrieved from http://www.thetakeaway.org/story/transcription-broadway-song sign-language-and-wheels/

Holcomb, T. (2013). *Introduction to American Deaf culture.* New York, NY: Oxford University Press.

Horn, J., Sperling, N., & Smith, D. (2012). *From the archives: Unmasking Oscar: Academy voters are overwhelmingly white and male.* Retrieved from https://www.latimes.com/entertainment/la-et-unmasking-oscar-academy-project-20120219-story.html

Hughes, R. O. (2015). *Hughes, Regina Olson, 1895–1993.* Retrieved from http://www.gallaudet.edu/library-deaf-collections

and-archives/collections/manuscript-collection/mss-175.html

IBFS. (2015). *The international breastfeeding symbol.* Retrieved from http://www.breastfeedingsymbol.org/history/

Jean-Philippe, M. (2019). *Natasha Ofili is the principal in the politician—and she's breaking barriers for deaf actors.* Retrieved from https://www.oprahmag.com/entertainment/a29232832/netflix-the-politician-deaf-principal-natasha-ofili/

Jejeune. (2019). *Jejeune magazine: I love you, by Mara.* Retrieved from https://www.jejunemagazine.com/home/bymara

Jordaan, B. (2015). *Braam Jordaan.* Retrieved from https://en.wikipedia.org/wiki/Braam_Jordaan

Katz-Hernandez, D. (2013). *Time displacement with signing hands.* Retrieved from https://www.facebook.com/daniel.katzhernandez/videos/vb.1216097028/10202566999355642/?type=2&theater

Kilpatrick, B. (2007). *The history of the formation of deaf children's theater in the United States* (Unpublished doctoral dissertation). Lamar University, Beaumont, TX.

Krassenstein, B. (2014). *Completely blind and deaf photographer can now "see" his own work, thanks to 3D printing.* Retrieved from http://3dprint.com/12671/3d-print-blind-deaf-photography/

Krentz, C. (2000). *A mighty change: An anthology of deaf American writing 1816–1864.* Washington, DC: Gallaudet University Press.

Lammle, R. (2010). *Roll over Beethoven: 6 modern deaf musicians.* Retrieved from http://mentalfloss.com/article/25750/roll-over-beethoven-6-modern-deaf-musicians

Lane, H. (2004). *A deaf artist in early America: The worlds of John Brewster, Jr.* Boston, MA: Beacon Press.

Lane, H., Hoffmeister, R., & Bahan, B. (1996). *A journey into the Deaf-World.* San Diego, CA: DawnSignPress.

Leigh, I. W. (2009). *A lens on deaf identities.* New York, NY: Oxford University Press.

List. (n.d.). *List of oldest and youngest academy award winners and nominees.* Retrieved from https://en.wikipedia.org/wiki/List_of_oldest_and_youngest_Academy_Award_winners_and_nominees

Loeffler, S. (2014). Deaf music: Embodying language and rhythm. In H. D. Bauman & J. J. Murray (Eds.), *Deaf gain: Raising the stakes for human diversity* (pp. 436–456). Minneapolis: University of Minnesota Press.

Maler, A. (2015). Songs for hands: Analyzing interactions of sign language and music. *Journal of the Society for Music Theory, 19*(1). Retrieved from http://www.mtosmt.org/issues/mto.13.19.1/mto.13.19.1.maler.php

Martin, H. (2011). *Writing between cultures: A study of hybrid narratives in ethnic literature of the United States.* Jefferson, NC: McFarland & Company.

McCaskill, C., Lucas, C., Bayley, R. & Hill, J. (2011). *The hidden treasure of Black ASL: Its history and structure.* Washington, DC: Gallaudet University Press.

McKay-Cody, M. (2019). *Memory comes before knowledge—North American Indigenous Deaf: Socio-cultural study of rock/picture writing, community, sign languages, and kinship* (Unpublished doctoral dissertation). University of Oklahoma, Norman.

McKinsey, R. (2014). *Bold details characterize deaf photographers' work.* Retrieved from http://www.timesofisrael.com/bold-details-characterize-deaf-photographers-work/

NAD Bilingual Position. (2015). *National association for the deaf: New bilingual position statement released.* Retrieved from https://nad.org/news/2015/6/new-bilingual-position-statement-released

NADvlogs. (2010). *The preservation of sign language by George W. Veditz.* Retrieved from https://www.youtube.com/watch?v=XITbj3NTLUQ

Nomeland, M., & Nomeland, R. (2012). *The deaf community in America: History in the making.* Jefferson, NC: McFarland & Company.

NTD. (2015). *National Theater of the Deaf: You see and hear every word!* Retrieved from http://www.ntd.org/ntd_history.html

Okrent, A. (2014). *3 awesome translations from this sign language rap battle on Jimmy Kimmel*

Live. Retrieved from http://theweek.com/ articles/447979/3-awesome-translations from-sign-language-rap-battle-jimmy-kimmel-live

Padden, C., & Humphries, T. (2005). *Inside Deaf culture*. Cambridge, MA: Harvard University Press.

Patterson, C. (2015). *Texas state DE Brian Guendling does "Uptown Funk" in sign language*. Retrieved from http://www.cbs sports.com/collegefootball/eye-on-collegefootball/25 236568/watch-texas-state-debrian-guendling-does-uptown-funk-insign-language

Peisner, D. (2013). *Deaf jams: The surprising, conflicted, thriving world of hearing-impaired rappers*. Retrieved from http://www.spin.com/2013/10/deaf-jams-hearing-impaired-rappers/

Peters, C. (2000). *Deaf American literature: From carnival to canon*. Washington, DC: Gallaudet University Press.

Pimentel, M. (2015). *Michael Pimentel photography: Biography*. Retrieved from http://michaelpimentel.com/photographer/?page_id=2

Puente, M. (2010). *In D.C. WORLDEAF presents a truly silent film festival*. Retrieved from http://usatoday30.usatoday.com/life/movies/news/2010-11-04-deaffilmfest04_ST_N.htm

Reed, R. (1993). The little paper family: A rich heritage and a promising future. In G. Olsen & F. Turk (Eds.), *Kaleidoscope of Deaf America* (pp. 48–53). Silver Spring, MD: National Association for the Deaf.

Richardson, S. (2008). *Bling-bling videophone necklace cartoon*. Retrieved from http://srid4 fun.blogspot.com/2008/01/bling-bling videophone-necklace-cartoon.html

RID Performing Arts. (2014). *Performing arts standard practice paper task force*. Retrieved from https://drive.google.com/file/d/0B3 DKvZMflFLdd0hnZC1BMjJvTlU/view

Rodriguez, K. (2015). *With a little "Uptown Funk," a college player is inspiring hearing-impaired*. Retrieved from http://www.si .com/more-sports/2015/07/11/texas-state brianguendling-asl-uptown-funk

Samaripa, M. (2015). *Michael J. Samaripa: Visual communicator*. Retrieved from http://www .michaeljsamaripa.com/about/

Sanborn, I. (2014). *Ian Sanborn's rooster*. Retrieved from https://www.youtube.com/ user/ICSCI/videos

Sayre, M., & Rankin, T. (1995). *Deaf Maggie Lee Sayre: Photographs of a river life*. Jackson: University Press of Mississippi.

Sonnenstrahl, D. (2002). *Deaf artists in America: Colonial to contemporary*. San Diego, CA: DawnSignPress.

Spring. (n.d.). *Spring Awakening (musical)*. Retrieved from https://en.wikipedia.org/ wiki/Spring_Awakening_(musical)

Suggs, T. (2001). *Fisher wins grand prize at festival*. Retrieved from http://www.trudy suggs.com/fisher-wins%E2%80%88grand %E2%80%88prize-at-festival/

Takeuchi, K. (2012, Spring). ASL Manga; Visual representations in storytelling. *Deaf Studies Digital Journal*, 3.

Torrance, S. (2014). *On the ethics of "my" art*. Retrieved from http://www.torrentsofthought .com/on-the-ethics-of-my-art/

Ugwu, R. (2020). *The hashtag that changed the Oscars: An oral history*. Retrieved from https://www.nytimes.com/2020/02/06/movies/oscarssowhite-history.html

Weisblum, V. (2015). *How we listen determines what we hear: Christine Sun Kim on her recent sound works, working with blood orange*. Retrieved from http://www.artnews.com/2015/09/28/how-we-listen-determines what-we-hear-christine-kim-on-her-recent-sound-works-teaming-with-blood-orange/

Westfall, M. (2015). *What do deaf people think of the "performance" of the sign-language translator in Sia's video below?* Retrieved from https://www.quora.com/What-do-Deaf-people-think-of-the-performance-of-the-sign-lan guage-translator-in-Sias-video-below

Whitworth, E. (2014). *Appropriate method for appropriation*. Retrieved from http://impactmind.com/appropriatemethodfor-appropriation/

Wilde, R. (2015). *ASL interpreters bring ACL fest's music alive for Deaf community*. Retrieved from http://www.twcnews.com/tx/austin/austin-city-limits-music-festival/2015/10/4/asl-interpreters-bring-acl-fests-music-alive-for-deaf-community.html

Witteborg, E. (2015). *ASL-Tut short story: Social media dystopia*. Retrieved from https://www.facebook.com/KissFist.Memes/videos

Wood, D. & Wood, H. (1997). Communicating with children who are deaf: Pitfalls and possibilities. *Language, Speech and Hearing Services in Schools, 28*, 348–354.

Young, T. (2015). *#Deaftalent, Avenged & Twitter*. Retrieved from http://silentgrapevine.com/ 2015/03/deaftalent-avenged-twitter.html

Zola, C. (2015). *Let's talk (or sign!) about the Deaf, not hearing interpreters*. Retrieved from http://www.slate.com/blogs/lexicon_valley/2015/06/10/sign_language_let_s_talk_or_sign_about_the_deaf_not_hearing_interpreters.html

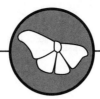

CHAPTER 12

Advocating and Career Opportunities

INTRODUCTION

At this point, you have learned quite a bit about Deaf people and issues impacting their lives. Is that learning going to stop here? Now that you know what the issues are, have you thought about advocating or supporting the Deaf community? Why might this be helpful?

The Deaf community needs your support as allies in ensuring their access to good education, training, jobs, medical care, and legal assistance. This is a social justice issue, as you can see from all the issues outlined throughout this book. In all fairness, the Deaf community wants to be treated in an equitable way. The Deaf community also seeks individuals such as yourself who can show everyone else how comfortable you can be with Deaf people. Your new understanding of Deaf culture makes you a more sensitive supporter. What if you get a petition to keep a school for the Deaf open when the state legislature threatens to close it due to budget problems? Will you support this petition and sign it or not? If you are a school administrator and a Deaf person

with appropriate qualifications applies to be a principal, will you support that person's application and hire that person? If you need legal advice, will you go to a qualified Deaf lawyer? Would you have supported the United Nations' effort to have the Convention on the Rights of Persons With Disabilities (CRPD, 2016) ratified? This is a document that protects the rights to full and equal access as members of their societies for persons with disabilities. The National Association of the Deaf supports this document. As of this book publication date, even though 161 other countries have ratified this document, the United States has not ratified it. The U.S. Congress feels that the U.S. government should control this process, not foreign countries. But this has the downside of sending a negative message about this country's support for individuals with disabilities having full and equal access despite the United States' support through laws ensuring the rights of this population.

Do you support the right of Deaf persons to live in specific senior housing where they can interact with other Deaf peers and receive information through ASL? The U.S. Department of Housing and Urban Development (HUD) tried to get Apache ASL Trails, a state-of-the-art senior housing in Arizona designed for Deaf access, to sign a compliance agreement that would prohibit this housing from allowing more than 25% of its residents to have a disability (Collom, 2013; National Association of the Deaf, 2014). This meant that not more than 25% of the residents can be Deaf. This also meant that not all Deaf people can benefit from living in a state-of-the-art senior citizen facility that was built to be accessible for deaf people, with doorbell light systems, flashing fire alarms, and so on. It took many letters and meetings before HUD finally agreed that this housing is indeed for Deaf people. In this case, do you support the Deaf people who want to be able to live there and enjoy a community of Deaf residents?

> Can you think of other ways you could provide support to deaf people?

All of the examples we have presented here show the need for ongoing advocacy. Advocacy refers to the act or process of pleading, supporting, or recommending a cause or a person (Dictionary.com, 2019). Even though Deaf people have come a long way, there are still instances when hearing people struggle to look at Deaf people as equals. Often, they will only listen to hearing people like themselves, so this is when hearing allies, like some of you, continue to be needed. The Deaf community has never ceased its efforts to eliminate discriminatory attitudes and behaviors, including barriers to communication. They appre-

ciate the assistance of hearing people in supporting their efforts to live full lives and have access to everything that hearing people have. It is important that these hearing people who endeavor to be allies do not participate in advocacy efforts out of pity or as interfering individuals but rather out of conviction that Deaf people can benefit from this collaborative advocacy in order to counteract discrimination and oppression ("How to be an Ally to the Deaf Community," 2016). This is a social justice effort.

However, there are times when Deaf-hearing cross-cultural conflicts can derail efforts at allyship. Gournaris and Aubrecht (2013) explain that successful Deaf-hearing partnerships in which hearing partners can be allies depend on sensitivity to one's biases, whether for Deaf or hearing cultural aspects, willingness to acknowledge cross-cultural conflicts and improve themselves, true commitment to achieving equality, and empathic understanding of hearing dominance tendencies.

DEAF-HEARING COLLABORATION

When Deaf and hearing people are able to collaborate on issues, there are benefits for both Deaf and hearing collaborators. Although the Deaf person is helped, particularly in cases involving access issues or discrimination, the hearing person also benefits from this type of collaborative advocacy. Through working with the Deaf person or with Deaf people, the hearing person has the opportunity to learn more about Deaf people and about being deaf. The hearing person also has the opportunity to learn more about attitudinal barriers that Deaf people all too often face and develop ways to combat these barriers. The hearing person has the opportunity to become aware of their hearing privileges and welcome dialogue in becoming a better ally. And the Deaf person can learn about hearing perspectives and therefore respond to or work with these perspectives. The four authors contributing to this book exemplify how hearing and deaf people can learn from each other. Three of us are Deaf, one is hearing, and each of us has diverse opinions and beliefs, and we have learned from each other while revising this book.

How did deaf and hearing collaboration start? In fact, there is a long history of deaf and hearing collaboration. We can go back to the time of the Abbe de l'Epee, who is mentioned in Chapter 3. He started his work with deaf children around 1760. In addition to founding the first school for the deaf in Paris, France, he was able to standardize the teaching of signs and present results with successful students who demonstrated they had a language and could communicate. He hired one of his top students, Laurent Clerc, as an assistant teacher and brought him to London, England, to demonstrate the competency of Deaf people to discuss complex issues (Rée, 1999). This is one of the early examples of how a hearing person worked together with a deaf person to advocate for how deaf people should be educated.

While in London, Clerc made the acquaintance of Thomas Hopkins Gallaudet, a hearing individual whose goal was to establish a sign language institution for the deaf in North America (Rée, 1999; Sayers, 2018). Gallaudet came first to London to see what deaf education was like and then went on to Paris to see the school there. While in Paris, he invited Clerc to accompany him to the United States and work with him to open the first school for the deaf in the United States. Clerc had an administrative role in the school for over 40 years. Without this early deaf-hearing collaboration, the history of deaf education in the United States might have been very different. Gallaudet University was named for Thomas Hopkins Gallaudet in recognition of his founding the first school for the deaf in the United States (Van Cleve & Crouch, 1989).

Fast-forward to more recent times, when hearing educators consistently took over the education of deaf children and disregarded the input of educators who were deaf, as exemplified by the result of the 1880 Milan Congress (mentioned in Chapter 1). This trend, an example of hearing superiority or audism attitudes that ignored the contributions Deaf people could make, continued for decades.

With the realization that deaf students on average were not making satisfactory progress in developing language and achieving academically, hearing educators of deaf students are now collaborating with educators who are deaf to develop more effective approaches. Many examples of positive deaf-hearing collaborative efforts can be found in research groups and schools for the deaf throughout the country. Marschark and Lee (2014) note evidence that the Deaf community is advocating for the use of sign language as an integral part of this linguistic-cultural minority community. This lends support for the use of a bilingual approach (see Chapters 4 and 5 for details). At schools such as the Maryland School for the Deaf (2019), there is a strong bilingual approach, spearheaded by its Deaf superintendent, James Tucker, working in collaboration with both Deaf and hearing staff. The school is accredited and can boast of outstanding graduates. This is one example of a successful deaf and hearing collective effort. Another example is that of Kathleen Treni, former principal of the New Jersey Bergen County Special Services School District Program for the Hearing Impaired. She is deaf and worked actively with hearing colleagues to ensure the success of her program, which offers a continuum of communication support services (Schmidberger, 2015). Treni is proud of the high graduation rate of students in this program.

In terms of research, one can point to the highly successful Visual Language and Visual Learning at Gallaudet University, a research center that is supported by the National Science Foundation (VL2, 2019). A primary goal of this center is to include teams of Deaf and hearing researchers from multiple disciplines to carry out its research agenda, a goal that has been admirably carried out. One critical criterion for successful Deaf and hearing research partnerships relies on the ability of hearing collaborators to embrace a Deaf epistemology, meaning that Deaf partners are truly viewed as equal partners, not as tokens, and their knowledge of what it means to be Deaf and critical areas for research is valued by hearing collaborators (Singleton, Jones, & Hanumantha, 2014; Wolsey, Dunn, Gentzke, Joharchi, & Clark, 2017).

What about advocacy? The Americans With Disabilities Act (also see Chapters 8 and 10) has provisions that lower barriers for deaf and hard-of-hearing people. This could not have happened without alliances between deaf and hearing advocates who worked hard to get Congress to pass this act (Lang, 2000; Peltz Strauss, 2006). The same is true for the Newborn and Infant Hearing Screening and Intervention Act of 1999 that requires babies to be tested for hearing at birth (National Association of the

Deaf, 2006). We now have video relay services and television captioning (see Chapter 9). This happened because of strong deaf-hearing collaboration and negotiation with industries providing telecommunication and television services as well as advocating for government regulations to require access (e.g., Ideal Group, 2012).

We need to acknowledge the importance of sign language interpreters in the development of healthy deaf-hearing relationships. After all, how can deaf and hearing people work together if communication access is different? Sign language interpreters serve as bridges to facilitate communication. Serious problems can occur if interpreting is not adequate. For example, if an interpreter incorrectly translates the ASL sign for "acquisition" to the English spoken word, "pick-up," the hearing audience or hearing person may see the deaf person as unsophisticated in the use of language. As the signs for both terms can be easily mistaken for each other, it is critical for the hearing interpreter to understand the context and use the appropriate vocabulary.

To make sure deaf-hearing communication is successful, it is very important to ensure that sign language interpreters are qualified and skillful in formulating accurate translations. If interpreters do not know the terminology in, for example, medicine, law, or engineering, how can they convey accurate information to deaf people? The books, *Deaf Professionals and Designated Interpreters* (Hauser, Finch, & Hauser, 2008) and *Deaf Eyes on Interpreting* (Holcomb & Smith, 2018), explain what interpreters need to do to ensure good collaboration between deaf and hearing people through following up on recommendations made by deaf people.

CAREER POSSIBILITIES

Another way of supporting Deaf people and being not just their advocate but also their ally is to enter careers that involve working with Deaf people and collaborating with them as partners. In that way, you can become effective ongoing advocates for Deaf people, who are often underserved or whose abilities are questioned. The next part of this chapter will highlight examples of different careers that have the potential to positively influence the lives of Deaf people. One important caveat is that in many of these careers, fluency in ASL is a requirement for success, especially in the education and health care/mental health fields, as has been demonstrated in this book. Individuals need to be sensitive to their own ASL fluency levels and accept their need for ASL interpreters when requested by Deaf people. Knowing some ASL is not sufficient in communication-intensive careers. Another important point has to do with ethical considerations in working with a culturally different community, in this case the Deaf community. Sensitivity to linguistic and cultural aspects as well as openness to becoming competent in Deaf culture ways of relating are critical in careers that involve working with culturally Deaf individuals or with Deaf communities.

ASL Interpreters

Deaf people typically do not have full access to spoken language, whether in terms of understanding others or being understood by others, and typically the system is not set to be fully accessible, whether it be in schools, at work, or else-where. Because of this, both Deaf and hearing people will often need sign language interpreters to communicate with each other. Sign language interpreters provide a form of access that helps Deaf and hearing people communicate with each other. There is a critical need for ASL interpreters throughout the United States who sign fluently and read sign language well (National Association of the Deaf, 2019a). ASL interpreters can do freelance interpreting or work for schools, universities, hospitals, agencies, the government, courts, private businesses, or other places in the community. There is also a need for qualified ASL interpreters to provide Video Relay Interpreting (VRS) and Video Remote Interpreting (VRI, equivalent to distance interpreting using a computer and Internet access) (see Chapter 9 for details). By working as an ASL interpreter, you are working to make sure that Deaf people have the same immediate access to information and communication that hearing people have. In that way, you can provide critical support to the Deaf community. Figure 12–1 shows an interpreter at work.

It is important to understand that even if you are fluent in American Sign Language, this does not qualify you to be an ASL interpreter. Many people think that sign language interpreting means that the sign language interpreter signs exactly what the hearing person is saying. That is a myth. Let us explain further. Elizabeth Winston (1994) writes that the process of understanding a language and then interpreting it into another language makes the result not exactly the same. ASL interpreters need to understand the process of translating from one language to another and how to convey the translation so that the meaning is not lost. They

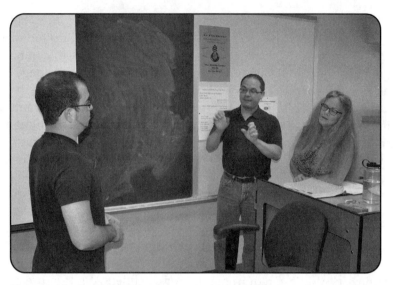

Figure 12–1. Interpreter at work. Used with permission. Photo courtesy of Brian Sattler.

also need to understand the cultures they work with and work to make sure cross-cultural communication between Deaf people, including Deaf people of minority groups, and hearing people is effective. They have to have cognitive, linguistic, and technical skills. They must be able to follow ethical practices, including confidentiality, professionalism, respect for the consumers, and appropriate business practices, and take continuing education courses to keep up to date with the profession. The ability to maintain confidentiality is especially necessary because of the small nature of the Deaf community, where many people know each other but may not always want their information shared. Further information can be found on the website of the Registry of Interpreters for the Deaf (RID, 2019).

All of the skills mentioned here need to be developed. That will require time and training. If you are interested in becoming an ASL interpreter, you can find training programs at community colleges and universities throughout the United States. A BA degree in ASL Interpretation is necessary prior to certification. The RID can help you locate training programs in your area. The RID certifies ASL interpreters basted on training, experience, and examination results.

As a point of information, Deaf individuals can also become interpreters, in this case Deaf Interpreter (DI; National Consortium of Interpreter Education Centers, 2016) or Certified Deaf Interpreter (CDI; RID, 2019). These Deaf interpreters work often with hearing interpreters to ensure that both the spoken and signed languages used by both parties are translated fully and comprehensively. DIs tend to have life experiences that facilitate various ways of communicating with Deaf individuals using a wide range of visual language and communication forms. Gallaudet University's Department of Interpretation and Translation provides training not only for ASL interpreters but also for Deaf Interpreters. Austin Community College was the first to offer a course for Deaf interpreters only.

DeafBlind interpreting, with training provided at Austin Community College and Western Oregon University, is a specialization that requires a different set of skills. DeafBlind interpreters are trained to use tactile or Protactile ASL interpreting. Again, this requires intensive training on how to convey language through tactile means. Protactile ASL was developed by DeafBlind individuals themselves as a means of communicating linguistically using various forms of touch to convey not only body cues but also encourage two-way communication (Morrison & Voight-Campbell, 2017).

Teachers

Teaching is a career that appeals to many individuals. Education is critically impor-tant in ensuring that all children grow up to be knowledgeable and literate. Deaf children have too often been undereducated because of systematic barriers in language and communication (see Chapters 3, 4, and 5). On the other hand, there are many deaf adults who remember excellent teachers in their lives, teachers who were able to reach out to these individuals, communicate with them, and inspire them to do their best in whatever they were doing. What was special about these teachers?

We like to think that these teachers were excellent because they truly cared about the deaf children and youth they were teaching. They made sure their students got the language and the knowledge the students needed. They wanted to make sure their deaf students could maximize their potential and fully contribute to society. Those teachers certainly were on the forefront in advocating for their students by helping them reach their potential.

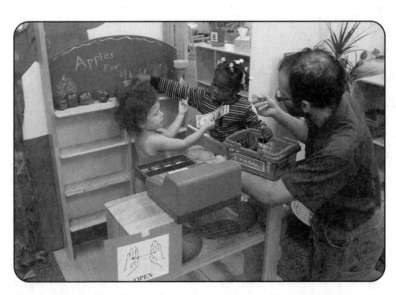

Figure 12–2. Teacher with students. Used with permission.

John Harrington, who taught at P.S. 47 in New York City, thought that one of his students, Alfred "Sonny" Sonnenstrahl, pictured in Figure 12–3, was knowledgeable enough in math to get into Stuyvesant High School, the best high school in New York City at that time (and in the United States as well). But Sonny would have to take an exam to gain admission to Stuyvesant High School. Other teachers were not so sure he could pass because he was Deaf and even expressed that belief to him. Harrington stayed after school every day to tutor Sonny in math and other areas that would be on the exam. Sonny complained as he wanted to play with his friends after school. But he still kept on attending the tutoring sessions. Because of this, he passed among the top 100 out of 2,400 boys who took the test for Stuyvesant. He later became an engineer and eventually an advocate. Many years later, Sonny spoke about John Harrington and how he challenged Sonny to do his very best. He never forgot Harrington and wished he could show his appreciation. (Alfred Sonnenstrahl, personal communication, June 18, 2019)

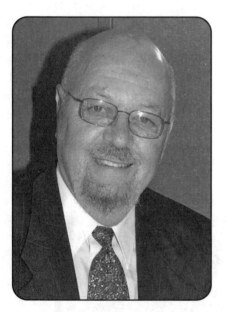

Figure 12–3. Alfred "Sonny" Sonnenstrahl. Used with permission.

Have you thought about teaching deaf students as a career? Understanding Deaf culture and history will help you better understand how to support students who are Deaf. You will be aware of what Deaf students need, especially access to information. If you are hearing, you would be willing to work alongside Deaf teachers, and if you are Deaf, you could guide hearing teachers. Being fluent in sign language is really important if you are interested in teaching deaf children. Administrators of schools for the deaf often need teachers and teacher aides who are fluent in ASL, and deaf students often appreciate these teachers. Not only that, ASL itself is also beneficial for children who can hear but are mute and do not speak, children with autism, and children who respond better to sign language than to spoken language.

If you like children and adolescents, teaching could be your future. You could work as a teacher or teacher's aide in a school for the deaf, or in the mainstream, at public schools with deaf classes or deaf students. Or you can teach in private schools that have deaf students.

Teacher training programs and programs that train teachers' aides, including those programs that focus on deaf students, are eager to recruit future teachers or teacher aides, Deaf and hearing, who have diverse backgrounds. The goal of these programs is to teach future teachers and teacher aides how to effectively help children develop emotionally, socially, and intellectually into adults who can be productive citizens with good quality of life. It takes less than 1 year to learn how to be a teacher's aide, while becoming a teacher requires a college education. But it takes about 7 years to become conversationally competent in ASL, so if you are interested in teaching deaf children, the earlier you can immerse yourself in ASL, the better.

Programs that train teachers for the deaf will also teach about language learning issues and ways of communicating with deaf students. Teachers must be certified. Each state has its own certification requirements. Students who are learning how to be teachers of the deaf must also meet these certification requirements. You also need to be competent in the basic academic areas, including mathematics, science, social studies, and English at the elementary level. The curriculum for deaf students should be the same as that for hearing children. Teacher training programs will help with this. If you want to teach deaf students in high school, you need to be trained also in the content area you plan to teach.

If you want to see more Deaf teachers in the field, you need to be aware that state teaching licensure-certification/Praxis[1] requirements have posed an obstacle for many Deaf teachers. Laurene Simms (2019) argues that there is a need to fight to change the teaching licensure system so that it is more accessible for Deaf teachers. This is something ASL students can try to do as allies.

Early Childhood Educators

Another career possibility is that of early childhood educator. The National Education Association (2019) has claimed that early childhood education is one of the best investments our country can make. Early childhood education covers nursery, prekindergarten, and kindergarten education. Young children who go through early childhood education tend to do better in school later on, get better jobs, and avoid trouble with the law.

There are programs at the community college level to prepare students for early childhood education jobs in a variety of settings, not only schools but also child care settings. There are also undergraduate programs with majors in early childhood education. If you love young children, this is the place for you. And if you want to work with young deaf children, here are some things you need to know.

The Individuals With Disabilities Education Act (IDEA) includes the provision that families are entitled to services for children with disabilities from birth onward (Raimondo & Yoshinaga-Itano, 2016). Deaf children who are enrolled in early intervention programs have a far better chance at developing language, whether signed or spoken, and also the ability to learn many things through using their brain in different ways, guided by caregivers and early childhood intervention specialists (Bosso, 2011). As an early childhood educator working with deaf children and their parents or caregivers, you would be in a unique position to foster the deaf child's language and social development in addition to helping the parents learn how to best communicate with their child. You would probably be

---

[1]Praxis tests measure academic skills and subject-specific content knowledge needed for teaching.

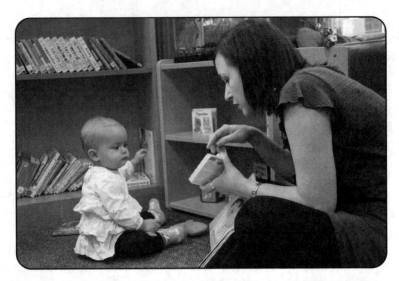

Figure 12–4. Early childhood educator. Used with permission.

working in public school districts, day/residential schools for the deaf, or agencies serving deaf people that have early intervention programs.

To become an early childhood educator working with deaf children, you will need to take courses that cover basic education, early childhood development, language development, audiology, parent issues, the educational nature of play, and so on in addition to an internship experience in working with young deaf children. There are programs in different states that offer both BA and MA degrees in early childhood education. Being fluent in ASL is necessary if you are in programs that encourage a bilingual approach to language learning. Fluency not only in English but also in ASL (just knowing a few signs is not enough) will help the cognitive development of babies and children (see Chapters 4 and 5). Because young deaf children are often fitted with hearing aids or cochlear implants, you will need to make sure these instruments are working properly and being used, and

help parents understand this as well. You will also be using various communication strategies in your work with deaf children and their parents. These strategies include nonverbal communication, directing attention, linking language and meaning, and reducing the need for divided attention (Mohay, 2000).

Audiologists

Most of you probably never heard of the word *audiology* before reading this book. It is well known that people are living longer and longer due to improvement in treating diseases and more healthy living. However, as people age, the possibility of their becoming hard of hearing or deaf increases. The population of people with hearing loss is growing fast. When they need help in checking their hearing, they may go to an otologist (ear doctor) or ear, nose, and throat (ENT) doctor. Often the doctor will refer them to an audiologist for further evaluation. Because of this, the word *audiology* should be more familiar with the general population, but that is not the case.

Exactly what do audiologists do? They evaluate hearing loss and make recommendations about the best way to work with what hearing is left. This is called "aural rehabilitation." If you have read Chapter 2, you now have some idea of what auditory technology is. Audiologists are trained to be experts in auditory technology. They do hearing screening to determine if there is a possible hearing loss. They also do hearing evaluations using various tests to find out the hearing level and the extent of difficulty a person may have in understanding speech. If necessary, they will follow up with a hearing aid evaluation to determine which hearing aid is best for the type of hearing loss the client may have. If the person meets the criteria for cochlear implantation (see Chapter 2), the audiologist may discuss cochlear implant options and ask if the individual is interested. Audiologists often work in hospitals, schools, audiology clinics, rehabilitation centers, and private practices.

When a baby is identified as deaf after undergoing universal newborn hearing screening in the hospital shortly after birth and being followed up by the otologist or ENT, the audiologist is usually the next person to meet with the parents or caregivers. The audiologist is a very important member of the early intervention team (St. John, Lytle, Nussbaum, & Shoup, 2016). If the audiologist is an ally to the Deaf community, the audiologist will be very careful to explain all types of language and communication opportunities to the parents or caregivers. The audiologist can explain about the role of ASL in English language development and about resources in the Deaf community as well as resources for spoken language. The audiologist can help parents and caregivers feel comfortable about having a child who may eventually become part of the Deaf community. The audiologist can also advocate for better hearing services for the larger community as well as better

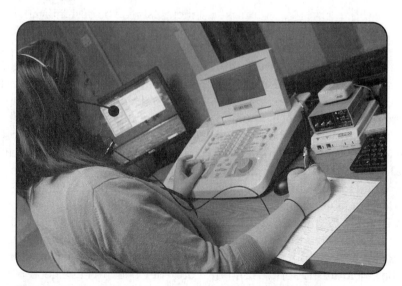

Figure 12–5. Audiologist at work. Used with permission.

access to resources for parents of deaf children. This is especially important in rural areas where services are few and far apart. Attending EHDI (Early Hearing Detection and Intervention) meetings will help the audiologist develop effective strategies to advocate for more quality early intervention programs at the state level, emphasize the importance of follow-up when babies are first identified as deaf, and increase awareness of how to create quality services.

To become an audiologist requires 4 years of graduate training and a doctoral degree called the AuD (Doctor of Audiology). You can have a bachelor's degree in any field to enter a training program in audiology (All Allied Health Schools, 2019). You have to be very interested in technology and relate well with people in order to succeed as an audiologist. If audiologists are fluent in ASL, culturally Deaf people will appreciate their services as long as they feel that audiologists respect their decisions about hearing amplification and communication.

Speech and Language Therapists

You may ask why this category is in a book about Deaf culture and sign language! Speech and language pathologists, often known as speech and language therapists, often collaborate with audiologists in treatment planning for young deaf and hard-of-hearing children who are expected to have difficulty in producing understandable speech. However, speech and language therapists can be of help if they recognize the importance of Deaf culture and support a bilingual program that includes not only ASL but also spoken English. Case in point: Culturally Deaf mothers have decided on

cochlear implants for their deaf children, and several of them agreed to participate in an interview study (Mitchiner, 2015; Mitchiner & Sass-Lehrer, 2011). These Deaf mothers saw the need to expose their Deaf children to spoken language as well as ASL. They wanted their children to be fluent in both languages. They knew there was a need to expose their Deaf children to more spoken language than what they could provide in the home. It was a challenge for them to find services and programs that exposed their children to both ASL and spoken English. They had to scramble to get help from hard-of-hearing or hearing family members, hearing teachers, peers, and speech therapists. One mother stated that her hearing son's first language was ASL, and he could learn spoken language outside the home. Why couldn't her Deaf child have the same experience? In the end, those mothers felt their children did well in developing spoken language because they already had ASL as a means to help them transition to spoken language.

This is where speech and language therapists can be of significant help in supporting this process. If they are comfortable working within a bilingual approach, they will be of great service to the slowly increasing number of children from culturally Deaf families who now have cochlear implants. Their job is to evaluate speech, language, and communication and work with children (and adults, too) to improve their spoken language (American Speech-Hearing-Language Association, 2019). They can be found in public or private schools, hospitals, rehabilitation centers, community clinics, university speech and hearing centers, and so on. They need to have good people skills, patience, and imagination in developing good treatment plans. There are numer-

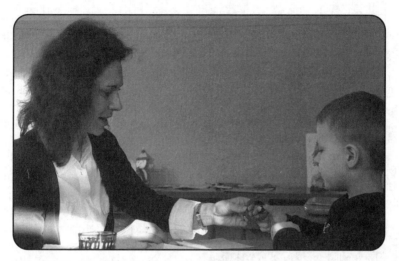

Figure 12–6. Speech therapist at work. Photo by Pixabay.com/ CC by 1.0.

ous job opportunities after training at the graduate level as a master's degree is required. At the undergraduate level, a strong general liberal arts background is good preparation for graduate study in speech and language pathology.

Vocational Rehabilitation Counselors and Job Coaches

Who helps Deaf people get jobs? Yes, friends and family can be helpful. Vocational rehabilitation counselors are also key players in helping Deaf people prepare for and obtain employment. Their job is to assess the individual's capabilities and limitations, help the client set goals for employment and independent living, arrange the necessary training and therapy to meet these goals, and finally facilitate training and placement (Price, 2018). A desire to help people fulfill their goals, good listening skills, patience, and compassion are necessary in order to do a good job as a vocational rehabilitation counselor.

The vocational rehabilitation counselor is in an excellent position to advocate for Deaf people, especially Deaf students. This counselor is also in an excellent position as an ally to help Deaf clientele develop self-advocacy skills, thereby empowering them to take charge of their work situations (Schoffstall, Cawthon, Tarantolo-Leppo, & Wendel, 2015). Many state governments have rehabilitation services for deaf and hard-of-hearing clients. These services include audiological evaluation and assessment, assistive devices, telecommunication devices, speech and language therapy, and interpreter services.

Vocational rehabilitation counselors may be assigned to schools for the deaf or get referrals of deaf students in the mainstream. With their knowledge about what Deaf people can do, they are in a good position to assess the potential for each Deaf client, develop goals with the client, and advocate to ensure that the Deaf client can get good training, a college education, or entry into jobs. Many Deaf people appreciate the support their vocational rehabilitation counselor gave

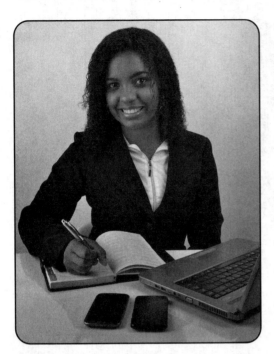

Figure 12–7. Vocational rehabilitation counselor at work. Photo by Pixabay.com/CC by 1.0.

them when they were starting to explore careers and training/education possibilities. They especially appreciate those counselors who know ASL, can communicate with them, and help them with their goals. Without these services, it is easy for many Deaf people to fall through the cracks and not receive the best preparation for careers and jobs. This leads to these individuals applying for and receiving Social Security Disability Insurance benefits rather than work, particularly if this income is greater than what they may obtain with minimum wage jobs.

Although there are vocational rehabilitation counselors with BA degrees who can do case management, it is best to get a master's degree in rehabilitation counseling. This degree takes 2 years of full-time enrollment to complete. Graduates can obtain jobs in the educational system, including high schools, state government agencies that focus on rehabilitation services, hospitals, and nonprofit or community agencies. The Division of Deaf Studies and Professional Studies at Western Oregon University offers a graduate specialization in rehabilitation counseling.

Job coaches are part of vocational rehabilitation services. Their primary function is to help vocational clients learn how to do jobs and accurately carry out job functions, usually on a one-on-one basis. They develop plans that will help them train the new employees to perform their jobs adequately (Inge, Green, & Targett, n.d.). Job coaching requires a high school diploma. Different states may have different certification requirements for job coaches.

Even if you are not interested in this type of career, here is how you can get involved. You could meet with your state vocational rehabilitation services office to learn more about how you can support their efforts to serve Deaf people and increase employment opportunities. This is another good advocacy opportunity. If you ever have your own business or manage a business, such as a Subway franchise, you can think about hiring qualified deaf people or training deaf people to do the jobs that are part of the business. After all, venues like Kuala Lumpur in Malaysia's and DC's Signing Starbucks or San Francisco's Mozzeria (a pizza restaurant) are staffed by Deaf employees.

Mental Health Service Providers

The majority of Deaf people do get through life just fine. But, just as for the hearing population, there are Deaf people who need mental health services, as mentioned in Chapter 8. However, it has been documented that this special population is woefully underserved (e.g., Glickman, 2013). Outside of the major cities in the United States, there are very few places such as community agencies and private practices where culturally Deaf people can receive assessment, psychotherapy, or medications and experience direct communication in ASL. There are also significant problems with incorrect diagnoses. Hearing professionals who know very little about Deaf culture or how Deaf people communicate may mistakenly diagnose Deaf people as having intellectual disabilities, developmental delays, or mental illness. Because of this, there is a strong need for advocacy to make sure Deaf people who need mental health support get linguistic and culturally accessible assessment and treatment from professionals who know Deaf culture (National Association of the Deaf, 2019b). On its website, the NAD addresses the need for state and federal agencies as well as mental health centers to understand the needs of Deaf children and adults with mental health issues, especially regarding linguistic and cultural affirmation. This website also mentions what to do in case of discrimination in providing services, such as not providing qualified ASL interpreters. One way in which mental health service providers who are fluent in ASL can broaden service delivery is through telepsychiatry and teletherapy (Wilson & Schild, 2020). The 2020 coronavirus pandemic has highlighted the importance of using this technology to help with mental health issues with the population being sequestered at home to prevent the spread of COVID-19.

Even with the increased use of telehealth services, again, the problem is that we do not have enough qualified mental health professionals who understand Deaf culture and are fluent in ASL. Just

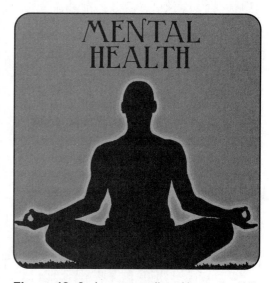

Figure 12–8. Image credit to Alexander Wilkins. Used with permission.

taking an ASL course is not enough. But some professionals do take an ASL course and think they are fluent after taking a few courses. It takes a long time to become fluent in ASL. So that should give you an idea of how important advocacy for this group of Deaf people is, so that they can get the help they need. This includes not only advocating for accessible services that individuals need but also for increasing employment opportunities at mental health and rehabilitation agencies.

So, what are mental health career possibilities? An overview of training needs for these careers can be found in a chapter written by Brice, Leigh, Sheridan, and Smith (2013). Here, we describe a volunteer opportunity and several career tracks for mental health service providers.

Hotline Volunteer

Being a hotline volunteer is a good way to gain the skills that are needed for mental health career training opportunities. Good listening and communication skills are important and part of the training that usually takes several weeks. This is an opportunity for personal growth. You can volunteer for crisis lines or sexual assault support service hotlines if you are fluent in ASL. There are hotlines specifically designated for deaf callers, such as the one provided by ADWAS (see Chapter 8 for a discussion of domestic violence). After you gain experience providing hotline services, you can provide training to new volunteers. This type of experience can help you decide if you are interested in becoming a mental health service provider.

Clinical Mental Health Counselor

This is a profession that focuses on combining psychotherapy with practical, problem-solving approaches to help clients change their approach to the problems they face if they are having difficulty dealing with these problems (CounselorLicense.com, 2019). Clinical mental health counselors do assessment, diagnosis, crisis management, brief and solution-focused therapy, alcoholism and substance abuse treatment, and psychoeducation/prevention programs. They work in a wide variety of settings, including community agencies, hospitals, substance abuse treatment centers, and behavioral health organizations. Training is at the graduate level and a master's degree is required. To be licensed requires that one pass a national or state-level licensing examination.

There are two training programs that prepare students to become mental health counselors who work with deaf and hard-of-hearing people. One is at Gallaudet University and the other is at Western Oregon University. These programs have as their goal that of preparing counselors who are highly skilled at communicating with Deaf people and are knowledgeable about the culture of Deaf people.

School Counselor

This career track involves doing counseling in schools or other educational settings. The goal of the school counselor is to help students focus on academic, personal, social, and career development so that they can do well in school and be prepared to function well after school is completed (American School Counselor Association, 2019). They also help coordinate students, parents, and teachers when it comes to issues related to goals, abilities, and areas that need improvement. Gallaudet University's counseling department adds a mental health component to the school counseling training in order to provide more support to students as needed. You can see how a school counselor can provide support by helping the student solve problems, such as family or emotional problems, which make it hard to achieve academically. In the mainstream, where most Deaf students are, the school counselor will not know much about what the Deaf student's life is like or understand the needs of the Deaf student. Advocating by helping the school counselor to understand what is needed can be very helpful for Deaf students who are alone in the mainstream.

Social Work

This is a broad career that has opportunities for different types of social work activities. These activities include helping people obtain services that they need; counseling and psychotherapy with individuals, families, and groups; helping organizations or communities provide or improve social and health services; and working on legislative efforts (National Association of Social Workers, 2019). Overall, there needs to be a commitment to social justice and social change.

Areas of practice include, for example, adolescent health, aging, behavioral health, end of life, children/youth/families, clinical social work, and school social work, and we can add Deaf and hard-of-hearing individuals and their families! Because of their training in legislative work and advocacy, social workers may be well prepared to advocate for the needs of Deaf populations, as well as other underserved populations. The Social Work program at Gallaudet University is in an excellent position to train students to do exactly that. There are many general social work programs throughout the United States, but Gallaudet University's Social Work program is the only one in the country that includes the Deaf component. This program offers both bachelor's- and master's-level training.

Clinical Psychology

Clinical psychologists focus on mental health and do assessment, diagnosis, psychotherapy, and prevention of mental health problems (American Psychological Association, 2019). These problems include, for example, depression and anxiety. Clinical psychologists also promote positive adjustment, personal development, and the ability to adapt to different life situations. In working with individuals, families, and groups, clinical psychologists can work in a variety of specialty areas, including child or adult mental health, learning disabilities, emotional disturbances, substance abuse, geriatrics,

health psychology, and neuropsychology. With appropriate training, some states allow clinical psychologists to prescribe medication for psychiatric disorders. Similar to the above disciplines, clinical psychologists also work in hospitals, medical centers, private practice, community agencies, academic settings, or private practice. It is important to have good communication skills and be creative in terms of treatment planning.

For this career, a doctoral degree is required, either a PhD or a PsyD. The training is challenging and intensive. There are many clinical psychology doctoral programs to choose from, but again Gallaudet University offers the only PhD program in clinical psychology that includes specialization in working with and researching Deaf populations. This program requires that graduates be competent in communicating with and treating Deaf people in need of mental health services. It also emphasizes the need to partner with Deaf people as a way of helping them achieve a positive quality of life.

If thinking about a doctorate is too far off, you can take psychology courses at the undergraduate level. There are psychology career opportunities with an undergraduate degree in psychology. This degree can be obtained at many colleges and universities. If you do major in psychology and are not sure you want to continue right away with graduate study, there are several jobs that you could consider exploring that relate to mental health (Cherry, 2019). These jobs include case management, career counselor, rehabilitation specialist, sales representative, and psychiatric technician. Skills required for these jobs cover the ability to assess client needs, keep good records, express care and empathy, and advocate for the client.

Emergency Medical Technicians

Emergency medical technicians (EMTs) are health service providers who initially evaluate patients in emergencies and determine what to do next. They respond to all kinds of emergencies such as heart attacks, pandemics, accidents on land, criminal violence, and natural disasters such as hurricanes. If patients need to go to the hospital, what EMTs do is provide medical support while getting the patients into ambulances and rushing them to hospitals.

Deaf people are able to call 911 using video relay services, captioned telephones, or TTYs (see Chapter 9). If EMTs can communicate with them, the process of evaluating the emergency and making decisions becomes easier. There are basic, intermediate, and paramedic levels of training that go from weeks to months. You can Google EMT training to get more information about training. There are deaf people who work as EMTs, including ASL users (Harvey, 2017).

Other Career Possibilities

Frankly, in any career that you may choose, knowing ASL may strengthen your application for any type of work because you most likely will encounter Deaf people in your line of work. Think about, for example, hairdresser, computer technician, cafeteria worker, police officer, sanitary worker, Park Services ranger, sales clerk, dental hygienist, funeral director, paralegal, day care worker, auto mechanic, and so on. These are jobs that do not require more than a high school or community college education, depending on the field. Your ability to use ASL with Deaf people, whatever your career choice is, will make a difference, and feedback from them will show their appreciation. There is a quote by Nelson Mandela (2008): "If you talk to

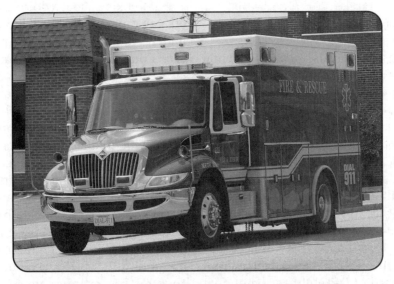

Figure 12–9. An emergency vehicle. Photo by Morguefile.com/ CC by 1.0.

a man in a language he understands, that goes to his head. If you talk to him in his language, that goes to his heart."

CONCLUSIONS

We have covered just a few of the career possibilities in working with Deaf people. We have also emphasized the need to be advocates for Deaf people and to support them so that they can have similar access to services and events, just as hearing people do. We have also discussed the importance of deaf and hearing collaboration as well as fluency in ASL. You can be creative and find ways in which you can advocate for or support Deaf people, depending on the areas you are interested in.

REFERENCES

All Allied Health Schools. (2019). *How to become an audiologist: Education, licensing, and certification.* Retrieved from https://www.allalliedhealthschools.com/physical-therapy/how-to-become-an-audiologist/

American Psychological Association. (2019). *Clinical psychology.* Retrieved from https://www.apa.org/ed/graduate/specialize/clinical

American School Counselor Association. (2019). *School counselors: Our impact.* Retrieved from https://www.schoolcounselor.org/school-counselors-members/careers-roles

American-Speech-Language-Hearing Association. (2019). *Your career is calling.* Retrieved from https://hearingandspeechcareers.org/

Bosso, E. (2011). Letter from the Vice President, Early childhood intervention: Foundations for success. *Odyssey, 12,* 2.

Brice, P., Leigh, I. W., Sheridan, M., & Smith, K. (2013). Training of mental health professionals: Yesterday, today, and tomorrow. In N. Glickman (Ed.), *Deaf mental health care* (pp. 298–322). New York, NY: Routledge.

Cherry, K. (2019). *Entry-level job options for psychology majors.* Retrieved from https://www.verywellmind.com/what-can-you-do-with-a-bachelors-degree-in-psychology-2794943

Collom, L. (2013). Feds target Arizona complex for hearing-impaired. *The Arizona Republic.* Retrieved from https://www.usatoday.com/story/news/nation/2013/05/29/feds-target-complex-for-hearing-impaired/2368573/

Counselor-License.com. (2019). *Mental health counselor.* Retrieved from https://counselor-license.com/careers/mental-health-counselor/

CRPD. (2016). *Convention on the Rights of Persons With Disabilities.* Retrieved from https://www.un.org/development/desa/disabilities/convention-on-the-rights-of-persons-with-disabilities.html

Dictionary.com. (2019). Retrieved from https://www.dictionary.com/browse/advocacy

Glickman, N. (Ed.). (2013). *Deaf mental health care.* New York, NY: Routledge.

Gournaris, M. J., & Aubrecht, A. (2013). Deaf/hearing cross-cultural conflicts and the creation of culturally competent treatment programs. In N. Glickman (Ed.), *Deaf mental health care* (pp. 69–106). New York, NY: Routledge.

Harvey, A. (2017). Being Deaf in EMS. *EMSWorld.* Retrieved from https://www.emsworld.com/article/218355/being-deaf-ems

Hauser, P., Finch, K., & Hauser, A. (2008). *Deaf professionals and designated interpreters.* Washington, DC: Gallaudet University Press.

Holcomb, T., & Smith, D. (Eds.). (2018). *Deaf eyes on interpreting.* Washington, DC: Gallaudet University Press.

How to be an ally to the deaf community. (2016). Retrieved from https://store.treehousevideo.com/contents/read-how-to-be-an-ally-to-the-deaf-community/

Ideal Group. (2012). *Steve Jacobs and the history of video relay services in the United States.*

Retrieved from http://www.ideal-group .org/?p=91

Inge, K., Green, H., & Targett, P. (n.d.). *Supporting individuals with significant disabilities: The roles of a job coach.* Retrieved from https://vcurrtc.org/research/printView.cfm/630

Lang, H. (2000). *A phone of our own.* Washington, DC: Gallaudet University Press.

Mandela, N. (2008). *Mandela in his own words.* Retrieved from http://edition.cnn.com/2008/WORLD/africa/06/24/mandela .quotes/

Marschark, M., & Lee, C. (2014). Navigating two languages in the classroom. In M. Marschark, G. Tang, & H. Knoors (Eds.), *Bilingualism and bilingual deaf education* (pp. 213–341). New York, NY: Oxford University Press.

Maryland School for the Deaf. (2019). Retrieved from http://www.msd.edu

Mitchiner, J. (2015). Deaf parents of cochlear-implanted children: Beliefs in bimodal bilingualism. *Journal of Deaf Studies and Deaf Education, 20*(1), 51–66.

Mitchiner, J., & Sass-Lehrer, M. (2011). My child can have more choices: Reflections of Deaf mothers on cochlear implants for their children. In R. Paludneviciene & I. W. Leigh (Eds.), *Cochlear implants: Evolving perspectives* (pp. 71–94). Washington, DC: Gallaudet University Press.

Mohay, H. (2000). Language in sight: Mothers' strategies for making language visually accessible to deaf children. In P. Spencer, C. Erting, & M. Marschark (Eds.), *The deaf child in the family and at school* (pp. 151–166). Mahwah, NJ: Erlbaum.

Morrison, S., & Voight-Campbell, R. (2017). *What is ProTactile and what are its benefits?* Retrieved from https://www.tsbvi.edu/tools-items/573-tx-senseabilities/fall-2017/5651-what-is-protactile-and-what-are-its-benefits

National Association of Social Workers. (2019). *Practice.* Retrieved from https://www.social workers.org/Practice

National Association of the Deaf. (2006). *Nationwide hearing screening for deaf infants.* Retrieved from http://www.infanthearing .org/resources_home/positionstatements/docs_ps/National%20Association%20of% 20the%20Deaf.pdf

National Association of the Deaf. (2014). *The battle for accessible housing.* Retrieved from https://www.nad.org/2014/01/30/the-battle-for-accessible-housing/

National Association of the Deaf. (2019a). *Interpreting American Sign Language.* Retrieved from http://www.nad.org/issues/ameri can-sign-language/interpreting-american-sign-language

National Association of the Deaf. (2019b). *Mental health services.* Retrieved from http://www.nad.org/issues/health-care/mental-health-services

National Consortium of Interpreter Education Centers. (2016). *Deaf interpreter.* Retrieved from http://www.interpretereducation.org/%20specialization/deaf-interpreter/

National Education Association. (2019). *Early childhood education.* Retrieved from http://www.nea.org/home/18163.htm

Peltz Strauss, K. (2006). *A new civil right.* Washington, DC: Gallaudet University Press.

Price, E. (2018). *How to become a vocational rehabilitation counselor.* Retrieved from https://www.innerbody.com/careers-in-health/how-to-become-a-vocational-rehabilitation-counselor.html

Raimondo, B., & Yoshinaga-Itano, C. (2016). Legislation, policies, and the role of research in shaping early intervention. In M. Sass-Lehrer (Ed.), *Early intervention for deaf and hard-of-hearing infants, toddlers, and their families* (pp. 105–134). New York, NY: Oxford University Press.

Rée, J. (1999). *I see a voice.* New York, NY: Metropolitan Books.

RID. (2019). *Registry of Interpreters for the Deaf.* Retrieved from https://rid.org/rid-certi fication-overview/available-certification/cdi-certification/

Sayers, E. (2018). *The life and times of T. H. Gallaudet.* Lebanon, NH: ForeEdge Press.

Schmidberger, S. (2015). A New Jersey partnership that works! *Volta Voices, 22,* 30–31.

Schoffstall, S., Cawthon, S., Tarantolo-Leppo, R., & Wendel, E. (2015). Developing consumer and system-level readiness for effective self-advocacy: Perspectives from vocational rehabilitation counselors working with deaf and hard of hearing individuals in post-secondary settings. *Journal of Developmental and Physical Disabilities, 27*(3), 533–555.

Simms, L. (2009, July). *Beyond the L2 profession.* Paper presented at the American Sign Language Teachers Association Conference, San Diego, CA.

Singleton, J., Jones, G., & Hanumantha, S. (2014). Towards ethical research practice with deaf participants. *Journal of Empirical Research on Human Research Ethics, 9*(3), 59–66.

St. John, R., Lytle, L., Nussbaum, D., & Shoup, A. (2016). Getting started: Hearing screening, evaluation, and next steps. In M. Sass-Lehrer (Ed.), *Early intervention for deaf and hard-of-hearing infants, toddlers, and their families* (pp. 169–197). New York, NY: Oxford University Press.

Van Cleve, J., & Crouch, B. (1989). *A place of their own.* Washington, DC: Gallaudet University Press.

VL2. (2019). *Visual language and visual learning.* Retrieved from http://vl2.gallaudet.edu

Wilson, J. & Schild, S. (2020). Provision of mental health care services to deaf individuals using telehealth. *Professional Psychology: Research and Practice, 45*(5), 324–331.

Winston, E. (1994). An interpreted education: Inclusion or exclusion? In R. C. Johnson & O. P. Cohen (Eds.), *Implications and complications for deaf students of the full inclusion movement* (Gallaudet Research Institute Occasional Paper 94-2, pp. 55–62). Washington, DC: Gallaudet Research Institute.

Wolsey, J.-L. A., Dunn, K. M., Gentzke, S. W., Joharchi, H. A., & Clark, M. D. (2017). Deaf/hearing research partnerships. *American Annals of the Deaf, 161*(5), 571–582.

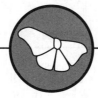

CHAPTER 13

Final Thoughts on
Deaf Culture and Its Future

In this book, you have noticed how vibrant and alive the Deaf community in the United States is. Our "take-away" to you is this: Deaf culture is more than signing, separate schools, and a past history and heritage. Although all of these are fundamental, still Deaf culture is much more. *Deaf culture reflects a diverse group of people who may have different perspectives but have in common the understanding of what it means to be Deaf, and incorporating visual and tactile ways of connecting with their environment. For them, being Deaf often includes the use of signed languages and written languages in visual and tactile senses, and the ability to enjoy productive lives and connect with others who are Deaf, DeafDisabled, and DeafBlind.*

Within today's modern Deaf culture, there is so much going on in the Internet, the arts, and the development of ASL courses as well as bilingual programs in various schools for the deaf, plus research on the linguistics of ASL. Either annually or every two years, there have been large gatherings of Deaf people at conventions held by, for example, Deaf Seniors of America, the National Association of the Deaf, National Black Deaf Advocates,

International Catholic Deaf Association and other religious associations, Council de Manos, and TDI (Telecommunications for the Deaf). During the 2020 coronavirus pandemic, in-person gatherings were not possible to minimize the spread of the virus. Instead, Deaf organizations created opportunities for online meetings and gatherings thanks to technology (see next paragraph). Deaf people have organized cruises and tours to go overseas and learn about other countries and cultures. In many communities, Deaf festivals and Deaf expos are popular. Deaflympics, an international winter and summer sports event held every 4 years, attracts Deaf people from all over the world.

Technology, in particular videophones, texting, FaceTime and Skype, YouTube, and so on, has greatly improved access to information and has provided more connections among Deaf people themselves. Thanks to the Internet, people can open an iPad and with a click get into Deaf-based websites, authentically told and seen through the lens of Deaf people themselves rather than being filtered through hearing people's perspectives.

Thinking back to the Deaf gain concept presented in Chapter 1, you can see the benefits to being Deaf when you consider the visual and tactile aspects of ASL and the use of eyes and touch to connect with the world. The recently developed concept of DeafSpace is one example (Bauman, 2013; Hurley, 2016). DeafSpace focuses on architecture or areas with open vistas, open rooms, eye contact, visual attention, and creativity, as well as a different way of experiencing the environment. It is a type of space that is also popular in newly built homes with more open spaces. Yet, with all of these developments, various writers have expressed fears about the future of Deaf culture and the Deaf community. Why?

Some Deaf children are born to Deaf parents and often are born into the culture of Deaf people. Most deaf children born to hearing parents are not exposed to historical and social aspects of Deaf culture from birth onward, but still these children are experiencing their world as Deaf people, using their senses in a different way compared with hearing peers. That has been true for centuries. With the increasing number of deaf children in mainstream education programs rather than in specialized schools for the deaf, the pathways to Deaf culture are not as straightforward compared to previous years. Back then, in schools for the Deaf, Deaf children absorbed Deaf culture as they interacted with Deaf peers and Deaf adult role models. And technology has increasingly made it possible for Deaf people to access hearing societies in ways they never could have imagined in years past. With advances in hearing technology, including FM systems, digital hearing aids and cochlear implants, access to the Internet, improvements in telecommunications and signaling devices, and legisla-

tion such as the ADA protecting the rights of people with various disabilities, the opportunities for Deaf people to immerse themselves in hearing society have greatly increased. For example, increasing numbers of Deaf students opt to go to hearing colleges instead of colleges with specialized teaching for Deaf students, such as Gallaudet University, Ohlone College, Southwestern College for the Deaf, California State University at Northridge, and the National Technical Institute for the Deaf at Rochester Institute of Technology. The plus here is that these Deaf college students are bringing their ASL and Deaf culture to mainstream universities and their communities, thus increasing awareness among hearing administrators, faculty, and students who may previously have never met a Deaf person.

Moving on, the number of deaf children and adults with cochlear implants continues to increase. Research results indicate that these individuals have the potential to significantly improve their ability to understand spoken language and speak the language, but see comments below regarding those who do not benefit from their cochlear implant. Parents are less inclined to encourage their deaf child to be part of a community of Deaf people when they see the child communicating with hearing family and friends. Medical advances have resulted in more deaf children surviving illness and trauma, but with additional disabilities that may make it difficult for them to be part of Deaf culture. Stem cell research has strengthened the possibility for hearing nerve cell regeneration. There is ongoing genetic research to separate deaf genes and in this way minimize the possibility of deaf children being born. Some see this as a gift to society, while others describe this effort as a form of eugenics to eliminate Deaf people. So what does all this mean for Deaf culture? Is Deaf culture as a way of life doomed to fade away?

> Perhaps you can have a discussion on whether it is a good idea for scientists to continue to find ways to eliminate genes that affect the ability to hear. What are your thoughts about this issue?

Carol Padden (n.d.) writes that even back in 1913, Deaf people were wondering if the Deaf community would survive. This was because of the decision at the 1880 International Congress on the Education of the Deaf in Milan, Italy, to stop the use of sign language in schools for the deaf (see Chapter 1). Fast-forward to 2004, when Trevor Johnston of Australia wrote the following article: "W(h)ither the Deaf Community? Population, Genetics, and the Future of Australian Sign Language." In this article, he forecast a diminishing of the signing Deaf community and loss of Auslan (Australian Sign Language) due to improved medical care, mainstreaming, cochlear implants (in Australia, approximately 90% of deaf children have cochlear implants), and genetic engineering. In a later interview, Johnston continued to fear the loss of Auslan (White, 2014). However, he stated that the fear of losing a sign language, in his case Auslan, is less because of FaceTime and Skype, which allow Deaf people separated by geography to communicate regularly. Not only that, interestingly, users of Auslan have increased compared to 2002, when Johnston was doing the research for his 2004 article. But he still predicts the loss of sign languages in smaller developed countries such as in Australia. He feels that signing through

FaceTime and Skype is not the same as face-to-face signing, and thus the sign language may be altered because of these different modes of transmission. How sign language is adapting to these different modes, including the use of handheld mobile phones, has been assessed (e.g., Keating, Edwards, & Mirus, 2008; Lucas, Mirus, Palmer, Roessler, & Frost, 2013).

We four authors say Deaf culture is alive and well. Why do we think this is so? We do recognize that Deaf culture continues to evolve, as it has evolved through the centuries of its existence. If you google Deaf culture on the Internet, what will you find? Lots and lots of listings related to Deaf culture and what it is like today compared to what it was like in the past. Because of the Internet, Deaf culture is now being transmitted to a much larger audience of interested people, not only in the United States but all over the world as well. The ways Deaf people interact on a daily basis are different, thanks to the Internet, a rising educated Deaf middle class that focuses on small gatherings, and organizations and associations that provide legal, advocacy, and social services to Deaf people. Also, Deaf people continue to attend ASL services at religious settings that are sensitive to their needs. There are Deaf ministers, priests, and rabbis who conduct services in ASL, and the Internet shows an imam signing as well. During the 2020 coronavirus (COVID-19) pandemic, press conferences held by governors in 47 different states showed ASL interpreters conveying health-related updates, thanks to the advocacy efforts of Deaf people who see themselves as deserving equal access to health-related information.

A most surprising development in recent times is that enrollment in ASL and Deaf Studies classes has grown by leaps and bounds in public schools and universities. Following close behind is an explosion of research on the pedagogical practices of the teaching of ASL as a L1 (first language) and L2 (second language) (Rosen, 2020). Today, schools, universities and colleges are uniquely positioned to utilize ASL and Deaf Studies classrooms to increase the presence of Deaf and DeafDisabled individuals on campus as teachers and as students (Robinson & Henner. 2018).

ASL signs are also taught to hearing babies to jumpstart early communication. ASL signs are expanding. Academic ASL is now differentiated from the everyday use of ASL, just as Academic English is differentiated from everyday spoken English. ASL, similarly to Auslan, is also evolving, with new vocabulary and with changes in use as individuals from the mainstream come in contact with the Deaf community or communities.

Deaf mentors are now trained to teach babies who are recently implanted to use signs first, so that these deaf children can "piggyback" their speech onto the signs that they use, believing that this may be one way to develop spoken English (Yoshinaga-Itano, 2006). Published research continues to investigate this process to determine how the interface between spoken and signed languages can facilitate language development (e.g., Giezen, Baker, & Escudero, 2013; Goodwin, Davidson, & Lillo-Martin (2017). VL2 (Visual Language and Visual Learning), a large research program housed at Gallaudet University, has produced research into how ASL can facilitate English learning in creative ways that will expand the usefulness of ASL and English bilingual instruction in public schools. Another research team, the CERP (Center for Education Research Partnerships) at the National

Technical Institute for the Deaf at Rochester Institute of Technology, has conducted studies to explore the cognitive and language underpinnings of deaf students' learning, including those who use ASL, use sign communication, and have cochlear implants. They have published numerous books for researchers, teachers, and parents that synthesize hundreds of studies in deaf education, including the use of ASL. The National Deaf Center on Postsecondary Outcomes at the University of Texas at Austin, directed by Dr. Stephanie Cawthon, a hard-of-hearing educational psychologist, regularly publishes monographs about diversity and Deaf persons in higher education and employment.

Research into ASL as a language has expanded from investigations of the structure and form of ASL into brain studies that teach us how sign languages as well as visual-spatial stimuli are processed in the brain. Studies using brain scans of infants, children, and adults are providing insights into the development of the bimodal bilingual brain, thereby deepening our understanding of the psycholinguistics and neurolinguistics of both spoken and sign languages.

VL2, mentioned above, also has a brain laboratory, called BL2 (Brain and Language Laboratory for Neuroimaging), where research is being conducted on the deaf bimodal bilingual brain.

Dr. Poorna Kushalnagar, who herself is Deaf, directs the Deaf Health Communication and Quality of Life Research Lab at Gallaudet University. She is the principal investigator of grants funded by the National Institutes of Health (NIH) that total close to $3 million. These grants support studies aligned with her primary interests in culturally Deaf health communication and culturally Deaf patient-reported outcomes research, all of which involve collaborations between Deaf and hearing researchers and community members. All of these research activities are evidence of how fertile the field is in the research of signed languages and Deaf culture.

We underscore the point that not all children with cochlear implants are lost to Deaf culture. Although there are many cochlear-implanted children who are using only spoken language, large-scale results continue to be variable. This means that there are too many who continue to struggle with learning to listen and speak. More and more of them are being exposed to sign language to support their development of spoken language. And schools for the deaf are becoming more bilingual and bimodal with the goal of helping deaf children develop competency in both languages. This is in large part in response to a glaring need for change since too many deaf children are lagging in educational achievement. Additionally, there are successful charter schools for the deaf that focus on bilingual and bicultural education.

Roberta "Bobbi" Cordano, pictured in Figure 13–1, the first female Deaf president of Gallaudet University, is a founding member of two successful charter schools for the deaf, the Metro Deaf School, a pre-K through eighth-grade school, and the Minnesota North Star Academy, for high school students, both of which are located in St. Paul, Minnesota. These charter schools, which have now merged into one entity, are both bilingual and bicultural. This shows her belief in and commitment to bilingual, bicultural education for Deaf children.

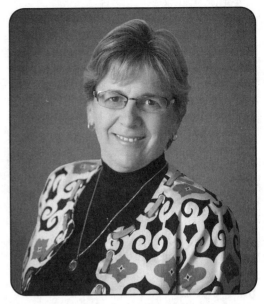

Figure 13–1. Roberta "Bobbi" Cordano, 11th president of Gallaudet University. Used with permission.

Following the tradition of Clerc and Gallaudet, who set up one of the first hearing/Deaf bilingual working teams, Deaf professionals and their colleagues have led major language reform movements in bilingual/bicultural and bimodal/bilingual education, not only in charter schools but in early education by providing training to early childhood educators and also training for teachers in K–12 and at university teacher-preparation programs. Over the past 50 years, Deaf scholars have entered doctoral programs, have written dissertations on language and literacy to explore alternative frameworks to use ASL and fingerspelling to learn to read, and now have joined faculties at community colleges and universities (Andrews, Byrne, & Clark, 2015; Kusters, De Meulder, & O'Brien, 2017).

Deaf professionals have also led the way in ensuring that parents of newly identified deaf infants are told about different opportunities and avenues for language learning, including ASL. If they choose ASL, the Joint Committee on Infant Hearing has released a 2019 position statement that emphasizes the importance of well-trained professionals fluent in ASL to work with these parents. Parents are affirming that sign language is helpful particularly when children do not have their cochlear implants on, such as during swimming time or at bedtime (Christiansen & Leigh, 2002/2005).

Deaf professionals and their hearing colleagues at CEASD (Conference of Educational Administrators of Schools and Programs for the Deaf) have initiated a national campaign, called Child First, to ensure that ASL is included on the continuum of language opportunities provided to parents of deaf children. The Child First group introduced the Alice Cogswell and Anne Sullivan Macy Act, on September 17, 2015, in the U.S. House of Representatives. This bill was sponsored by both House representatives and senators in 2017 but was not acted on. There are plans to reintroduce this bill. This act hopes to amend the Individuals With Disabilities Education Act to make sure the unique communication and language needs of deaf children are addressed during the IEP meeting, including the use of ASL. And on the state level, there is a strong effort by Deaf advocacy groups to pass bills to ensure that deaf children have the language skills (e.g., either signed or spoken language or both) to be ready for kindergarten by age 5.

As deaf children in the mainstream, including cochlear-implanted children, get older, they find opportunities to go to Deaf festivals, Deaf sports events, Deaf conferences, and other Deaf places where they interact with culturally Deaf adults. As Breda Carty (2006) writes, there has been a steady stream of latecomers to Deaf communities throughout the decades, individuals who are curious about and want to connect with Deaf people, and this has not stopped. Some of the reasons for this curiosity include difficulties in communicating with hearing people, feelings of isolation within noisy environments, and not liking the feeling that they are the only deaf person in their world.

Culturally Deaf people are succeeding in careers related to the worlds of education, business, medicine, law, social services, education, and many other employment opportunities. Increasing numbers of Deaf people with MD (medicine), PhD/EdD (linguistics, anthropology, psychology, counseling, social work, administration, education, the sciences, and so on), and JD (law) degrees have gone on to impact their fields and increase opportunities for other Deaf people. The field of Deaf Studies has been impacted by this influx of professionals who live the culturally Deaf experience (e.g., De Clerck, 2018; Kusters et al., 2017). These Deaf scholars are increasingly defining Deaf Studies and leading this discipline away from hearing-centric perspectives toward perspectives based on their lived experiences and scholarly analyses. They are developing new models or alternative Deaf-led theories for explaining what Deaf culture is about, even as the culture is going through changes fueled by social media and increased connections between Deaf people. There is significantly more focus on cultural and language diversity. Robinson (2016, 2019), however, notes the presence of a significant gap in the scholarship on intersectional Deaf experiences, with most of it having been produced by white Deaf scholars. Robinson notes that we need to focus more on social justice issues and the rich diversity of social identities and experiences among Deaf people. This translates into the need for more study of diverse Deaf communities such as those mentioned in Chapters 6 and 7. There is also a need for more Deaf scholars who are representative of these diverse Deaf communities who can expand on the richness of the diverse Deaf experiences.

Many Deaf people continue to marry other Deaf people, and the chances of their having Deaf children remain a possibility, particularly due to the connexin 26 gene. Believe it or not, in the late 1800s, there was a movement to legally forbid deaf people to marry, but that failed to become law. This cannot happen today because the legal and human rights of Deaf people are now recognized.

What about the international scene? Deaf communities all over the world are using their own sign languages. These communities, particularly in less developed countries, are not dying out and their sign languages are still in use. Researchers have gone to these communities, including, for example, the Adamorobe community (Kusters, 2015) and the Bedouin village of Al-Sayyid (Fox, 2007; Kisch, 2012). Other sign languages are emerging when different deaf communities come together and interact as in the case of Israeli Sign Language (ISL). ISL evolved within the deaf community in Israel around the 1930s, with the establishment of the first Israeli School for the Deaf in 1932 in Jerusalem. Immigrants across the globe contributed to the signing used by a small number of deaf Jews and Arabs already in Jerusalem. Immigrants from Germany and from other countries in Europe, North Africa, and the Middle East brought their sign language and home signs, which blended with ISL. From here, a conventional local sign language evolved, and today, ISL is used in a wide range of settings, including the educational system, deaf social and cultural institutions, interpreting programs, and the media (Dachkovsky, Stamp, & Sandler, 2018). Sign language continues to spawn other innovative research projects about how Deaf individuals communicate and maintain contact with each other. Joe Murray (2008) writes about transnational Deaf spaces where Deaf people from different countries interact. This definitely has been facilitated by the availability of the Internet and in this way strengthens the connections of Deaf people.

Let's not forget the arts. Plays such as the Deaf West Theater's 2015 Broadway production of *Spring Awakening* opened to rave reviews by theater critics. This production had both ASL and spoken English fully incorporated into the performance. And an art exhibit, *Let There Be Light: De^ARTivism*, had a successful run at the Pepco Edison Gallery during August and September 2015. The artwork in this exhibit focused on the themes of darkness versus light—the darkness of communication barriers versus the light of access to language (Mansfield, 2015). Black Deaf art has been showcased at the Dyer Arts Center in Rochester, New York, under the heading, *Unfolding the Soul of Black Deaf Expressions* (McGrain, 2015). And not only that, Deaf literature and poetry continue to be published. *Deaf American Prose* (Harmon & Nelson, 2012) and *Listening Through the Bone* (Conley, 2018) are excellent ways to get a taste of Deaf culture and the lives of Deaf people through Deaf authors' writings. Similar to Deaf literature, ASL literature, which incorporates the linguistic structures of ASL in its form and meaning, is expanding via the use of visual technology.

So we leave you, the reader, hopefully with optimistic feelings about Deaf culture, ASL, and the future of the Deaf community. The Deaf community of the future will not look like the Deaf community of today. Nor will the size of the Deaf community be the same. But then, today's Deaf community does not look like the Deaf community of a century ago, and it likely was smaller back then than it is today. Deaf culture is an important part of the diversity that we find not only in the United States but also internationally. On the practical side, Deaf culture provides expertise and support to the many hearing families who look for effective ways to communicate with and educate their deaf child. If you are able to learn ASL and communicate with Deaf people, you will have progressed in the ability to learn even more about the culture of Deaf people and how it has contributed to the richness of their lives.

REFERENCES

Andrews, J. F., Byrne, A., & Clark, M. D. (2015). Deaf scholars on reading: A historical review of 40 years of dissertation research (1973–2013): Implications for research and practice. *American Annals of the Deaf, 159,* 393–418.

Bauman, H. (2013). DeafSpace: An architecture toward a more livable and sustainable world. In H.-D. Bauman & J. Murray (Eds.), *Deaf gain* (pp. 375–401). Minneapolis: University of Minnesota Press.

Carty, B. (2006). Comments on W(h)ither the Deaf community. *Sign Language Studies, 6,* 181–189.

Christiansen, J. B., & Leigh, I. W. (2005). *Cochlear implants in children: Ethics and choices.* Washington, DC: Gallaudet University Press. (Original work published 2002)

Conley, W. (2018). *Listening through the bone.* Washington, DC: Gallaudet University Press.

Dachkovsky, S., Stamp, R., & Sandler, W. (2018). Constructing complexity in a young sign language. *Frontiers in Psychology, 9,* 2202.

De Clerck, G. (2018). A sustainability perspective on the potentialities of being Deaf: Toward further reflexivity in Deaf Studies and Deaf Education. *American Annals of the Deaf, 163*(4), 480–489.

Fox, M. (2007). *Talking hands.* New York, NY: Simon & Schuster Paperbacks.

Giezen, M., Baker, A., & Escudero, P. (2013). Relationships between spoken word and sign processing in children with cochlear implants. *Journal of Deaf Studies and Deaf Education, 19*(1), 107–125. doi:10.1093/deafed/ent040

Goodwin, C., Davidson, C., & Lillio-Martin, D. (2017). English article use in bimodal bilingual children with cochlear implants: Effects of language transfer and early language exposure. In M. LaMendola & J. Scott (Eds.), *Proceedings of the 41st annual Boston University Conference on Language Development* (pp. 283–295). Somerville, MA: Cascadilla Press.

Harmon, K., & Nelson, J. (Eds.). (2012). *Deaf American prose: 1830–1930.* Washington, DC: Gallaudet University Press.

Hurley, A. K. (2016, March 2). How Gallaudet University's architects are redefining deaf space. *Longform.* Retrieved from https://www.curbed.com/2016/3/2/11140210/gallaudet-deafspace-washington-dc

Johnston, T. (2004). W(h)ither the Deaf community? Population, genetics, and the future of Australian Sign Language. *American Annals of the Deaf, 148,* 358–375.

Joint Committee on Infant Hearing. (2019). Year 2019 position statement: Principles and guidelines for early hearing detection and intervention programs. *The Journal of Early Hearing Detection and Intervention, 4*(2), 1–144.

Keating, E., Edwards, T., & Mirus, G. (2008). Cybersign and new proximities: Impacts of new communication technologies on space and language. *Journal of Pragmatics, 40*(6), 1067–1081.

Kisch, S. (2012). *Deafness among the Negev Bedouin: An interdisciplinary dialogue on deafness, marginality and context* (Doctoral dissertation). Retrieved from https://pure.uva.nl/ws/files/1761078/114760_thesis.pdf

Kusters, A. (2015). *Deaf space in Adamorobe: A village in Ghana.* Washington, DC: Gallaudet University Press.

Kusters, A., De Meulder, M., & O'Brien, D. (Eds.). (2017). *Innovations in Deaf Studies.* New York, NY: Oxford University Press.

Lucas, C., Mirus, G., Palmer, J., Roessler, N., & Frost, A. (2013). The effect of new technologies on sign language research. *Sign Language Studies, 13*(4), 541–564.

Mansfield, E. (2015, June 26). *Let there be light: De^ARTivism exhibition.* Washington, DC: PRWeb. Retrieved from http://www.prweb.com/releases/2015/06/prweb12808727.htm

McGrain, V. (2015). *Dyer Arts Center exhibits Black deaf innovators.* Retrieved from https://www.rit.edu/news/dyer-arts-center-exhibits-black-deaf-innovators

Murray, J. (2008). Coequality and transnational studies: Understanding Deaf lives. In H.-D. Bauman (Ed.), *Open your eyes: Deaf Studies talking* (pp. 100–110). Minneapolis: University of Minnesota Press.

Padden, C. (n.d.). *The future of Deaf people.* University of California San Diego. Retrieved from http://www.seattlecentral.edu/faculty/cvince/ASL125/125_future_of_deaf_people carol.htm

Robinson, O. (2016). Seeking that which might constitute our common humanity: Deaf Studies, social justice, and the liberal arts. *Sign Language Studies, 17*(1), 89–95.

Robinson, O. (2019, July 2). *Discovering the nerd within: Elevating our praxis as a field.* Paper presented at the American Sign Language Teachers Association Conference, San Diego, CA.

Robinson, O., & Henner, J. (2018). Authentic voices, authentic encounters: Cripping the university through American Sign Language. *Disability Studies Quarterly.* Retrieved from http://dsq-sds.org/article/view/6111/5128

Rosen, R. (2020) (Ed.). *The Routledge handbook of sign language pedagogy.* New York, NY: Routledge.

White, M. (2014, November 13). Cochlear implants, technology, and vaccinations diminish use of Australian Sign Language. *The Sydney Morning Herald, Digital Life.* Retrieved from http://www.smh.com.au/technology/technology-news/cochlear-implants-tech nology-and-vaccinations-diminish-use-ofaustralian-sign-language-20140514-zrc3j

Yoshinaga-Itano, C. (2006). Early identification, communication modality, and the development of speech and spoken language skills: Patterns and considerations. In P. Spencer & M. Marschark (Eds.), *Advances in the spoken language development of deaf and hard-of-hearing children* (pp. 298–327). New York, NY: Oxford University Press.

Index

Note: Page numbers in **bold** reference non-text information.